Physiology of Fitness

Third Edition

W9-AZC-350

Brian J. Sharkey, PhD
University of Montana

Human Kinetics Books
Champaign, Illinois

Library of Congress Cataloging-in-Publication Data

Sharkey, Brian J.
  Physiology of fitness / Brian J. Sharkey. -- 3rd ed.
    p. cm.
  Includes bibliographical references.
  ISBN 0-87322-267-9
  1. Sports--Physiological aspects. 2. Physical fitness.
3. Exercise--Physiological aspects.   I. Title.
RC1235.S52 1990
613.7--dc20   89-24466
                                         CIP

ISBN: 0-87322-267-9

Photo credits: p. 163, by Gary Eifert; p. 235, by Stephen Warmowski, courtesy of *The Daily Illini*, University of Illinois at Urbana-Champaign

Developmental Editors: Marie Roy and Holly Gilly
Copyeditor: Julie Anderson
Assistant Editors: Julia Anderson, Valerie Hall, Robert King, and Timothy Ryan
Proofreader: Laurie McGee
Production Director: Ernie Noa
Typesetter: Yvonne Winsor
Text Design: Keith Blomberg
Text Layout: Jayne Clampitt
Cover Design: Hunter Graphics
Cover Photo: Dave Black and Quinton Instrument Co.
Illustrations: Gretchen Walters, Keith Blomberg
Printer: Versa Press

Printed in the United States of America   10 9 8 7 6

Human Kinetics Publishers
Box 5076, Champaign, IL 61825-5076
1-800-747-4457

Canada: Human Kinetics Publishers, P.O. Box 2503, Windsor, ON N8Y 4S2
1-800-465-7301 (in Canada only)

Europe: Human Kinetics Publishers (Europe) Ltd., P.O. Box IW14
Leeds LS16 6TR, England
0532-781708

Australia: Human Kinetics Publishers, P.O. Box 80, Kingswood 5062,
South Australia
618-374-0433

New Zealand: Human Kinetics Publishers, P.O. Box 105-231,
Auckland 1
(09) 309-2259

CONTENTS

To Barbara—
The perfect companion
for the long run

PREFACE

After only 4 months of training, there I was poised on the starting line for the longest run of my 35 years, a 7-mi road race. As the gun went off and the crowd surged forward on a wave of adrenaline, I was swept along by a series of sensations, ranging from excitement . . . to control . . . to concern . . . to impending exhaustion. When I plodded around the last corner and headed for the finish line, I reached for the finishing "kick" I once knew as a high school runner—but it wasn't there. Obviously I had lost it somewhere along the way. But during that run and in the months preceding it, I had literally discovered myself. As I sought fitness along the roads and trails, I made progress in other areas as well. Today, years later, I am confident that the passage to fitness marked a turning point in my life.

Those words appeared in the prefaces of the first and second editions of this book. The second edition published in 1984 went on to say

Today, several passages and turning points later, I continue to learn about fitness and life. The medium of discovery these past few years has been cross-country skiing. Some time after I passed the age of 40 I sought new challenges, experiences, and a new way to seek the rewards of fitness, so I took up cross-country skiing. In addition to training for the sport, I studied cross-country skiing in the laboratory and in the field. This intense personal and professional involvement with one of the most demanding of sports has provided new information and insights concerning fitness and how it can be achieved.

Now as I begin this third edition, I feel compelled to reveal the experiences and events that influenced my approach to this revision. Age and job demands made the maintenance of fitness more difficult and performance less gratifying. A major career and geographic change challenged me to be adaptable and to enjoy new friends and activities instead of lamenting the loss of old ones. And, as I approached my 50th year, I watched as illness temporarily subdued some vigorous friends, and I realized again the values and limits of fitness and other health habits.

These experiences were integrated with new research on fitness and health; new findings concerning cholesterol and heart disease; prudent approaches to diet and nutrition; new perspectives on aging; and a bright prognosis for fitness, health, wellness, and longevity. Age, experience, and 3 decades of research have tempered the unabashed enthusiasm of the first edition, softened the performance orientation of the second, and produced a more balanced approach, with understanding, empathy, and opportunities for all to enjoy. Above all, I'm even more convinced of the value of the active lifestyle.

So join me again as we continue to explore the developing story of fitness. *Physiology of Fitness* is an up-to-date guide to the prescription of exercise for health, fitness, and performance. You've seen other fitness books and may have read a few, but if you're still starved for information and explanations, I think you've found what you have been seeking. This book is for the individual who wants to develop a deeper understanding of fitness, for the enthusiast who wants to know why and how the body responds, for the newcomer who needs more motivation, or for the skeptic who needs more proof. I set out to write the thinking person's fitness book—I hope you'll say I succeeded.

The book is divided into five parts that explore the dimensions of fitness. Each part is subsequently divided into chapters, and each chapter begins with a list of objectives that outlines the territory covered in the text. Figures and tables provide technical and practical information. The practical information will help you determine your best avenue to fitness and the technical material will help you probe the physiological dimensions of fitness.

This book is about fitness and its relationship to health and performance, but it is concerned with other things as well—things like self-discovery, experience, understanding, achievement, and the quality of life. Invest in fitness and you will earn immediate health dividends. In time you'll reap more substantial rewards—the capital gains of vitality, high-level health, and performance. And as your interest in fitness continues to grow and mature, you will harvest the accumulated wealth of your endowment—your potential. You should by all means spend time developing your intellectual, artistic, emotional, and spiritual gifts, but if you ignore the physical you may never experience all that life has to offer.

Proceed in good health, and soon you will begin to experience what an eloquent friend has termed that "state of grace" called fitness.

ACKNOWLEDGMENTS

Thanks go to Rainer Martens and the professional staff at Human Kinetics Publishers, to past and present colleagues and graduate students, to Art and other co-workers in the U.S. Forest Service, and to colleagues in the American College of Sports Medicine for inspiration, advice, and review of the ideas and interpretations contained herein.

Special thanks go to Marie Roy of Human Kinetics Publishers for her help in the preparation of the manuscript and to Diane Krogh for assistance in word processing.

INTRODUCTION TO FITNESS

This chapter will help you

become familiar with the terms, definitions, and benefits of fitness,

understand the relationships between fitness, health, and wellness, and

compare your current level of fitness to recommended and typical values.

We can approach the study of fitness in at least two distinctly different ways. One is objective and physiological; the other is subjective, emotional, and psychological. The former is concerned with calories, heartbeats, and quantifications of exercise, whereas the latter "tunes in" on sensations, "turns on" with activity, and "gets high" on hormones. I will begin with the physiological approach to help you understand how fitness provides the foundation for high-level health and contributes to the joy of living. I will then move from the objective to the subjective, from the physiological to the psychological. As you become involved in the active lifestyle you will certainly experience both. After months of systematically working toward your fitness goals you may relish a mellow period, when you seek the sheer joy of movement. Months later you may feel the need to train intensively again. Feelings, moods, and motives change and you should not ignore them.

Exercise physiology explores the immediate and long-term effects of exercise on the function of muscles, organs, and systems of the body and the relationship of activity and fitness to health. Although scientists studied some aspects of exercise before the turn of the century, and

1

German, French, and English researchers did landmark work in the early 1900s, modern exercise physiology probably had its roots in Scandinavian laboratories and at the Harvard Fatigue Lab in the 1930s (Horvath & Horvath, 1973). As you can see, exercise physiology is a relatively young science.

The physiology of fitness began to receive serious scientific attention in the 1950s, when studies of British bus drivers and civil servants linked regular exercise to a lower risk of heart disease (Morris, Heady, Raffle, Roberts, & Parks, 1953). Before that the major incentive for fitness was military preparedness. During the two world wars and the Korean War, U.S. military leaders, concerned about the fitness levels of draftees, called for greater attention to fitness in the schools. Today, we value fitness for its relationship to health and for its contributions to performance in work or sport.

Fitness Components

Although fitness means many things to many people, in this book it refers to specific components—aerobic and muscular fitness.

Aerobic Fitness

Aerobic means in the presence of oxygen, as contrasted with **anaerobic**, meaning in the absence of oxygen. Aerobic fitness is defined as the capacity to take in, transport, and utilize *oxygen*. Aerobic fitness is developed and maintained through large-muscle activities such as walking, jogging, cycling, swimming, and others that allow sustained metabolism.

Because aerobic fitness involves so many important organs and systems (respiration, heart and circulation, muscles), it tells a lot about the health of these components and about health in general. That is, when aerobic fitness improves, physical and mental health are enhanced. The benefits of aerobic exercise and fitness include

- improved circulation, respiration, and fat metabolism;
- reduced stress levels, body fat, and risk of heart disease;
- stronger bones, ligaments, and tendons;
- weight control;
- more energy and less fatigue;
- enhanced mood, self-concept, and body image;
- greater emotional stability; and
- a more positive outlook.

The increased capacity and adaptability associated with aerobic fitness can add life to your years, not just years to your life.

In the early 1960s less than 5% of the adult population in the United States engaged in regular aerobic exercise. At that time heart disease was epidemic and getting worse. But times have changed. Recent polls show an increase in the number of active adults and a decline in the incidence of heart disease. Walkers, runners, cyclists, and aerobics participants are everywhere, exercising for health, for weight control and appearance, for performance, or for the fun of it. Many are active year-round, swimming and cycling in the summer and alpine and cross-country skiing in the winter. Doctors encourage patients to exercise for preventive health or rehabilitation, and many are taking the advice.

Even psychiatrists have discovered fitness. They prescribe physical activity, and some even run with their patients. Aerobic exercise reduces anxiety and depression; it serves as a tranquilizer and can even help you fall asleep. Some think it makes one more productive, even more creative. Yes, we are caught up in a veritable mania for fitness, a bona fide trend, not a fad (Naisbitt, 1984). Fitness and other aspects of the healthy lifestyle are beginning to lower health care costs. However, some segments of society have ignored the trend. Later in this chapter we'll examine the status of fitness and see that there is still much work to be done.

Some authorities include body composition, the proportion of fat and lean tissue, as a component of fitness. Although I agree with the need to maintain a relatively low percentage of body fat and believe that aerobic exercise is the best way to lose unwanted fat, I treat body composition and body fat in a separate section. Why? Exercise, by itself, may not be enough to control body weight and fat. Food intake is also an important part of the energy balance equation. You'll learn more about body fat and body composition in Part III, Fitness and Weight Control.

Muscular Fitness

Strength, muscle endurance, and flexibility—the components of muscular fitness—were once viewed as the essence of fitness, but lost some favor during the rise of aerobic exercise. Today they are making a comeback based on sound health benefits and on what they do for appearance, self-concept, and performance.

Muscle tone and flexibility contribute to good posture and can help prevent the lower back problems that plague millions of Americans. As the years pass and strength and flexibility decline, your ability to engage fully in life diminishes. Countless senior citizens face retirement unable to enjoy the fruits of their labor. They paid attention to fiscal fitness but failed to prepare physically.

Muscular fitness helps in other ways. It can help you cope with the demands of your job. It can improve your performance in an activity or sport. It can boost your ego and improve your figure (or physique). When combined with aerobic fitness it may even improve your sex life! "Ridiculous," you say. "Fitness is not a panacea, a cure-all.'' Of course it isn't. But in a society dedicated to the automobile, remote control devices, and robots, fitness may be just what the doctor ordered. In an age when we face the threat of a genuine energy crisis, who will be better able to adapt and survive? The fittest, that's who!

Fitness, Health, and Wellness

Are fitness, health, and wellness synonyms, words with the same or nearly the same meaning? Although they are often used interchangeably in casual conversation, and although there is some overlap, the words have distinctly different connotations to exercise physiologists and other health professionals.

Fitness and Health

A positive relationship exists between fitness and health. As fitness improves, health risk declines and life expectancy inches upward. However, that doesn't imply that continued increases in fitness will continue to yield improvements in health status. On the contrary, excessive amounts of exercise can cause health to decline. The path to fitness carries risks as well as benefits. The proper amount yields optimal health, yet too much promises illness or injury. Too much exercise leads to muscle and skeletal injuries, suppression of the immune system, and a decline in resistance to infection. Too much weight loss can lead to hormonal problems and mineral deficiencies. So to be accurate we say that regular, moderate *activity* is associated with health. Fitness, which is partially inherited, is less likely to be correlated to health than is the amount of regular, moderate activity. Of course, regular activity improves fitness—to a point.

Other health-related aspects of fitness include greater attention to a healthy diet, improved weight control, reduction or elimination of cigarettes, reduced stress, better sleep patterns, and other manifestations of the healthy lifestyle. So fitness contributes to health in many ways, and we'll explore them throughout this book.

Health and Wellness

For many years health was defined as the absence of disease, and that is how many people still use the term. But in recent years the definition of health has been expanded to include a state of complete physical, mental, and emotional well-being, not merely the absence of disease or infirmity. In that context the relationship of fitness to health becomes more clear. The relationship of health and wellness is equally clear. Ardell (1984) defined wellness as ''a conscious and deliberate approach to an advanced state of physical and psychological/spiritual health'' (p. 5). So wellness is *movement* toward an advanced state of health, also called optimal or high-level health.

Although the old view of health placed illness on one side of a line and health on the other, with doctors and the treatment-oriented health care system defending the latter against the former, wellness is viewed as a dynamic, fluctuating state of being, a process where you—the individual—are responsible for your health (see Figure I.1). The health care system and traditional medicine are treatment oriented, and workers in the system focus on correcting the problems brought on by illness, injury, or disease. Wellness involves health promotion and disease prevention, focusing on behaviors that lower the risk of illness or injury. The treatment system employs an army of high-priced professionals and costs billions of dollars. Wellness depends on individual responsibility, low-cost helpers, and reduced reliance on health professionals. Because "preventive health" sounds silly and "health promotion" sounds like advertising, the term **wellness** has caught the public fancy, and fitness/wellness programs are catching on at every level of society and in every age group, from kids to senior citizens.

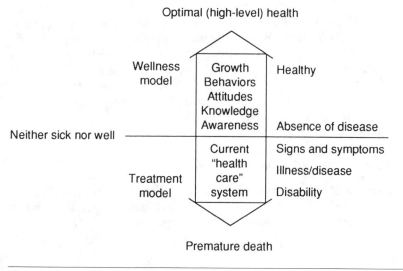

Figure I.1. The health continuum.

Fitness and Wellness

The first version of this book preceded all but the earliest stages of the wellness movement (Sharkey, 1974). But optimal health, or wellness, is what this book is all about. Fitness is an essential component of high-level health or wellness. Fitness requires individual initiative, and it helps prevent disease, leads to better physical health, and provides the springboard to enhanced psychological health. But excess emphasis on the physical side of wellness can interfere with health and with the balance of the physical, emotional, spiritual, social, occupational, and intellectual components of wellness. In fact, fitness is but one part of the physical dimension, which also includes nutrition, health habits, environmental concerns, and safety. But fitness can contribute to other dimensions of wellness, such as the emotional, social, and occupational, and some would add that fitness has the potential to enhance the intellectual and spiritual dimensions as well. Subsequent chapters explore these relationships in more detail.

Fitness and the Active Lifestyle

My goal in writing this book is to help you achieve an active lifestyle, in which vigorous physical activity is an important part of every day. To achieve that end we'll muddle through some facts and figures and present an objective, factual approach to fitness, but we won't stop there. Before you've finished the book I hope you will be hopelessly addicted to physical activity. When that happens you will plan each day around your activity—the most important part of the day. And if for some reason you are unable to participate, you will sense something essential is missing. When you experience withdrawal symptoms after a day or more of inactivity, you will know you are hooked on physical activity, compelled to live an active lifestyle for the rest of your years.

But what if you become injured or ill, what then? There are a few valid excuses to avoid regular activity, including acute illness, fever, or serious injury that requires immobilization. In most other cases there is an activity suited to your condition.

Exercise and fitness can be used for

- **prevention of degenerative conditions brought on by inactivity,**
- **rehabilitation following injury, operation, or chronic disorder, and**
- **performance and enjoyment in work, recreation, or sport.**

Prevention

Some years ago Kraus and Raab (1961) wrote a book entitled *Hypokinetic Disease*. They contended that lack of activity was a major factor in the development of heart and other degenerative diseases. Today, health experts agree that sanitation and medical science have achieved about as much as can be expected in the war against sickness and death. Additional dollars for health care cannot and will not achieve what can be earned if each of us adopts better health habits, including an active lifestyle. Every major epidemiological study lists regular physical activity as an essential component of health and longevity. Because so many adults are inactive, it is likely that increases in the level of activity in the population would have *more* effect on lowering the incidence of heart disease than would modification of any other heart disease risk factor (Caspersen, 1987). And the famous Harvard alumni study has shown that exercise and fitness are associated with lower death rates for other degenerative diseases, including stroke, cancer, and respiratory disease, as well as for suicide. To top it all off, the active alumni even lived longer (Paffenbarger, Hyde, & Wing, 1986).

Rehabilitation

Exercise and fitness are now accepted approaches in rehabilitation. Instead of long periods of bed rest, early ambulation is the rule for conditions ranging from knee repair to coronary bypass surgery. Within days, rehabilitation exercises begin. In most cases the exercises are an essential factor in the long-term success of the procedure. Therapists employ exercise following most forms of surgery (including orthopedic and cardiac), as part of the ongoing treatment for chronic disorders such as diabetes and multiple sclerosis, for kidney and lung patients, and to help patients return to the work place. Failure to continue the exercises means a return of the problem, as is the case with many low back disorders. So the smart approach is to employ preventive exercise to avoid the burdens of rehabilitation.

Performance in Work, Recreation, and Sport

Exercise and fitness can enhance performance and enjoyment in recreation and sport. But for many it can also improve performance or the enjoyment of work. Workers in physically demanding occupations, like construction, logging, or fire fighting, profit from conditioning as much as those who participate in demanding sports. And less physical work, such as cutting hair, can be more enjoyable with regular attention to exercises for the back. Future chapters will help you improve your performance in work and sport.

The Activity Index

Now it's time to assess your level of activity using the procedures in the activity index (see Table I.1). If you don't score at least 80 you may need more activity to achieve all the benefits of exercise and fitness. As you increase the intensity, duration, and frequency of exercise, the score and your fitness level go up while the risk of heart disease goes down.

Health and longevity suffer when regular physical activity is missing. But sedentary individuals miss other things as well. They miss the joy of movement, the thrill of change as fitness and performance improve, and the senses of discovery, achievement, and reaching their potential. Inactive individuals limit their life and their ability to adapt. Fitness allows a more creative adaptation to life.

Table I.1 The Activity Index

Based on your regular daily activity, calculate your activity index by multiplying your score for each category (Score = Intensity × Duration × Frequency).

	Score	Daily activity
Intensity	5	Sustained heavy breathing and perspiration
	4	Intermittent heavy breathing and perspiration—as in tennis, racquetball
	3	Moderately heavy—as in recreational sports and cycling
	2	Moderate—as in volleyball, softball
	1	Light—as in fishing, walking
Duration	4	Over 30 min
	3	20 to 30 min
	2	10 to 20 min
	1	Under 10 min
Frequency	5	Daily or almost daily
	4	3 to 5 times a week
	3	1 to 2 times a week
	2	Few times a month
	1	Less than once a month

Evaluation and Fitness Category

Score	Evaluation	Fitness category[a]
100	Very active lifestyle	High
80 to 100	Active and healthy	Very good
40 to 60	Acceptable (could be better)	Fair
20 to 40	Not good enough	Poor
Under 20	Sedentary	Very poor

Note. From *The Effects of Exercise and Fitness on Serum Lipids in College Women* (p. 46) by D. Kasari, 1976, unpublished master's thesis, University of Montana.

[a]Index score is highly related to aerobic fitness.

The Status of Fitness

Now that you've estimated your level of activity, you'll want to know how it compares with the levels of others. What is the status of activity and fitness among youth, adults, and senior citizens? Before I attempt to answer those questions, you should know how much activity is considered essential for fitness and health. One responsible organization, the American College of Sports Medicine (ACSM), says that to become aerobically fit in a health-related way, the average healthy adult should exercise 3 to 5 times per week, for 15 to 60 min, at a heart rate (HR) that ranges from 65 to 90% of the HR range: [(max HR − resting HR) × .65] + resting HR (American College of Sports Medicine, 1986). But these guidelines were designed to achieve fitness and high-level health; it may be that *less* intense activity is sufficient to lower the risk of degenerative diseases, if that is your only goal.

Youth Fitness

Youth fitness has long been a concern, first for military preparedness, then as preparation for sport, and now for its relationship to health. Regardless of the purpose or type of test, our youth have never looked good when compared with those of other nations. This is surprising considering our standard of living, quality of nutrition, and past performance in international sport. In 1980 the American Association for Health, Physical Education, Recreation and Dance (AAHPERD) introduced its Health-Related Fitness Test. For the first time our youth were tested on items that were related to health, not military or athletic performance. Items include a skinfold test for body fatness, flexibility and abdominal tone tests related to muscular fitness and low back health, and an aerobic fitness test.

A 1985 study of health-related fitness (Ross, Dotson & Gilbert, 1985) contrasted the results with objectives from a report outlining health objectives for the year 1990. *Promoting Health/Preventing Disease: Objectives for the Nation* (U.S. Department of Health and Human Services, 1980). Youth fitness objectives for the year 1990 include 60% attending physical education classes daily, 70% having periodic fitness tests, and 90% participating in activities that promote cardiorespiratory health. The 1985 data indicated that although 58.9% of 5th through 12th graders participated in appropriate physical activity year-round, 46.9% engaged in activity with carry-over potential, and 41% knew the signs of adequate activity, we were still a long way from reaching the stated objectives (Ross et al., 1985). In fact we are losing ground as many schools drop physical education to achieve fiscal fitness. Interestingly, a recent fitness survey (Pate & Ross, 1987) found a relationship between parental physical activity and the child's body fat, with children of active parents tending to have lower levels of body fat. Parental example is important in molding a child's attitude toward activity.

Adult Activity

How many adults achieve the level of activity called for by the ACSM or participate in any activity for that matter? A major study of adult exercise habits conducted by the President's Council on Physical Fitness and Sport (1973) found that 45% of all adult Americans reported *no* job-related or leisure activity. Have things improved? A January 1988 survey conducted by the *New York Times* found that 54% did not exercise on a regular basis (70 to 80 million Americans are almost totally sedentary), and only 15% said that they exercised daily. In spite of the enthusiastic estimates of increased activity, many experts feel that only 10 to 20% of the adult population meets or approaches the ACSM activity guidelines. Other adults may be active occasionally, but occasional activity doesn't insure the health benefits associated with regular moderate activity. That is why scientists at the U.S. Public Health Service Centers for Disease Control say that increasing the level of physical activity in the population may have more effect on reducing the incidence of heart disease than modifications of either blood pressure, cholesterol, or cigarette smoking (Centers for Disease Control, 1987).

Senior Fitness

If adult activity is poor it will get worse as adults become senior citizens. Longitudinal and cross-sectional aging studies show that fitness declines 8 to 10% per decade (e.g., your fitness could decline 40 to 50% in 5 decades). But this data shows what is, not what could be. Studies of active adults indicate that the decline can be slowed to 4% or even 2% per decade. And some studies prove that fitness can be maintained or slightly increased over a 10-year period. The major factors involved in fitness are modifiable, that is, they can be influenced with regular activity (Sharkey, 1987). So ignore population studies and look at active seniors; they will show you the benefits of the active lifestyle.

Recommendations for Activity and Fitness

Does this mean that the fitness boom is a bust, that fitness was only a passing fad and not a bona fide trend? No, it doesn't; it means that few of us understand or appreciate the benefits of activity. It means that those of us dedicated to the values of fitness, health, and wellness still have a great deal of work to do, especially with those groups that have traditionally ignored the health and fitness message. The implications of inactivity are more degenerative disease, higher health care costs, and the staggering burden of maintaining an aging, sedentary population. And yet the solutions are not that difficult. In most cases they are inexpensive, energy conserving, and easy on the environment.

Youth

Kids need more activity, in school and out. In addition to regular (daily) physical education, they could receive physical education homework that requires parental involvement. Parents need to be better role models for the active lifestyle. They need to schedule active weekends and vacations that promote health-related fitness. Communities need to encourage active recreation, as do other local, state, and federal agencies. Public policy can be used to foster or inhibit activity.

Adults

Colleges, the military, business and industry, and other parts of the private and public sector need to promote health and fitness. We need to adopt a national health ethic that influences public policy and makes it easy to be active. We need to reward activity with lower health and life insurance rates and perhaps tax those things that reduce activity or diminish health and the quality of life.

Seniors

If we do the job with youth and adults, the growing numbers of senior citizens will not be a problem. Instead they will be a robust, self-sufficient group capable of living a happy, healthy life of 8 decades or more (see chapter 16). In the meantime we should do all we can to help senior citizens remain active. Fitness definitely extends the prime of life.

The Public Health Service has set a series of health objectives for 1990:

90% of children and adolescents should participate in fitness activities that can be carried into adulthood.

Over 60% of children ages 10 to 17 should participate in daily physical education programs.

Over 60% of adults ages 18 to 64 should participate regularly in vigorous activity.

50% of adults 65 years and above should engage in appropriate physical activity.

Also, for 1990, over 70% of adults should be able to identify exercise that promotes fitness; over 50% of primary care physicians should include an exercise history in their examination of new patients; over 25% of large companies and institutions should offer fitness programs; 70% of children should be tested with an appropriate fitness test; data should be available to evaluate short- and long-term effects of physical activity on health, health care costs, and job performance; and data should also be available for monitoring national trends and patterns of participation in physical activity.

Although we have been slow in making progress toward these goals (U.S. Public Health Service, 1987), it is nice to know that the U.S. government has recognized the value of exercise and fitness and is beginning to articulate a national health ethic with the potential of lowering health care costs and improving the quality of life.

In reality, the key to a solution is *individual responsibility*. The active lifestyle is a cost-effective way to prevent disease and to promote robust health. We are all responsible for our own health habits and lifestyle. Each must do his or her part to lower health care costs and avoid becoming a burden on family, friends, and society. We can't rely on doctors and medicine—the responsibility is our own.

By now you are acquainted with the meanings and benefits of fitness and have assessed your current level of activity. I hope you are motivated to learn more and to undertake a personal program, convinced that fitness and the active lifestyle pave the way to a healthy, productive, and enjoyable life. Remember, when you feel the need for more information on the physiology of fitness, consult Appendix A.

In this text, we use the term *calorie* (abbreviate *cal*) when talking about energy expenditure and intake. Technically, the correct unit is a *kilocalorie* (*kcal*). Here, we are following popular usage, so calorie = kilocalorie.

PART
I

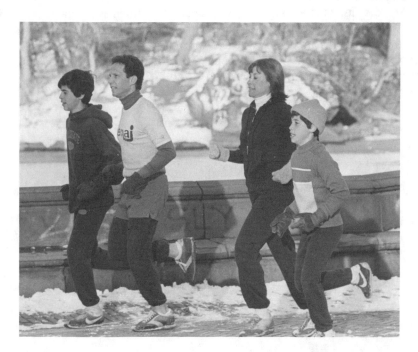

AEROBIC FITNESS

Somewhere above the pace of your normal daily activities but well below maximal effort you will find aerobic exercise. If you do aerobic exercise almost every day you will improve your level of aerobic fitness, and as fitness improves you'll enhance your health, vitality, and the quality of your life.

Aerobic fitness describes how well you are able to take oxygen from the atmosphere into the lungs and blood, then pump it to working muscles where it is utilized in subcellular organelles, called mitochondria, to oxidize carbohydrate and fat to produce energy. No other measure says more about the health of your oxygen intake, transport, and utilization systems.

The exercise you do to improve aerobic fitness reduces the risk of heart disease and other problems and adds years to your life as well. Rhythmic moderate exercise such as brisk walking, jogging, running, swimming, cycling, cross-country skiing, and rowing are aerobic. They demand increases in respiration, circulation, and muscle metabolism and allow the increases to be sustained long enough to promote adaptation of the systems. Remember, it is the activity, the aerobic exercise, that is most associated with health and longevity. And regular moderate exercise improves fitness.

Aerobic fitness is among the best preventive medicines available. In Part I you'll learn about aerobic fitness and how to develop aerobic exercise prescriptions for yourself, family, and friends. Appendix A provides an in-depth description of aerobic exercise, and Appendix B provides aerobic fitness tests and programs, as well as training tips and aerobic alternatives.

CHAPTER

1

UNDERSTANDING AEROBIC FITNESS

This chapter will help you

define aerobic fitness and understand how it is measured,

identify factors that influence or limit aerobic fitness, and

understand your aerobic potential.

Aerobic exercise involves moderate activity that utilizes oxygen-using, or oxidative, pathways to supply energy for muscular contractions.

AEROBIC FITNESS IS THE ABILITY TO

Take in
Transport —— OXYGEN
Utilize

If you do aerobic exercise several times a week you will begin to improve your aerobic fitness. Each time you do a little more you overload oxygen transport and utilization systems, and your body adapts to the increased requirements. This process of overload and adaptation is called training, and when you do aerobic training you improve aerobic fitness. To better describe the process, I'll first define aerobic exercise.

Aerobic Exercise

Dress for exercise, stretch, warm up, and then begin with a slow walk. Increase your pace a little as each minute passes, going from a slow to a fast walk (even

15

a jog or a run). Continue to increase your speed little by little until the effort becomes uncomfortable, your breathing is deep and rapid, and you begin to doubt your ability to continue. Everything up to this point has been aerobic, which means in the presence of oxygen. If you continue to increase exercise intensity you will change to anaerobic or nonoxidative exercise, which involves intense effort of necessarily short duration and an accumulation of lactic acid in the blood.

Lactic acid is both an energy carrier and a metabolic by-product of intense effort that signals increasing intensity. It serves as a promissory note that insures the repayment of the oxygen debt incurred when effort exceeds your ability to produce all your energy needs via oxidative pathways. Lactic acid and the high levels of carbon dioxide produced in vigorous effort are associated with labored breathing, general discomfort, and a sense of distress. Aerobic exercise can be defined as exercise below the point where blood lactic acid levels begin to rise, below the so-called anaerobic threshold.

Aerobic metabolism of a molecule of glucose is far more efficient than anaerobic; aerobic metabolism yields 38 molecules of a high-energy compound called adenosine triphosphate (ATP), the energy currency, versus only 2 molecules by the anaerobic route, and aerobic metabolism produces less lactic acid. So aerobic exercise is relatively pleasant and relaxing, not unpleasant and painful. And the aerobic utilization of abundant fat reserves insures an adequate supply of energy for extended periods of effort. Aerobic exercise can be sustained comfortably for several minutes to many hours. You can carry on a conversation during moderate aerobic exercise.

Intensity of Exercise

Aerobic and anaerobic exercises differ in intensity; light to moderate activity is aerobic, whereas extremely vigorous or intense effort is anaerobic. Table 1.1 illustrates how heart rate and breathing increase with exercise intensity, and how we switch from mostly fat to mostly carbohydrate as exercise becomes more vigorous. The table also shows how the nervous system recruits different types of muscle fibers as the effort becomes more intense. Humans have three main types of muscle fibers: slow twitch (slow oxidative or SO) fibers that are efficient in the use of oxygen; a faster contracting type that uses oxygen and carbohydrate (muscle glycogen) and is called fast oxidative glycolytic (FOG); and a fast twitch fiber that isn't well suited for aerobic or oxygen-using metabolism (fast glycolytic or FG). As we go from a walk to a jog, faster fibers are recruited to help us go faster. Go from a jog to a run and even more fast fibers are needed. Recruit too many fast glycolytic fibers and the effort becomes predominantly anaerobic (see Figure 1.1). See Appendix A for more on slow and fast twitch muscle fibers, lactic acid, and other details.

Table 1.1 Levels of Exercise Intensity

	Exercise intensity		
	Light	Moderate	Intense
Example	Walking	Jogging	Running
Metabolism	Aerobic	Aerobic	Aerobic/anaerobic
Energy source	Fat and CHO	CHO and fat	CHO and fat
Heart rate	< 120	120-150	> 150
Breathing	Easy	Can talk easily	hard to talk
Muscle fiber recruited	SO	FOG	FG

CHO = carbohydrate.

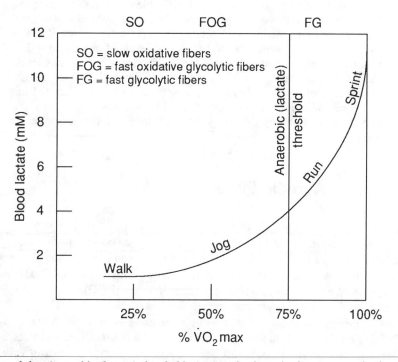

Figure 1.1. Anaerobic (lactate) threshold. As exercise intensity increases we begin to recruit FOG fibers. Continue to increase intensity (% $\dot{V}O_2max$) and FG fibers are recruited. More blood lactate accumulates because FG fibers produce more and because fewer fibers are idle and therefore are unable to remove (take up) lactate.

Anaerobic Threshold

When exercise becomes too intense, more energy is produced anaerobically, and lactic acid begins to accumulate in the blood. Carbon dioxide production also rises and the rate and depth of breathing increases. The labored breathing and the discomfort caused by acid metabolites and lactic acid (also called lactate) are signs that you have stepped over the anaerobic threshold. Aerobic exercise is that which remains below the anaerobic threshold. Why do I bother you with all this detail? Because I think that you may be interested in knowing the difference between aerobic and anaerobic exercise, knowing how much is enough to improve fitness, and knowing why aerobic exercise is better for the health (e.g., aerobic exercise burns fat).

Physiologists discourage the use of the term **anaerobic threshold**, because many muscle fibers may still be aerobic or oxidative during the transition. Physiologists prefer the term **lactate threshold** to designate the point of rising lactic acid. Lactate can be produced in one fiber and used as an energy source in another. Blood levels of lactic acid reflect both the production and removal of the 3-carbon molecule. Rising levels can indicate increasing production, decreased removal, or both. Recent studies suggest that trained muscles are better able to remove lactate from the blood and use it as an energy source. In fact, lactic acid's main role may be that of energy carrier—before, during, and after exercise.

Measuring Aerobic Fitness

Aerobic fitness, the capacity to take in, transport, and utilize oxygen, is best measured in a laboratory test called the **maximal oxygen consumption (VO_2max)**. The test requires a treadmill, bicycle ergometer, or some other exercise device; a metabolic measurement system that measures oxygen, carbon dioxide, and the volume of expired air; and an electrocardiogram (ECG) to keep an eye on the heart and measure heart rate during the test.

After a health risk assessment, the subject signs a consent form and is fitted with ECG electrodes. Following a warm-up on the treadmill, the subject takes a brief rest. He or she then begins the test wearing a nose clip and a valve to direct exhaled air into the metabolic analyzer. The test involves a walk (for the less fit) or run on the treadmill, which is programmed to increase grade every 1 to 2 min. Oxygen consumption is computed during each minute as the test proceeds from low to medium to maximal aerobic effort. The test is terminated when the values reach maximum (level off in spite of increased treadmill grade) or when the subject can no longer keep up with the treadmill. The highest level of oxygen used is called the maximal oxygen consumption, or aerobic fitness.

Scores in the range of 3 to 4 L of oxygen per minute (L/min) are common, and values of 5 to 6 L/min have been reported for endurance athletes. When reported in L/min (**aerobic capacity**), the score provides useful information about the total capacity of the cardiorespiratory system. However, because the value is related to body size, larger individuals tend to have higher scores. To eliminate the influence of body size, the maximal oxygen consumption score in liters is divided by the body weight in kilograms:

$$3 \text{ L/min} \div 60 \text{ kg} = 50 \text{ ml/[kg} \times \text{min]}$$

The resulting value (in milliliters of oxygen per kilogram of body weight per minute) allows a direct comparison of individuals, regardless of body weight. This measure, also known as **aerobic power**, is more related to endurance performance in running and other weight-bearing activities, and it is the most popular way to express aerobic fitness. If two individuals have the same score in liters, but one weighs 60 kg and the other 100 kg (220 lb), it is easy to see which is more fit:

$$3 \text{ L/min} \div 100 \text{ kg} = 30 \text{ ml/[kg} \times \text{min]}$$

I know which one I'd bet on in a 5-k race, how about you? The one with a score of 50 is better able to take in, transport, and utilize oxygen in each unit of muscle.

The average male college student scores from 45 to 50 ml/[kg × min], and the average female from 39 to 43, depending on his or her level of activity. Top male endurance athletes score in the 80s, and top females are in the 70s. On the other end of the scale, older, inactive individuals may score in the 20s or low 30s (see Table 1.2).

Table 1.2 Fitness Comparison

Subjects	Age	Men (ml/[kg × min])	Women (ml/[kg × min])
Untrained	18-22	45	39
Active	18-22	50	43
Trained	18-22	57	53
Elite	18-22	70	63
World class	18-22	80+	70+
Untrained	40-50	36	27
Active	40-50	46	39
Trained	40-50	52	44
Elite	40-50	60+	50+

Because laboratory tests are costly, time consuming, and not readily available, I recommend less complicated methods for the estimation of aerobic fitness (see Appendix B). Use the method best suited to your age and level of activity, but be sure to precede the test with the Pre/Fit questionnaire, Table 3.5 on page 57. In Appendix B you will also find a step-by-step laboratory protocol that I have used with success on subjects ranging from the sedentary to world class endurance athletes.

In spite of the fact that aerobic fitness is defined and tested with a $\dot{V}O_2$max test and almost all fitness training studies have used the $\dot{V}O_2$max to evaluate changes in fitness, this test may not be the best measure of fitness. In a $\dot{V}O_2$max test you only achieve that maximum level for 1 or 2 min, then you quit. In real life situations few of us ever work at the $\dot{V}O_2$ max level. Although the max test is related to exercise intensity, it is only moderately related to performance in endurance events. Endurance or duration is related to the muscle's ability to utilize oxygen. Different lab tests (e.g., oxidative capacity of muscle tissue or lactate threshold) or field tests (3,200-m run) may someday replace the $\dot{V}O_2$max as the standard test of fitness (Weltman, 1989). I'll say more about this important point in later chapters.

Factors Influencing Aerobic Fitness

Although training accounts for a large measure of fitness, other factors such as heredity, sex, age, body fat, and level of activity also influence the level of fitness.

Heredity

Is an aerobic fitness score of 80 the product of heredity or training? The answer is probably both. It takes tremendous natural endowment and years of training to achieve high-level endurance performances. I'll discuss training in the following chapters; for now I'll say that the influence of aerobic training is limited. Only adolescents can hope to improve aerobic fitness much more than 30%, and that would take months of training. Canadian researchers have studied differences in aerobic fitness among fraternal (dizygotic) and identical (monozygotic) twins. Young twins were studied to minimize the effects of variables in the environment, such as diet and training. Intrapair differences were far greater among fraternal than identical twins, with the largest difference between identical twins being smaller than the smallest difference between fraternal pairs. The author of one study concluded that variability in aerobic fitness was genetically determined, that heredity plays an important role in aerobic fitness (Klissouras, 1976). More recent estimates based on a wider range of subjects suggest that the heritability of aerobic fitness is about 40% (Bouchard, personal communication, 1988). So there are limits on genetic influence and on our ability to improve with training.

But what can we inherit that contributes to aerobic fitness? The definition of aerobic fitness (the ability to take in, transport, and utilize oxygen) provides some clues. In addition to a greater lung capacity, larger heart, more red cells and hemoglobin, and a better capillary supply, we may also inherit a higher percentage of oxidative (both slow and fast) muscle fibers. Some world class endurance athletes have 80% slow oxidative fibers. Because research on humans doesn't prove that fiber types can be changed dramatically, we can assume that the fibers are inherited. (*There is evidence that fibers become more oxidative with training and some animal evidence that fibers can be changed from fast to slow after extemely long periods of continuous electrical stimulation.*) Of course, what we inherit is far less important than how we use our natural endowment.

Sex

Before puberty, boys and girls differ little in aerobic fitness, but from then on girls fall behind. In general women average about three fourths of men's capacity. One reason may be hemoglobin; men average about 2 g more per 100 ml of blood (15 vs. 13 g/dl), and hemoglobin concentration and aerobic fitness are related in women (Haymes, Harris, Beldon, Loomis, & Nicholas, 1972). On the other hand, some women have hemoglobin values higher than the average man.

Women are generally smaller and have less muscle mass. Another reason women score lower on fitness is less complicated; women have more body fat (25% vs. 12.5% for college-aged women and men, respectively). Because aerobic fitness is usually reported per unit of body weight, the individual with less fat and more lean weight (muscle) has a decided advantage. Some researchers argue that aerobic fitness should be reported per unit of lean body weight. That method reduces the differences in fitness between men and women. Unfortunately, it doesn't remove excess fat or improve performance. There are good reasons why women have more fat, including sex-related differences, so women shouldn't try to become too thin. I only raise the issue to explain why the average values differ.

Until recently, women were prohibited from competing in races longer than the 1/2 mi; overprotective (or prejudiced) officials didn't think women could stand the strain. Today women are running marathons and beyond (100-mi races) and doing beautifully. And among the top endurance athletes in the world, aerobic fitness and performance differences between the sexes are diminishing. As more and more women have the opportunity to train and compete, who knows how well they may do?

Age

Aerobic fitness usually increases into the late teens or early 20s, and then declines slowly with the years. The rate of decline for inactive individuals seems similar (about 8 to 10% per decade) regardless of the initial level of fitness (see Figure 1.2). Those who decide to remain active can cut the decline in half (4% per decade), and those who train can cut that in half for a decade or more (Sharkey, 1987). One friend started training at age 30 and was able to increase his fitness from 46 to 54 in a few months. Thereafter his active lifestyle slowed the decline to less than 4% per decade. Now, at age 50, he is still above his fitness level at age 30.

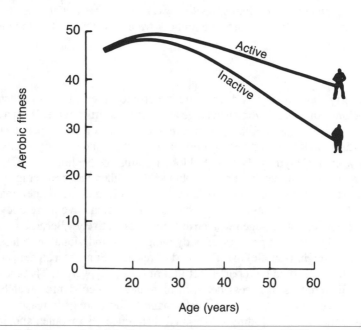

Figure 1.2. Age and aerobic fitness. Adapted from Sharkey (1977).

So in spite of the typical decline in fitness with age, ample evidence exists to support the effectiveness of training at all ages. Trainability declines with age, with the 30% improvements of adolescents declining to but 10% at age 70. Exercise gerontologist Dr. Herb deVries showed that aerobic fitness can be improved in both men and women, even after the age of 70 (deVries, 1986). Larry Lewis ran every day, well beyond his 100th birthday. Larry worked as a waiter in San Francisco; he ran 6 mi per day in Golden Gate Park, then put in a full day's work!

Do you think it is too late to start? Larry O'Neil, a lumberman from Montana, was in his late 50s when he began training as a competitive walker. Six years later he won a gold medal in the Senior Olympics. And even more dramatic is the case of Eula Weaver, who at 81 had a heart attack to add to her problems of congestive heart failure and poor circulation. Unable to walk 100 ft at first, she worked up to jogging 1 mi each day and riding her stationary bicycle for several more. She even lifted weights several days a week. At 85 she won the gold medal for the mile run in her age group at the Senior Olympics. It's never too late to start! (Learn more about age and performance in chapter 16.)

Body Fat

About one half of the decline in fitness with age can be attributed to the typical increase in body fat. Remember that we calculate the fitness score by dividing oxygen consumption by body weight. If body fat increases, your fitness declines. So the easiest way to improve fitness is to rid yourself of excess fat. For example, if Bob (at 100 kg or 220 lb and 20% fat) loses 10 kg (22 lb) or half of his body fat, his aerobic fitness score will go from

$$4 \text{ L} \div 100 \text{ kg} = 40 \text{ ml/[kg} \times \text{min]} \qquad \text{to}$$

$$4 \text{ L} \div 90 \text{ kg} = 44.4 \text{ ml/[kg} \times \text{min]}$$

Without any exercise, just weight loss, his fitness has improved 10%! Now if he receives a 25% improvement in fitness from training, as well as any additional weight loss, his fitness score could rise to 55 or more.

Impossible you say? Not at all. My old friend Earnie once smoked two packs a day, weighed over 250 lb, and bragged about his sedentary lifestyle. When he took the Forest Service fitness test, it was all he could do to finish with a score in the low 30s. Then Earnie got the message; he stopped smoking, started training, and paid attention to his diet. Today, some years later, you wouldn't recognize him. Under a layer of fat he found a trim, handsome body. Now he weighs around 170, and his fitness score is 58. He knows that the decision to change his lifestyle was the best he's ever made.

Activity

Finally, fitness is influenced by your level of activity. Most of us fall between two extremes, complete bed rest on one hand and excessive endurance training on the other. One study (Saltin et al., 1968) showed that 3 weeks of complete bed rest led to a fitness decline of 29% (almost 10% per week). Eight weeks of training restored fitness in previously trained subjects and led to improvements for previously sedentary individuals. Another study of highly trained athletes showed that cessation of training (detraining) was followed by a relatively rapid loss of fitness. In 12 weeks the gains of many months were lost (Coyle, Hemmert, & Coggan, 1986). The range of improvement from complete bed rest to vigorous training (62% in the Saltin study) provides some indication of the importance of regular physical activity.

As you will see in later chapters, regular physical activity has more to do with your health than with fitness per se. Because fitness is partially inherited and is related to sex and age, the current level of regular physical activity best correlates to health and longevity.

Potential for Fitness

Because aerobic fitness is influenced by how well you pick your parents, it seems unwise to emphasize comparisons between individuals. A better approach is to estimate how close you come to your potential for fitness. One way to do this is to be tested, at least annually, as you train to reach your potential. When your fitness score begins to plateau, you are probably approaching your potential. Exercise physiologist Dr. Jack Daniels tested some elite athletes annually for a number of years. One scored 82 when in top condition and below 80 when not training as seriously. He never exceeded 82, even when he was training 4 hours daily for the Olympics.

Someday we may be able to assess potential with a single laboratory test. Until then the only way to determine your potential is to begin training. Start working toward your potential. It takes time to achieve, and the odds are good that you have quite a way to go. In your quest you will learn a great deal about yourself as you improve your performance, health, and quality of life.

CHAPTER

2

AEROBIC FITNESS: THE TRAINING EFFECT

This chapter will help you

understand the effects of repeated aerobic exercise on the muscles, organs, and systems of the body,

differentiate among different types of aerobic training, and

define your own training goals.

Years ago, when I was just beginning serious study of fitness, we used the term **cardiovascular** to define fitness. Next came **cardiorespiratory**, and today we speak of **aerobic** fitness. The changes in terminology reflect the insights from several decades of research that have helped us focus on the important outcomes of training. We used the term cardiovascular when the best documented effects of training were on the heart and the circulation. Cardiorespiratory became popular when we began to understand the importance of oxygen intake as well as transport. And the term aerobic was adopted to indicate that oxygen intake, transport, *and utilization* were improved with training. Since 1967, when research first documented the effects of endurance training on the muscle's ability to use oxygen, there has been a growing awareness that some of the major effects of training are on the skeletal muscles themselves and their ability to carry out oxidative or aerobic energy production.

In other words, the *primary target organ* of training, the site where important structural and functional changes occur as a result of training, is *skeletal muscle*.

Of course, important secondary adaptations take place with training, such as changes in respiration, the heart, blood, circulation, the nervous system, the endocrine system, body composition, bones, ligaments, and tendons. But it is

25

impossible to improve the function of organs such as the heart without the use of the muscles. All these changes begin with muscular exercise. Train the muscles properly and the secondary benefits will follow; fail to train the muscles and the other changes are unlikely to occur. Keep that in mind and you'll have a better understanding of why and how fitness is good for your health and how you can achieve its benefits.

Training

When you repeat an exercise, such as walking or jogging, you recruit the same muscle fibers and energy pathways over and over again. When you do this on a regular basis, such as daily or every other day, your body begins to adapt to the new demands or overload by making adjustments. We call these adjustments the **training effect**. In a way not fully understood, the exercise signals the muscle fibers to undergo changes that permit more exercise in the future.

Changes only occur in the muscle fibers that are employed in the training, so training of the legs won't yield arm endurance, or vice versa. For this reason we say that exercise and training are *specific*; exercise should be tailored to involve appropriate muscle fibers in the fashion you intend to use them. Put another way, *you get what you train for*. We discuss specificity further in a later section of this chapter.

Training Studies

In this outline of the effects of training, I try to use studies conducted on human subjects. A typical training study involves pretesting for aerobic fitness and other measures; random assignment of subjects to experimental or control groups; weeks or even months of systematic and progressive training on a treadmill, laboratory bicycle, or in a supervised fitness program; and posttesting to determine the effects of training. Studies have ranged from low to high intensity, using low- to high-fitness subjects. After reviewing the effects of aerobic training, I will differentiate the effects of long, slow training versus high-intensity training and show how different types of training interact with various levels of fitness.

Detraining Studies

In recent years researchers have used another approach to study the training effect. They find subjects who have been steadily involved in a well-documented program and randomly select some of the subjects to interrupt training for a specified period (experimental group) while others continue the regime (controls). Then the researchers follow the decline of certain measures and relate the changes to decrements in performance. Although this approach has limits, it does eliminate the need for time-consuming training, especially in the case of highly trained athletes. I'll refer to both types of studies as I discuss the aerobic training effect.

Muscle Fibers

Muscle is the primary target organ of aerobic training. Therefore, our investigation of training shall begin with muscle, the motive force and recipient of many of the good things associated with regular exercise. The effects of aerobic training on muscle relate to the use of oxygen. (For more information on oxygen and energy production see Appendix A.) Oxygen is needed in the breakdown of carbohydrate and fat, the fuels that provide energy (in the form of ATP) for sustained contractions. What effect does training have on muscle? Training

- increases the levels of certain **enzymes** (proteins that speed metabolic reactions) that are needed for the aerobic breakdown of fuels to produce energy,
- increases the size and number (volume) of **mitochondria**, the cellular powerhouses that produce energy aerobically, and
- increases the muscle's ability to use fat as a fuel.

Before 1967, research had failed to demonstrate effects of training on muscle fibers. Dr. John Holloszy (1967) reasoned that earlier studies failed to overload the aerobic pathways. So he subjected rats to a very strenuous treadmill training program. Trained rats eventually were able to continue exercise for 4 to 8 hr, but untrained animals became exhausted within 30 min. Following the 12-week training program Holloszy sacrificed the rats to prepare the muscle tissue for chemical analysis. He found a 50 to 60% increase in mitochondrial protein (all oxidative metabolism takes place in the mitochondria) and a twofold rise in the oxygen consumption in the trained muscles. The muscles were better able to oxidize carbohydrate, and subsequent experiments (Holloszy, 1973) led to the fascinating conclusion that endurance-trained muscle fibers are better able to burn fat as a source of energy. His landmark experiments led the way to a better understanding of the effects and values of exercise. Incidentally, the changes found in animal experiments have all been confirmed in humans. (For a more recent discussion see Holloszy et al., 1986.)

Other studies confirmed and extended Holloszy's research. Gollnick and King (1969) put rats through a similar training program and studied the muscle with the electron microscope. The researchers found an increase in mitochondrial size and number.

Today we know that an increase in mitochondrial mass (and therefore mitochondrial enzymes) is due to branching of existing mitochondria and that the increase provides greater capacity for oxidation of energy sources, especially fat. Thus trained muscle is better able to utilize fat as the source of energy for sustained work. But the effects of enhanced fat metabolism extend beyond the realm of performance; following chapters discuss important health and weight control benefits.

Supply and Support Systems

The respiratory, circulatory, endocrine, and other systems supply and support muscles. How are they affected by aerobic training? Training

- increases the efficiency of respiration,
- improves the blood volume,
- improves the distribution of blood to the working muscles,
- enhances the delivery of blood to muscles via the capillaries, and
- increases the stroke volume and cardiac output while decreasing the resting and exercise heart rates; in other words, the heart becomes a more efficient pump.

Respiration and Oxygen Transport

Training improves the condition and efficiency of breathing muscles so the body can utilize more lung capacity during exercise. Aerobic training improves total lung capacity in at least two ways: by reducing the residual volume (that portion of lung capacity that cannot be used) and by increasing the inspiratory reserve and vital capacity. Residual volume increases with age and inactivity, and the decline in total lung capacity eventually reduces exercise capacity. Aerobic training can halt or even reverse the decline and insure adequate respiration throughout life.

Ventilation.   Training improves the maximum amount of air you can breathe per minute, the maximum pulmonary ventilation.

$$\text{Ventilation} = \text{Frequency} \times \text{Tidal Volume}$$

Training also enhances the efficiency of the process, so fewer breaths are needed to move the same volume of air. Compare a trained and untrained subject.

$$\text{Ventilation} = \text{Frequency} \times \text{Tidal Volume}$$

$$\text{Untrained } 60 \text{ L/min} = 30 \text{ breaths} \times 2 \text{ L}$$

$$\text{Trained } 60 \text{ L/min} = 20 \text{ breaths} \times 3 \text{ L}$$

The trained individual uses fewer breaths to move the same amount of air. Respiratory distress and the sense of fatigue are related to respiratory rate.

A trained person will also be able to move more air per minute (150 L/min or more, compared to 120 or less for the untrained). Slower, deeper breaths are more efficient, because they allow better penetration of air into the deep recesses of the lung (alveolar sacs) and more time for oxygen to enter the circulation. Training improves diffusion of oxygen from the lung into the capillaries of the pulmonary system. Diffusion depends on good ventilation and adequate blood flow in the pulmonary capillaries.

Blood Volume. Oxygen is transported via red cells and hemoglobin. We have long known that aerobic fitness is closely related to the total supply of hemoglobin in the blood. Both blood volume and total hemoglobin improve with training. And detraining studies (Coyle, Hemmert, & Coggan, 1986) show that the loss of blood volume with the suspension of training is closely correlated with the loss of important cardiovascular effects (such as a lower heart rate and increased stroke volume). Hence the effects of training on blood volume and hemoglobin may be more important to fitness and performance than to the effects on the heart itself.

Heart and Circulation

For years we have known that endurance training reduces the heart rate at rest and at a given work load and improves **stroke volume**, the amount of blood pumped with each beat of the heart. That is why we used the term cardiovascular to describe training effects. Training leads to an increase in the size of the left ventricle during the filling stage or diastole (increased left ventricular end diastolic volume, LVEDV). This increase takes place with little change in the thickness of the heart muscle (Morganroth & Maron, 1977). The trained heart pumps more blood each time it beats, at rest or during exercise. This is a normal reaction to training; it can't do harm and it certainly is related to improved performance.

When the pericardium sac, which encloses the heart, was removed from dogs, the animals were able to train and increase their cardiac output (Heart Rate × Stroke Volume) a whopping 20% (Stray-Gunderson, 1986). The ability to fill the ventricle with blood is highly related to performance. A large heart chamber or a heart without the restraint of the pericardium seems able to pump more blood. Of course, it also helps to have a greater blood volume to help fill the left ventricle.

The heart is a pump that ejects the blood that enters its chambers. Put more into the chamber and more comes out. Hence it is possible that changes in heart rate and stroke volume are related to improvements in blood volume, or other related factors, such as redistribution of blood.

If training doesn't have much effect on the thickness of heart muscle, what about the aerobic enzymes and mitochondria in the heart? Animal studies don't show much change in cardiac muscle enzymes; however, the trained heart does seem better able to use fat as an energy source for cardiac (heart) muscle. This improvement may be due to improved blood flow to the heart; evidence shows that training increases the diameter of the coronary arteries that supply the heart with oxygen and fuels.

So some of the major effects of endurance training seem to be the cardio-vascular effects, including decreased heart rate and increased stroke volume, which make the heart a more efficient pump. But what causes these changes? Does the heart rate go down because the stroke volume goes up, or does the stroke volume go up because the heart rate goes down? A likely answer emerges in coming sections.

Redistribution of Blood. Part of the answer may be related to the phenomenon called redistribution. Somehow, training teaches the body to route blood from less active tissue, such as digestive organs and kidneys, to active muscles and to the heart and eventually the skin for heat dissipation. This redistribution, caused by constriction of some blood vessels and dilation of others, increases blood flow to working muscles 20 times or more, even though cardiac output only increases 3 to 5 times. This important ability to regulate blood flow can be lost with several days of bed rest or weightlessness (as in space travel). But a few days of activity helps the body relearn this important ability.

Capillaries. Training even seems to enhance the delivery of blood to indi-vidual skeletal muscle fibers. Trained muscles have a higher capillary-fiber ratio (Blomqvist & Saltin, 1983). Because muscle fibers increase in diameter with training, the rise in the capillary-fiber ratio may be necessary to maintain a reason-able diffusion distance from the blood vessel to the interior of the muscle fiber. In other words, this may be an appropriate adjustment to the changing size of the fibers.

Cardiovascular Efficiency. Changes in cardiovascular efficiency may be due in part to changes in neural function that occur with training.

Nervous System

Training has several subtle but important effects on the nervous system, including

- improved efficiency and economy of motion and
- improved efficiency of the cardiovascular system.

Movement Efficiency and Economy

The economical athlete uses less energy to perform at a given speed. Hours of practice lead to relaxation and an efficient use of force to achieve results. This economy is especially evident in more complex activities such as swimming or cross-country skiing. But it is also found in running or cycling (Kearney & VanHandel, 1989).

Cardiovascular Efficiency

The nervous system participates in another adjustment that may help solve the question of why and how the heart rate and stroke volume change with training. In 1977 Saltin published a simple but elegant experiment. He directed subjects to train one leg on a bicycle ergometer, with the other leg serving as a control. He tested oxygen consumption and took muscle samples before and after training to test for oxidative enzyme activity. As you might imagine, the values increased only in the trained legs. The interesting finding was that the heart rate response to submaximal work was significantly lower for the trained legs (Saltin, 1977).

Saltin reasoned that the improvements in the trained muscle were responsible for the lower heart rate response. Mitchell, Reardon, McCloskey, and Wildnethal (1977) demonstrated that small nerve endings located in muscle are able to modify the heart rate response to exercise via connections to the cardiac control center in the brain. Thus it appears that training's influence on the muscles may alter cardiovascular function—the lower heart rate can be traced to the improved metabolic condition in the trained muscles. And when the heart beats more slowly it has more time to fill, allowing an improved stroke volume. This interpretation suggests that some of the well-documented cardiovascular effects of training are by-products of changes in the skeletal muscles. When we associate these changes with an increase in blood volume and redistribution of the blood, which together combine to put more blood into the heart, we understand why and how training allows a decrease in exercise heart rate and an increase in stroke volume. This suggests that some part of the time-honored cardiovascular effects are *specific* to the muscles being trained and that training doesn't necessarily transfer from one activity to another. I will elaborate on the significance of this point later in the chapter.

Endocrine System

The endocrine system includes the many glands whose secretions—hormones—are distributed by way of the bloodstream. The effects of training include

- changes in hormonal response and
- hormonal effects on fat mobilization.

Changes in Hormonal Response

Because the nervous and endocrine systems are functionally related, many physiology texts combine discussion of these systems in a neuroendocrine chapter. One example of this relationship concerns epinephrine (adrenaline), which is secreted by sympathetic nerve endings and by the adrenal gland. Animal studies show that the adrenal glands enlarge with training. But in animal studies subjects often train with a treadmill and receive a shock if they stop running. Obviously this method is stressful to the animals, so any increase in the size of the adrenal gland could be a reaction to stress, not just to the training.

Researchers have trained young men on the treadmill and measured stress hormones from the adrenal gland. Early exposure to strenuous treadmill training prompted a marked increase in stress hormones. As training progressed, the hormonal response returned to normal levels, in spite of a steady increase in daily work time on the treadmill. A large noisy treadmill and the subject's uncertainty regarding the difficulty of the task probably contributed to the initial stress response (Whiddon, Sharkey, & Steadman, 1969). Other studies show a decline in adrenal hormonal response with training (Docktor & Sharkey, 1971).

Many hormones are involved in the regulation of energy; epinephrine, cortisol, thyroxine, glucagon, and growth hormone raise blood sugar levels, whereas insulin is the only hormone capable of lowering blood sugar. Insulin secretion from the pancreas increases when blood sugar levels are elevated, such as after a meal, helping tissues take up the sugar. The other hormones are secreted when blood sugar levels are reduced, as in exercise. Epinephrine and growth hormone also are involved in the mobilization of fat from adipose tissue, whereas insulin leads to fat deposition. *Training seems to fine tune the body's secretion and response to hormones, leading to a more efficient use of hormones and energy sources.* Endurance training lowers the need for insulin because the muscle can take up sugar during exercise, even in the absence of insulin as in diabetes.

Fat Mobilization

Epinephrine is available from two sites, the adrenal gland and the nerve endings of the sympathetic nervous system. Epinephrine, like most hormones, acts on receptors in the membrane of its target organ, adipose tissue. The hormone activates a series of steps leading to the breakdown of triglyceride fat and the release of free fatty acids (FFA) into the bloodstream (see Figure 2.1). The FFA then travel to working muscles or to the heart where they can be used as a source of energy. During very vigorous exercise, lactic acid produced in the muscles

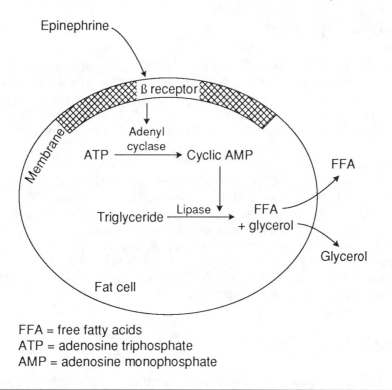

FFA = free fatty acids
ATP = adenosine triphosphate
AMP = adenosine monophosphate

Figure 2.1. Mobilization of free fatty acids from adipose tissue. Lactic acid inhibits the influence of epinephrine on the fat cell and blocks the mobilization of fat. *Note.* From Sharkey (1975).

seems able to block the action of the epinephrine, thereby reducing the FFA available for energy. Training improves the oxidative ability of muscle, leading to less lactic acid production, greater fat mobilization, and fat metabolism. Recent evidence shows that trained individuals are able to mobilize fat in spite of elevated lactate levels (Vega deJesus & Siconolfi, 1988).

Lactic acid is produced from a fragment of the carbohydrate molecule (called pyruvic acid) when there is too much pyruvic acid produced for the mitochondria to process oxidatively. Some of the pyruvic acid may be converted to the amino acid alanine instead of to lactic acid. The alanine is then released to the circulation, taken up by the liver, and converted to glucose, thus completing a glucose-alanine cycle. Training seems to increase this alternative pathway, leading to less lactic acid production (Mole, Baldwin, Terjung, & Holloszy, 1973). Whatever the cause, training leads to less lactic acid production and more fat mobilization and utilization, with profound implications for performance and health.

Body Composition

One of the most noticeable effects of training deals with the shape and composition of the body. What could be more vivid than a 40-lb weight loss revealing for the first time in years a trim and pleasing figure? Body composition refers to the relative amounts of fat and lean weight. Although the lean body weight (LBW) is relatively unchanged with endurance training, large fat loss is possible.

$$LBW = Body\ Weight - Fat\ Weight$$

Researchers usually employ underwater weighing or skinfold calipers to measure body fat. If you have 20% fat and weigh 120 lb, you have 24 lb of fat (and 96 pounds of lean weight). Lean weight may increase a bit with endurance training, especially if you had been sedentary before training. If you jog 3 mi a day, 5 days a week, you will burn about 1,650 calories per week (3 mi × 5 days × 110 cal/mi = 1,650 cal). In 2 weeks you'll burn 3,300 calories, almost a pound of fat (3,500 cal = 1 lb of fat). I'll say more about body composition and fat loss in chapter 8 and Appendix D.

Bones, Ligaments, and Tendons

Bones, ligaments, and tendons respond to the stresses placed upon them. Every change in function is followed by adaptive alterations. For bones, increased activity leads to a denser, stronger structure designed to counteract the new stresses. Inactivity leads to reabsorption of calcium and loss of supportive structures. Increasing age and inactivity create a dangerous combination for females. Bone demineralization, or osteoporosis, begins in early middle age (30 to 40 years) and becomes more serious after menopause. Inactivity hastens demineralization and weakening of bone. Although moderate activity causes bone tissue to become stronger and more dense, excessive training associated with weight loss and menstrual irregularities (amenorrhea, or absence of menstruation) can cause early osteoporosis. Calcium intake may be helpful, but it won't do much good without moderate exercise.

Moderate activity strengthens ligaments, tendons, and other connective tissue, such as the covering of muscles. By gradually increasing the work load you can make these tissues tough enough to withstand the normal demands of activity and to resist damage during accidents.

Specificity

In recent years research on training has led to an inescapable conclusion; the effects of training are *specific* to the manner in which the training is conducted. Let me explain what this means and how important it is.

Specificity of Exercise

An activity such as jogging recruits muscle fibers suited to the task. Slow muscle fibers are recruited for slow jogging. The metabolic pathways and energy sources are also suited to the task. So daily jogging recruits the same fibers and pathways over and over, leading to the adaptive response known as the **training effect**.

Specificity of Training

The outcomes of training are directly related to the activity employed as a training stimulus. Research shows that training has effects on muscle fibers as well as on the supply and support systems, such as the cardiovascular system. In general, effects on muscle fibers are likely to be very specific; that is, these effects will not transfer to activities unlike the training activity. So the effects of cycling or swim training on muscle fibers will not transfer to running nor to each other. *However, effects on the respiratory or cardiovascular systems are more likely to generalize or transfer to other activities* (Sharkey, 1988b).

Training leads to changes in enzyme systems in muscle fibers, so it is easy to see why those changes are specific. In the early stages of training the inability of muscle fibers to use oxygen limits performance. Later on, as the fibers adapt to the stimulus of training, the focus shifts to the cardiovascular system, including the heart, blood vessels, and blood. As muscles become better able to use oxygen, oxygen transport becomes the factor that limits performance (Boileau, McKeown, & Riner, 1981). The blood, blood vessels, and heart are essential factors in oxygen transport. It is easy to see why cardiovascular changes might transfer from running to cycling to swimming.

Endurance training increases blood volume and leads to changes in the distribution of blood flow. Both adaptations are likely to transfer from one activity to another. However, as noted earlier, some part of the heart rate (and stroke volume) change is due to conditions in muscle fibers that are relayed to the cardiac control center by small nerves. That means that *some part of the cardiovascular response is specific to the manner of training*. In other words, *most changes in muscle fibers and some of the cardiovascular effects will not transfer from one activity to another*. In spite of the widespread belief in the concept of *cardiovascular* fitness, the evidence suggests the concept is overrated.

Highly trained athletes learn that training is specific. They recognize that successful training must mimic the competitive event. Unfortunately many so-called fitness instructors have yet to understand the importance of specificity. They recommend circuit weight training to develop aerobic fitness, even though several studies show why the technique falls short of traditional approaches (Hempel & Wells, 1985).

Circuit weight training uses many muscle groups in an endurance weight training program. Circuit weight training fails to equal other types of aerobic training, because each muscle group is active for too short a period to produce changes in oxidative enzymes. Even though the heart rate is elevated throughout the training period, the heart rate elevations do not reflect metabolism or the need for oxygen. Arm work elevates the heart rate above that expected for the level of metabolism. It takes more than an elevated heart rate to produce changes in aerobic fitness.

Several extensive reviews show how specific training is best for specific results. Very little transfer occurs among activities such as running, cycling, swimming, or cross-country skiing. So for best results, train specifically. Of course you may engage in other activities for variety, to avoid overuse injuries (e.g., as in running), and to train other muscle groups.

Specificity of Testing

One implication of all this is that testing must be specific if it is to reflect all the changes due to training. In spite of what you see in some labs and many fitness clubs, cycling tests do not reflect the effects of running training, or vice versa. In fact, training effects are even more specific than that; hill runners are best tested on an uphill treadmill test, and hill-climbing cyclists are best tested with a standing bicycle test! Then how do we measure the effects of aerobic dance? We don't. In spite of the fact that some studies show that running is superior to aerobic dance (when tested on a treadmill), experience shows that runners poop out in aerobic dance and vice versa. As of yet we don't have a specific way to accurately assess the effects of aerobic dance, ballet, or any other dance form.

Implications for Training

What does all this mean for you and your training program? I've tried to show that individual muscle fibers undergo changes when they are recruited in exercise that lasts long enough to overload their oxidative capabilities. When aerobic metabolism is improved, the muscles use oxygen more efficiently. Training raises the anaerobic (or lactate) threshold, allowing more work to be done aerobically. This metabolic efficiency is relayed to the cardiac control center in the brain. As a result the heart can beat at a slower rate, providing more time for filling, which allows a larger stroke volume. Increased blood volume and redistribution of blood both help by providing ample blood for the heart to pump. Because so much depends on the effects of training on muscle fibers, training should be specific to its intended use.

Because training is specific, you must decide why you are training. Many train for all-around fitness, and that is fine. Others train to improve performance in a sport or activity. If you are training to run 10-k races or longer, consider the following. Long slow distance (LSD) training improves the ability of muscle fibers to use fat as an energy source. Engage in faster and necessarily shorter training and you recruit and train more muscle fibers. Do very fast but still aerobic training (such as interval training just below the anaerobic threshold) and even more fast twitch fibers improve in oxidative ability. Faster training may also elicit greater improvements in the cardiovascular system. The choice of training depends on the training goals. Train slower for distance, faster for speed. Elite athletes do both kinds of training so they can sustain speed over longer distances. (See Appendix A for more on slow and fast twitch muscle fibers.)

My choice? I like to do both in a single running workout. Start at an easy pace and cover most of the distance you've chosen. As you approach the end increase your pace to recruit and train fast fibers and achieve the extra benefits of high-intensity training. In this way you can get the best of both worlds with less risk of injury, and—here is the big bonus—the experience is more enjoyable. During slower portions of the workout you don't develop increased levels of lactic acid, so you feel comfortable. Carbon dioxide levels are lower, so breathing is less labored. You can even carry on a conversation. *One good gauge of pace is the* **talk test***; if you can't talk when you train, you're going too fast.*

As you near the end of the training session and speed up, the going gets tougher. But the distance is short and you are almost home, so it is easy to tolerate. Famous German training authority Dr. Ernst Van Aaken (1976) provided a simple way to estimate the amount of high-speed effort. He found that a 20:1 ratio of slow to fast training was sufficient to achieve results with elite distance athletes. If you run 5 mi pick up the pace for the last 1/4 mi. This short distance is enough to get the benefits of speed training, which is safer and easier after you are well warmed and relaxed.

Later chapters provide more ideas for your personalized training. Now let's see how exercise is prescribed to develop and maintain aerobic fitness.

CHAPTER

3

AEROBIC FITNESS PRESCRIPTIONS

This chapter will help you

use your fitness score and heart rate to develop an individualized fitness prescription,

achieve and maintain the level of fitness you desire,

select aerobic alternatives for use when your regular program can't be followed, and

decide if you should see your physician before beginning the program.

As with any treatment or drug, exercise must be prescribed and taken with care if its benefits are to be realized and if potentially harmful side effects are to be avoided. The dose of aerobic exercise that safely promotes the training effect (dose response) is usually expressed in terms of the **intensity, duration,** and **frequency** of exercise. Research and clinical experience are adding to a growing "pharmacopoeia of exercise," a carefully developed methodology for the safe and effective prescription of exercise.

Throughout history people have sought the health benefits believed to be associated with exercise. The Chinese practiced health-related exercise for centuries, and they continue to this day, with millions doing daily Tai Chi or riding bicycles. In Rome the physician Galen prescribed exercise for health maintenance more than 1,500 years ago. In the late 1800s, Dr. Dudley Sargent, physician and director of the Harvard College Gymnasium, tested students and *prescribed* exercises to rectify weaknesses. Exercise prescriptions improved only slightly until the 1950s when researchers established the link between physical inactivity and coronary heart disease. Since then, we have become more aware of the benefits and limitations of exercise as a modality for prevention and re-habilitation of disease. And we have gained in our ability to prescribe exercise for health, fitness, and performance in work and sport.

To best determine how hard (intensity), how long (duration), and how often (frequency) you should exercise to achieve the aerobic training effect, you should take one of the aerobic fitness tests found in Appendix B (step test or 1.5-mi run), unless you have been completely sedentary. If so, take the Pre/Fit questionnaire at the end of this chapter and assume you are in the low-fitness category (you may decide to see your physician, take an ECG-monitored exercise test, and use the results of that test to predict your level of fitness). You can take the submaximal step test after several weeks of activity. Young or active individuals may prefer the more demanding 1.5-mi run test to predict aerobic fitness. This test demands a maximal effort, so be sure that you are prepared for the challenge.

Use the fitness test to determine your fitness score and category, as shown in Table 3.1.

Now you are ready to develop a fitness prescription tailored to your age, sex, and level of fitness.

Table 3.1 Fitness Score and Category

Fitness score (ml/[kg × min])	Fitness category
Over 45	High
35-45	Medium
Under 35	Low

The Exercise Prescription

Years ago, before we knew how to prescribe exercise, we were faced with a number of unproven systems. The systems were based on the ideas and experience of well-known coaches, fitness experts, or physicians, but not on research. Then we began to recognize the factors associated with improvements in fitness. Hundreds of research studies have examined these factors and provided a safe and effective way to prescribe exercise. What are these factors?

▎**Intensity—how hard to exercise**
▎**Duration—how long to exercise**
▎**Frequency—how often to exercise**

Let's examine these factors and see why they are important.

Intensity

Intensity is important for many reasons. It determines the energy needs of the exercise, the energy source or fuel to be utilized, the amount of oxygen consumed, and the calories of energy expended (see Table 3.2). Early laboratory work defined intensity as the oxygen consumed or as a percent of the maximal oxygen consumption (e.g., 70% of maximum).

Table 3.2   Measures of Exercise Intensity

(For 70-kg individual, fitness score = 45)

Intensity	Heart rate (bpm)	$\dot{V}O_2$ (L/min)	Cal/min[a]	METs[b]
Light	100	1.0	5	4.0
Moderate	135	2.0	10	8.1
Heavy	170	3.0	15	12.2

[a]1 L of oxygen is equivalent to 5 cal/min.

[b]The MET or metabolic equivalent simply is a multiple of the resting metabolic rate. The resting rate is 1.2 cal/min (1 Met), so 12 cal/min = 10 METs.

The number of cal burned per min depends on body weight; therefore, a heavier individual burns more during a given exercise. Each MET equals 3.5 ml/[kg × min], so the MET is adjusted for body weight. The aerobics point system popularized by Dr. Kenneth Cooper is a close relative of the MET. Each aerobic point is worth 7 ml/[kg × min]) or 2 METs.

When it came time to translate these studies for use in the real world, researchers used the heart rate, which is related to oxygen consumption, as an indicator of intensity. *Today many people believe that fitness is attained by raising the heart rate, but that is a **mistake**. Aerobic fitness is achieved when the metabolic rate and oxygen consumption of muscles are elevated and the elevation is sustained long enough to overload the aerobic enzyme systems.* The heart rate is only a convenient external indicator of oxygen consumption. Sustained metabolism is the cause, and the heart rate is only a by-product.

Training Threshold.   Early training studies agreed that training had to exceed a certain minimum threshold if significant changes in aerobic fitness were to occur (see Figure 3.1).

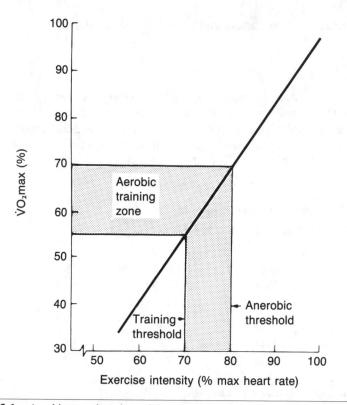

Figure 3.1.   Aerobic exercise: the training zone. Aerobic fitness improves when you exercise within the aerobic training zone.

One study trained young men at heart rates of 120, 150, or 180 beats/min. The higher intensity groups improved similarly, but the low-intensity subjects did not (Sharkey & Holleman, 1967). This and other studies seemed to agree that intensity had to exceed 130 beats per minute, which led to the realization that the effects of training were influenced by the level of fitness. Less fit individuals made progress at a lower intensity, whereas highly fit subjects had a higher training threshold (Sharkey, 1970). So each of us has a training threshold that depends on our level of activity or fitness.

Anaerobic Threshold.   Studies also suggest an upper limit to training intensity; training above that level doesn't yield extra benefits. When training becomes too intense, when the heart rate is too high, the exercise becomes predominantly anaerobic. Training above that point doesn't lead to additional improvements in aerobic fitness because it doesn't overload aerobic systems. Thus there seems to be an **aerobic training zone** that ranges from the training threshold (minimum training heart rate) to the anaerobic threshold (point of diminishing return). Training at the lower end of the zone leads to changes in slow oxidative muscle fibers. Training at the high end of the zone recruits and benefits fast oxidative glycolytic fibers and leads to central circulatory (cardiovascular) benefits. (See Appendix B for a test to determine your anaerobic, or lactate, threshold.)

Aerobic Training Zone.   Both the training threshold and anaerobic threshold are related to your level of activity and fitness. For inactive individuals the training threshold is lower, as you would expect. If normal daily activity seldom exceeds a slow walk, a brisk walk will elicit a training effect. Highly active and fit individuals have a higher training threshold. They also have a higher anaerobic threshold, especially if they regularly participate in high-intensity activity. Thus the training zone for the fit is far too strenuous for the unfit. You can use Figure 3.2 to calculate your aerobic training zone.

Simply take your age and fitness score and determine an appropriate zone. The training zone is based on a percentage of your estimated maximal heart rate. Because the maximal heart rate declines with age, it is important to use both age and fitness level to find your training zone. (Estimated maximal HR = 220 − age; e.g., for a 40-year-old, 220 − 40 = 180 maximal HR.)

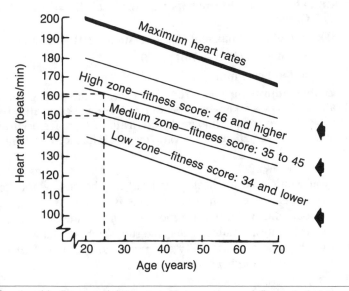

Figure 3.2.   Aerobic fitness training zones. Use your age and fitness to locate your training zone. For 25 years of age and a medium fitness score, zone = 151-162. *Note*: Percentages are percent of maximal heart rate. *Note*. From Sharkey (1977).

Heart Rate. Each of us has a resting and a maximal heart rate, which are influenced by activity and age. Your resting rate is highly influenced by your level of activity. As you do more exercise and become more fit, the resting rate declines. Although you can't estimate fitness from heart rate alone, the resting rate is a good way to measure your progress. The maximal rate is the highest possible rate for each person. The maximal rate declines with age, and it is influenced by fitness (see Table 11.1 in chapter 11). Because both the resting and maximal heart rates vary greatly, exercise prescriptions cannot be viewed as exact unless both values have been measured. The resting rate is easy to measure, but the maximal rate is usually determined at the end of a maximal exercise test on the treadmill or bicycle ergometer.

If your maximal heart rate hasn't been measured, you may have to adjust your training zone prescription. If the training zone for your age and fitness feels uncomfortably high, don't despair. Try working at the lower edge of the zone. If it still feels too high, your maximal heart rate probably is lower than the average for your age, and you should lower the zone. If the exercise feels too easy, work near the top or raise the zone—your maximal heart rate may be higher than average. The talk test is another way to determine if you are within your zone. You should be able to carry on a conversation while you train; exercise doesn't have to hurt to be good.

KARVONEN FORMULA

This formula allows the calculation of a training heart rate percent that is equivalent to the percent $\dot{V}O_2$max (percent maximal HR = percent $\dot{V}O_2$max). For 70% $\dot{V}O_2$max

$$HR = [70\% \times (\text{maximal HR} - \text{resting HR})] + \text{resting HR}$$
$$= [70\% \times (170 - 70)] + 70$$
$$= 140 \text{ beats/min}$$

This method adjusts for measured differences in the resting and maximal heart rates and avoids errors in estimation of training heart rates. It requires actual measurement of the maximal heart rate to be more accurate.

Note: With cardiac patients heart rates may be influenced by drugs or other factors.

In time you won't need to check your heart rate because you'll know how it feels to be "in the zone." The training zone is a place to begin, but as you learn more about your body, become more fit, and decide on your goals, you will outgrow heart rates, training zones, and stopwatches. You will know what it takes to get high on exercise. (Try the perceived exertion chart in chapter 13 as an alternative to the heart rate.)

Duration

Exercise duration and intensity go hand in hand. An increase in one requires a decrease in the other. Exercise duration can be prescribed in terms of time, distance, or calories. I'll use all three to show how they relate, but I prefer to use the calorie because it is so educational. The calorie (technically a kilocalorie) is the basic measure of energy intake (diet) and expenditure (exercise). You probably know how many calories you gain by eating (doubleburger = 550) or drinking (beer = 150). And you should also know how much exercise it takes to balance your energy intake (a little over 100 calories per mile of slow jogging [11-1/2 minutes per mile], or about 10 calories per minute).

Caloric expenditure during exercise is influenced by body weight. For example, a 150-lb individual burns 113 calories to run an 8-min mile, whereas a 180-lb person burns 136 calories. In this book caloric expenditures are based on the 150-lb example: Add or subtract 10% for each 15 lb over or under 150 lb. For example, add 20% to 113 calories to get the cost for the 180-lb example (113 × .20 = 22.6 + 113 = 135.6 calories). See Part III and the tables in Appendix D for more information on the caloric cost of exercise.

Years ago it was shown that low-fit individuals can improve with as little as 100 calories (5 to 10 min) of exercise per workout (Bouchard, Hollman, Venrath, Herkenrath, & Schlussel, 1966). Low-fit subjects do not respond to long duration or high-intensity training. But after several weeks of training, as fitness improves, subjects should aim for higher caloric expenditures (200 to 300 calories per workout). Early studies by fitness pioneer Dr. Tom Cureton showed that higher expenditures (over 300 calories) were needed to bring about changes in cholesterol levels (Cureton, 1969). And although 15-min sessions don't differ much from 30-min sessions, longer workouts (over 35 min) produce greater benefits in fitness (Wenger & Bell, 1986).

A study of 17,000 Harvard graduates provided another way to assess the importance of duration. Paffenbarger (1978) found a significant reduction in the risk of heart disease for graduates who averaged more than 2,000 calories of exercise per week. That translates into about 300 calories daily, 400 calories in 5 days, 500 calories in 4 days, and over 600 calories in 3 days. Longer duration training leads to improved fat metabolism in the muscles, so I recommend longer duration training (300 calories or more per session) to gain significant fitness as well as weight control and fat metabolism benefits. Although we have reasons to recommend over 30-min (or 300-calorie) sessions, no evidence indicates enhanced health from workouts that exceed 60 min (or 600 calories). Endurance athletes participate in longer workouts to achieve the stamina needed in distance events.

PROGRAM RECOMMENDATIONS

If you're in the low-fitness category, your exercise should last long enough to burn 100 to 200 calories; the medium category 200 to 400 calories; and the high category 400 calories or more (see Table 3.3). Begin at the low range for your category and work your way to the top. By the time you get there your fitness will have improved. If you are overweight and wish to burn more calories, exercise at a lower intensity and increase the duration. If you want to reduce your cholesterol and increase your high density lipoprotein (HDL) cholesterol, extend the duration of your workouts. Be willing to vary intensity and duration to avoid boredom in training. The prescription is a guide, not a rigid rule. If things get dull, change some aspect of your workout or take a day off.

Table 3.3 Exercise Duration

Fitness level ($\dot{V}O_2$max)	Duration (cal per exercise session)
Low (under 35)	100-200
Medium (35-45)	200-400
High (over 45)	Over 400

As you develop your program remember this: Paffenbarger found that exercise needs to exceed 7.5 calories per minute if it is to reduce heart disease risk. And studies show that individuals who do vigorous exercise have higher levels of HDL cholesterol and a lower risk of heart disease (Sharkey, Simpson, Washburn, & Confessore, 1980). Does that mean that walking or other moderate activities are without benefit? Of course not. Low-fit or previously inactive individuals will profit from walking. As fitness improves, the walking should become more vigorous *if continued improvements in fitness are desired*. Long walks will certainly burn lots of calories and aid in weight control. Some even think that long-duration walking will prove to have the same value for the reduction of heart disease as shorter, more intense types of effort. Time will tell, because millions are now involved in walking and other forms of moderate activity.

Frequency

For those in the low-fitness range, two or three sessions per week are sufficient to improve fitness (Jackson, Sharkey, & Johnston, 1968). But as training progresses in intensity and duration, it must also increase in frequency if continued improvements are to be achieved (Pollock, 1973). A recent review confirmed the fact that changes in fitness are directly related to the frequency of training when they are considered independent of the effects of intensity, duration, program length and initial level of fitness (Wenger & Bell, 1986). Six days per week is more than twice as effective as 2 days per week. So for fitness or weight control, consider more frequent exercise.

Athletes often engage in long sessions or they train 2 or more times each day. But smart athletes remember to observe the **hard-easy principle**, and follow hard or long sessions with short or easy ones. The hard-easy principle recognizes the fact that failure to allow adequate recovery from training nullifies its effects. The body needs time to respond to the training stimulus; some find they need more than 24 hr. Experiment with schedules to find the one that suits you best. Work out daily if you prefer, or try an alternate-day plan and increase the duration of the sessions. Whatever you do, be sure to plan at least 1 day of rest or diversion each week. A colleague and training partner once wrote, "We should approach running not as if we are trying to smash our way through some enormous wall, but as a gentle pastime by which we can coax a slow continuous stream of adaptations out of the body" (Frederick, 1973, p. 20).

Additional Considerations

The goal of the fitness prescription is to find the amount of exercise required to achieve optimal improvement. Too much exercise nullifies the purpose of the training and risks injury and even illness from suppression of the immune system. A comprehensive review of the interaction of training factors (Wenger & Bell, 1986) showed that maximal gains in aerobic fitness were achieved with high intensity (90% of $\dot{V}O_2max$), a duration of 35 to 45 min, and a frequency of 4 times per week. But lesser intensities still produced very respectable results, with much less risk of injury. And remember, improved fitness isn't the only goal. Health benefits may be achieved with less intensity, duration, or frequency, and I'll discuss this further in later chapters. Now let's develop a personalized prescription for fitness.

Your Prescription

Earlier in this chapter you used your age and level of fitness to arrive at a training zone (as shown in Figure 3.2) for exercise intensity. Now you will use this information to choose exercise duration and frequency. Using the nomogram developed by my colleague Dr. Jeff Broida (see Figure 3.3), you can determine the details of your prescription. Simply choose a heart rate within your training zone and, on the HR intensity graph, draw a horizontal line to connect that rate with the line closest to your level of fitness. Then drop straight down to the lower graph and intersect the line that describes the daily caloric expenditure for your level of fitness (100 to 200 for low fitness, 200 to 400 for medium, and over 400 for high). Finally continue your line to the left until it intersects the axis for exercise duration in minutes.

For example, a 40 year old with a fitness level of 45 and a training HR of 140 needs 400 calories of exercise; the nomogram indicates the 400-calorie level can be accomplished with just under 35 min of exercise at that heart rate. The nomogram also shows how you can get at least 2,000 calories per week using more days and shorter sessions or fewer days and longer sessions (the person

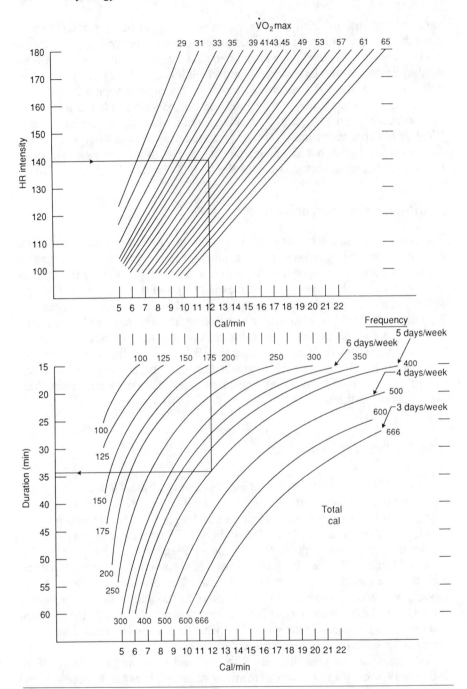

Figure 3.3. Nomogram for calculation of exercise duration. Begin with intensity, move across to fitness level ($\dot{V}O_2$max), then move down to total calories and across to duration (min). See explanation in text. From Broida, personal communication 1989.

in our example would need 57 min each day to get 2,000 calories in 3 days). Although beginners need not concern themselves with the 2,000-calorie target at first, they should work toward this exercise threshold, which has been associated with a lower risk of heart disease.

Mode of Training

Now that you have a fitness prescription, it's time to decide on a mode of training, set your training goals, and get going. People often ask me, "What is the best exercise?" Some think running or jogging is best; others argue the merits of swimming, saying it involves all the muscles of the body. Recently bicycling and cross-country skiing have been promoted, along with aerobics and walking. You've heard the arguments: You can jog anywhere anytime; cycling reduces pollution and provides transportation; cross-country skiing uses even more muscles and gets you back to nature; aerobic dance has social benefits; and walking is good anywhere, anytime, and at any age. What is the best exercise? The one you *enjoy*.

Some years ago, Dr. Mike Pollock and his associates (Pollock, Dimmick, Miller, Kendrick, & Linnerud, 1975) compared the fitness and weight control benefits of walking, running, and cycling. Sedentary middle-aged men trained at the same intensity, duration, and frequency for 20 weeks. Tests administered at the conclusion of training indicated that all three groups improved similarly in fitness, body weight, and fat. Thus, no one mode of training is superior to the others when the training prescription is the same. The best exercise is the one you enjoy and will continue to do regularly. Walking, jogging, swimming, cycling, and cross-country skiing are all good; they are rhythmic and moderate and are not likely to cause an injury. All can produce a training effect and, with skill, can lead to high levels of fitness (see Table 3.4). But remember, the caloric cost of swimming, cycling, and cross-country skiing depends on your level of skill as well as some other factors.

The caloric cost of swimming is influenced by skill, stroke, speed, and even water temperature. Unskilled swimmers tire quickly, regardless of their fitness for other sports—remember specificity? But for skilled athletes, swimming is an excellent way to train.

The cost of cycling is influenced by bicycle weight, gearing, terrain, and weather. Experienced cyclists need to pedal fast, ride uphill, or use a high gear to sustain a training heart rate. One approach is to work at a lower intensity for a longer duration. Another is to work hard on hills and, where safety permits, to use more speed. In time you'll be taking extended trips. A general rule is to cycle at a high cadence (80 or more revolutions per minute) to avoid knee soreness.

The calories expended in cross-country skiing depend upon skill as well as a multitude of other factors (e.g., stroke, snow conditions, and skis). Skilled skiers cover the ground using half the energy used by the unskilled. Ski weight,

Table 3.4 Sample Aerobic Activities

Fitness category (ml/[kg × min])*	Running		Jogging		Cycling		Walking	
	Distance (mi)	Time (min)	Distance (mi)	Time (min)	Distance (mi)	Time (min)	Distance (mi)	Time (min)
High (over 45)	3.4+	27+	3.4+	40+	7.8+	47+	4.2+	72+
Medium (35-45)	1.7-3.4	14-27	1.7-3.4	20-40	3.9-7.8	24-47	2.1-4.2	36-72
Low (under 35)	0.8-1.7	7-14	0.8-1.7	10-20	1.9-3.9	12-24	1.0-2.1	18-36

Note. Adapted from Sharkey (1977).

*Distance and time remain the same regardless of age.

width, and camber affect the energy cost. And the wrong wax for the conditions can make the sport downright difficult. But for those willing to learn the many skills of the sport, there is no more enjoyable way to achieve the benefits of fitness.

Popular games—tennis, racquetball, and basketball—are fine for maintaining a moderate level of fitness, but no serious student of fitness or sport considers them adequate for aerobic training. They don't provide the sustained metabolism needed to elicit changes. You should already be aerobically fit before you compete in these sports.

Don't play sports to get in shape!
Get in shape to play sports.

Finally, if you are preparing for a specific event, such as a distance run, bike trip, or ski tour, remember the principle of specificity and train using the exercise you will use in the event.

Cross Training

Triathlon training gave rise to the concept of cross training, with the suggestion that running and cycling could help enhance swim performance, and so forth. Unfortunately cross training doesn't work; running doesn't enhance swimming or vice versa (Sharkey, 1988a). However, you should consider using two or even three modes of training for other reasons. The repetition of running can lead to minor or even major problems. But when you take days off or switch to another form of exercise, the minor problems disappear. I run year round, but in the spring and summer I add cycling, in the fall I may roller ski, and in the winter I also swim and enjoy cross-country skiing. In some seasons I add a third mode like paddling, and I frequently participate in activities such as alpine skiing, tennis, and hiking. Try more than one training mode to exercise some muscles while resting others.

The Aerobic Training Program

Now that I've discussed aerobic fitness and described how you can develop your personal prescription, let's see how it all fits into an aerobic training program.

Each training session includes a warm-up, aerobic training, and a cool-down (see Figure 3.4). The warm-up, which should last about 5 min, gradually prepares the body for vigorous exercise. Begin with easy stretching, and as body temperature, circulation, and respiration adjust to the increased activity, move to more vigorous calisthenics. During the warm-up pay particular attention to (a) stretching lower back, hamstring, and calf muscles to prevent soreness and reduce the risk of injury, (b) gradually increasing exercise intensity, and

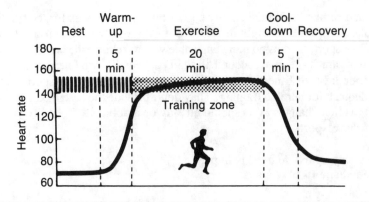

Figure 3.4. The aerobic training session. *Note.* Adapted from Sharkey (1977).

(c) stretching previously sore muscles. Some advocate stretching after several minutes of walking or easy jogging, saying it is easier to stretch a warmed muscle.

Let's take a closer look at a typical session for a 35-year-old man with a fitness score of 40. His prescription would be the following.

Intensity: 145 to 157 training zone
Duration: 200 to 400 calories (25 min at 12 calories per min = 300 calories)
Frequency: 5 to 6 days per week

The subject selects jogging as his mode of training. After the warm-up, he jogs at a comfortable 150 beats/min for 25 min to burn 300 calories. He can begin at the low end of the zone and speed up as he approaches the end of the run. After the run, he cools down with easy jogging, walking, and stretching. High levels of the hormone norepinephrine are present after vigorous exercise, making his heart more subject to irregular beats. The cool-down helps to lower excess norepinephrine and lower body temperature.

To vary the program, our friend can jog different routes, work at the upper edge of the zone for shorter periods (i.e., hard-short), or work at the lower edge for longer runs (i.e., easy-long). He can use another activity such as aerobics, swimming, or cycling for variety. No program should be the same day after day.

After a few sessions the effects of training will begin to emerge. The same pace or distance will feel easier and more enjoyable. As this occurs it is necessary to make adjustments that ensure *continued* progress. Our subject could

- jog the same distance at a faster pace (caloric expenditure remains about the same),
- cover more distance at the same pace (calories increase but intensity falls below the training zone), or
- gradually increase both pace and distance, thereby adjusting intensity and duration as his level of fitness improves.

In practice the third suggestion occurs naturally. You run faster without a greater sense of effort and fatigue, and extending the duration of a session becomes easier.

As you improve in fitness your prescription changes. The training zone moves higher along with duration (caloric expenditure) and frequency of training. Some training systems advocate increasing speed (intensity) at the expense of duration or distance. Remember that these studies used the $\dot{V}O_2$max test to determine aerobic fitness, and that this test isn't the best indicator of endurance performance. Although high-intensity training improves fitness ($\dot{V}O_2$max) and provides some central circulatory benefits, it isn't the best way to develop submaximal endurance (oxidative capacity of muscle) and it has serious drawbacks, especially for beginners. The drawbacks include risk of injury (muscle or tendon pulls), discomfort (leading some people to quit), and poor psychology. Exercise should not be something you do in a hurry to get it over with; it is a rich experience and deserves an important place in your day. Furthermore, long-duration exercise burns more calories and fat, allowing you to lose weight, lower cholesterol, and reduce heart disease risk. And the effort is more enjoyable, so you are likely to continue for months, years, or even for life.

Move to a higher level of intensity if you are interested in continued improvements in aerobic fitness. But if you are satisfied with your fitness, switch to a maintenance program. Now we'll consider the achievement, maintenance, and loss of fitness.

Achievement

The key to the achievement of fitness goals is to make haste slowly. Rush the process and the results could be painful, injurious, or worse. It takes time to coax that slow, continuous stream of adaptations from the body. You will experience improved energy and vigor within weeks, but these signs of success should not be viewed as a license for imprudent behavior. Athletes train 12 months a year for many years. Why then do older, less adaptable adults attempt to undo years of inactivity or try to remove a decade's accumulation of fat in a few short weeks?

What progress can you expect when you follow your prescription? Although the ultimate achievement will depend on your genetic endowment, with time and work you can achieve your potential. *The rate of improvement is influenced by two factors: age and initial level of fitness.* The greatest changes in your ability to take in, transport, and utilize oxygen take place when training begins during and just after puberty. Training during this phase of intense growth and development is more effective than subsequent training. *Adolescent training may lead to a 30 to 35% improvement in fitness. Young adults are able to improve as much as 25%. Trainability declines slowly thereafter,* but even a 70 year old can expect a 10% improvement (greater improvements in fitness can occur at any age when significant weight loss is involved.)

Active individuals are closer to their potential, their genetic limitation. There-fore, they will not improve as much as their less-active and less-fit contemporaries. Complete inactivity, such as prolonged bed rest, provides a clean canvas for the demonstration of dramatic changes, perhaps as much as 100% improvement above bed rest levels after several months of training. So sedentary folks may improve more than 30%, whereas trained athletes may have to be satisfied with 3 to 5% improvement or none at all, depending on the nature of their age, prox-imity to the genetic limit, and current and previous training.

The rate of improvement is dramatic at first, 3% per week for the first month, 2% per week for the second, and slowing to 1% or less thereafter. But even though the improvements in fitness begin to plateau after several months, the capacity to perform submaximal work continues to improve (see Figure 3.5). And most of our lives are spent far below the maximal level of effort.

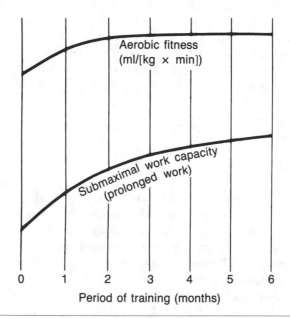

Figure 3.5. Training, aerobic fitness, and submaximal work capacity. With prolonged training, aerobic fitness begins to plateau, but the capacity to perform submaximal work continues to improve. *Note.* Adapted from *Textbook of Work Physiology: Physiological Bases of Exercise* (2nd ed.) by P.O. Åstrand and K. Rodahl, 1977, New York: McGraw-Hill; and from Sharkey (1977).

If you are a normally active adult, 20 to 40 years old, with a fitness score of 40, you may expect to achieve a score of 50. And continued activity will slow the rate of decline thereafter. Most important is the improvement in sub-maximal capacity, which is likely to improve until it approaches 70 to 80% of the maximal oxygen consumption. This means that you will be able to sustain once-fatiguing tasks for extended periods, without fatigue or discomfort. And the benefits will extend beyond your regular mode of exercise to all your daily tasks. Fitness expands your horizons!

Maintenance

Once you achieve the aerobic fitness and submaximal work capacity that meets your needs, you may want to switch to a maintenance program. That doesn't mean you will exercise less often, only that you will be free to utilize your new-found fitness in a variety of enjoyable activities. You will be able to maintain fitness with three sessions per week, leaving time and energy for tennis, alpine skiing, or other enjoyable pursuits. Or you may decide to improve performance in another aerobic activity. The choice is yours.

Researchers have approached the problem of maintenance in several ways. One is to train subjects to a level of fitness, then cease training to see how quickly the improvements recede. With some activity fitness doesn't decline that quickly, but with complete bed rest it may drop as fast as 10% per week (Greenleaf, Greenleaf, VanDerveer, & Dorchak, 1986). Another way is to try various frequencies for the maintenance of fitness (e.g., one, two, three, or four workouts per week). *Most studies show that you can maintain fitness with two or three sessions weekly, but the activity must be of the same intensity and duration used to achieve the improvements* (Brynteson & Sinning, 1973). Exercise of lower intensity but longer duration also seems to work, but it won't keep you tuned for a race. And it may be that one very long workout may help retain fitness for a while. But a combination of activities plus two to three sessions of training is sure to do the job.

More recently, researchers have used a more complex approach to study maintenance. By studying specific effects of training, such as the increase (or decrease) in the activity of aerobic enzymes, the researcher is able to plot the ''influence'' of a training bout.

From such studies, it appears that two to three sessions weekly are necessary for maintenance. Meet that requirement and you will avoid significant loss of fitness.

Estimates for the **half-life** of a training effect, the time it takes to lose one half of the benefit, range from 4.5 to 9.4 days (Watson, Srivastava, & Booth, 1983). The half-life is used because it is difficult to tell when the biological effects, such as levels of enzymes, finally return to pretraining levels. So researchers measure the total change and take half of that value. If half of the training effect is lost in 6 days, you'll want to train more often to maintain or improve fitness.

Does a previously fit individual regain lost fitness more quickly? Although the limited research in this area says probably not, common sense and observation argue for a tentative "maybe." The answer may depend on factors such as the initial level of fitness, genetic potential, and the extent of previous training. An extended period of serious training may result in structural changes that are not lost as quickly as enzyme activity and blood volume. And the repetition of training will certainly lead to skill and an economy of motion that makes subsequent activity seem easier.

But instead of worrying about the minimum amount of exercise necessary, I encourage you to find activities you enjoy and to integrate them into your lifestyle. Before long you'll view activity as an enjoyable and essential part of your day. You'll be hooked on exercise, and maintenance will take care of itself.

Medical Examination

Should you have a medical examination before you embark upon an aerobic fitness program? Per Olaf Åstrand, MD, the noted Swedish physician and physiologist, once said,

> The answer must be that anyone who is in doubt about the condition of his health should consult his physician. But as a general rule, moderate activity is less harmful to the health than inactivity. You could also put it this way: A medical examination is more urgent for those who plan to remain inactive than for those who intend to get into good physical shape!

The ACSM once called for a medical examination and a maximal exercise test prior to a major increase in exercise for any adult above the age of 35 years. More recently, the guideline has been relaxed to age 45 or above (American College of Sports Medicine, 1986). Chapter 11 includes more about medical examinations and exercise tests.

If you are older, are concerned about your health, or have several risk factors, by all means consult your physician for a medical examination prior to a major increase in exercise habits. But if you are asymptomatic (free of symptoms), reasonably active, and free of major risk factors (e.g., high blood pressure, a high cholesterol level, a smoking habit, or a family history of disease), an increase in activity does not represent an unreasonable risk. The benefits of exercise are so important for individuals and for society, we should not price exercise beyond the means of the average citizen. The cost of a preexercise medical exam may deter many from undertaking a moderate program: For some it is all the excuse they need.

To see if you should see your doctor, and to reduce doubts you may have concerning your readiness to undertake a fitness program, use the Pre/Fit Physical Readiness Exam to guide your decision (see Table 3.5). This simple questionnaire was adapted from materials published by the British Columbia Ministry

Table 3.5 Pre/Fit* Physical Readiness Exam for Fitness Test or Program

Pre/Fit is designed to help you help yourself. Many health benefits are associated with regular exercise. Completing Pre/Fit is a sensible first step if you plan to increase your physical activity. It will tell you whether you are ready for an exercise test or a graduated exercise program.

For most of us, physical activity poses no problem or hazard. Pre/Fit has been designed to identify that small number of individuals who should seek medical advice concerning the extent and activity most suitable for them.

Yes	No	
☐	☐	Has your doctor ever said you have heart trouble?
☐	☐	Do you frequently have pains in your heart and chest?
☐	☐	Do you often feel faint or have spells of severe dizziness?
☐	☐	Has a doctor ever said your blood pressure was too high?
☐	☐	Has your doctor ever told you that you have a bone or joint problem that has been aggravated by exercise, or might be made worse with exercise?
☐	☐	Is there a good physical reason not mentioned here why you should not follow an activity program even if you wanted to?
☐	☐	Are you over age 65 and not accustomed to vigorous exercise?
☐	☐	Are you using any drugs that might alter your response to exercise?

If you answered **YES** to one or more questions:

Consult with your doctor by telephone or in person *before* taking a fitness test or increasing your physical activity. Tell your doctor what questions you answered YES on Pre/Fit or show the doctor your copy.

After medical evaluation, seek your doctor's advice about your suitability for

• unrestricted physical activity, on a gradually increasing basis or

• restricted or supervised activity to meet your specific needs.

If you answered **NO** to all questions:

You have reasonable assurance of your suitability for

• a fitness test (the step test is a safe, submaximal test that measures aerobic fitness) and

• a fitness program—a *gradual* increase in exercise promotes fitness and minimizes discomfort.

_____
Signature

*Pre/Fit is adapted from the Physical Activity Readiness Questionnaire developed by British Columbia Ministry of Health.

of Health. As you can see, the Canadians have a less conservative view of exercise than do Americans. Answer no to all eight questions and you have reasonable assurance of your suitability for a fitness test and program.

PART
II

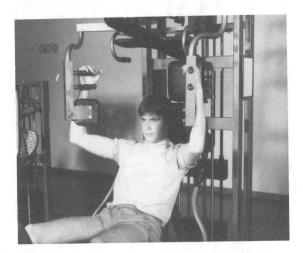

MUSCULAR FITNESS

For many years muscular fitness occupied a rather awkward position on the fringe of the fitness movement. We recognized its importance in athletics and for some physically demanding jobs, but we lacked conclusive evidence linking muscular fitness with health or the quality of life. But that has all changed. Now we can honestly say that aerobic and muscular fitness both contribute to health, but they do so in different ways.

Muscular fitness is essential if you are to avoid the low back problems that plague millions of Americans. And in recent years we have learned that muscular fitness training (e.g., weight training) is a good way to avoid the crippling bone demineralization known as osteoporosis. So if you intend to remain active beyond your 50th birthday, you should add muscular fitness training to your fitness program.

The primary components of muscular fitness are strength, muscular endurance, and flexibility. Other important components include speed, power, agility, balance, and coordination. The chapters in Part II describe each component and explain how to train for each with a safe, proven exercise prescription. People of all ages may utilize muscular fitness to improve performance in a favorite sport or activity or to look good in a bathing suit. Middle-aged individuals also rely on abdominal tone and flexibility exercises to prevent or minimize low back problems. And, those over 55 years of age employ strength and endurance activities to retain bone density and to remain active and independent. Integrate muscular activities into your program and you'll reap additional benefits of fitness throughout life. (See Appendix C for muscular fitness tests and exercises.)

CHAPTER

4

UNDERSTANDING MUSCULAR FITNESS

This chapter will help you

identify the primary components of muscular fitness,

recognize other uses of muscular fitness, and

understand how muscular fitness contributes to health and total fitness.

Primary Components of Muscular Fitness

This chapter begins with a consideration of the primary components of muscular fitness: strength, muscular endurance, and flexibility. These are called primary components because they are the ones most related to health. Other components, such as speed, power, agility, balance, and coordination, are covered later in the chapter.

Strength

Strength is obviously important for those whose occupation demands it or who participate in certain sports; surprisingly, strength is also important for those over 55 years of age. As we age our strength declines slowly. But somewhere after age 55 it begins to decline more rapidly. Throughout life we need some strength to avoid acute or chronic injury, to meet emergencies, and to engage fully and independently in life. It takes strength to change a flat tire, to shovel the walk, and to lift and carry infants, the laundry, or the groceries. Lack of muscular fitness leads to lack of activity, which hastens the loss of strength. But you can reverse this vicious cycle and remain strong and independent well into your 8th decade.

Definition. Strength is defined as the maximal force that can be exerted in a single voluntary contraction. Most of us possess more strength than we are able to demonstrate. In a fascinating experiment, Ikai and Steinhaus (1961) showed that significant increases in strength could be elicited by gunshot, shouting, drugs, or hypnosis during the contraction. Untrained individuals inhibit the full expression of strength. Inhibitions reside in the brain and in inhibitory muscle receptors. One effect of training is to reduce inhibitions and allow a fuller expression of available strength.

So strength is not an absolute value. It is subject to change, and this is what makes the subject of strength training so interesting. When strength improves, how much is due to reduced inhibitions and how much due to changes in the muscle tissue? Can we find a way to increase strength without spending a lot of time with weights?

Factors Influencing Strength. The force you exert in a maximal voluntary contraction depends on a number of factors, such as inhibitions, the number of contracting fibers, their contractile state (length and fatigue), and the mechanical advantage of the bony lever system. Most of these are easy to explain. More fibers equal more force; the stretched muscle exerts more force (probably because of elastic recoil and a favorable alignment of contractile proteins); the unfatigued muscle exerts more force; and mechanical factors conspire to magnify force or speed. Several other factors, including sex, age, and fiber type deserve more attention.

Sex. Until 12 to 14 years of age, boys are not much stronger than girls. Thereafter, the average male gains an advantage that persists throughout life. Is the difference due to the increase in the male sex hormone **testosterone** at puberty? Perhaps—the average male has 10 times the testosterone found in the average female. Testosterone is an anabolic (growth-inducing) steroid that helps muscles get larger. College women have half the arm and shoulder strength and 70% of the leg strength of men. But a relationship doesn't imply cause and effect. The relationship of strength and testosterone could be related to a third factor. For example, the hormone may make one more aggressive and willing to train harder.

Consider another confounding possibility—body fat. Young women have twice the percentage of fat (25%) as men (12.5%). When you look at strength per unit of lean body weight (body weight minus fat weight), women have slightly stronger legs, whereas arm strength is 30% below the men's values. Wilmore (1983) suggested that because women use their legs as men do (e.g., walking, running, and cycling), men's and women's leg muscles are similar in strength. However, because few women use their arms in heavy work or sport, their strength lags behind in this area. Thus it is too early to judge women the weaker sex. As more women engage in upper body strength activities for occupational purposes (police work, firefighting, or construction) or for sport, women's arm strength may approach that of men.

However, muscle size and strength do go together, and the average male is larger than the female. Most studies indicate a force of 4 to 6 kg per square centimeter of muscle girth. To estimate muscle girth in the upper arm, you should measure subcutaneous fat and bone size as well, because they will be part of the total circumference. The larger muscle is generally the stronger one but not necessarily the most successful in work or sport.

Age. Strength reaches a peak in the early 20s and declines slowly until age 55 or above. Thereafter the rate of decline usually accelerates, but it doesn't have to. When strength is used it hardly declines at all, even into the 60s. World class weight lifters have achieved personal records in their 40s. Training before puberty leads to improvements that are mostly due to changes in the nervous system (neurogenic factors include reduced inhibitions and learning how to exert force). Training after puberty combines nervous system changes with changes in the muscle tissue (myogenic changes). However, because testosterone levels decline in old age, senior citizens may be limited to neurogenic changes. Training at any age improves or maintains strength, especially when the diet is adequate. I'll say more about both later on.

Muscle Fiber Types. Earlier I noted the presence of two muscle fiber types— slow twitch and fast twitch. The larger, faster contracting fast twitch fibers have a greater potential for the development of tension. People with a higher percentage of fast twitch fibers have a greater potential for force development. Studies of human muscle tissue reveal that weight lifters have twice as much fast twitch fibers as nonlifters. The size can partially be attributed to training, partially to heredity. The effect of strength training on muscle fiber types has yet to be completely resolved; current evidence indicates that both types grow larger with training, but growth of the fast fibers is more pronounced. Strength training improves the capabilities of both types (see Appendix A for more on muscle fiber types).

Types of Strength. Strength can be measured and developed in several ways, each of which is highly specific. How the strength will be used should dictate the mode of training and testing.

Isotonic, or dynamic, strength is defined as the maximal weight that can be lifted one time. This is actually a measure of strength at the hardest part of the lift, usually the beginning. Because the mechanical advantage of your muscle-lever system changes, the lift becomes easy after you overcome the initial resistance and bad angle of pull. Dynamic strength measurements are related to performance in sport and work. Weight lifting with machines or free weights is the common form of isotonic training. (*Iso* means same, *tonic* means tone; *isotonic* means same tone.)

Isometric, or static, measures of strength are achieved when a subject exerts maximal force against an immovable object. Isometric strength is specific to the angle at which the muscle is trained and doesn't measure strength throughout the range of motion. You train by exerting near-maximum force against an immovable object. (*Metric* means length; *isometric* means same length.)

Isokinetic strength is measured by an expensive electronic or hydraulic apparatus that allows display of force output throughout the range of motion. Although such devices seem to be valuable testing and training aids, we don't yet know to what extent we need strength throughout the range of motion. (*Kinetic* means speed; *isokinetic* means same speed.)

Popular variations of these methods include **variable resistance** (resistance varies with speed) and **accommodating resistance** (resistance accommodates to available force). Although each type of apparatus has some interesting features, no method or system has proven superior in the development of strength in subjects with little previous muscular fitness training. More experienced lifters use the method suited to the task or activity. Athletes may use free weights, isokinetic machines, and even isometric contractions in an effort to improve performance. Strength is specific to the method of training, to the speed of contractions, and to the angle employed in training. And the method of testing should be specific to the mode of training if you want to accurately assess the effects of training. In other words, don't use an isometric test to reflect changes due to isotonic or isokinetic training, or vice versa.

Muscular Endurance

Muscular endurance means the ability to persist. It is defined and measured as the repetition of submaximal contractions or submaximal holding time (isometric endurance). Muscular endurance is essential for success in many work and athletic activities. Once you have the strength to perform a repetitive task, additional improvement in performance depends on muscular endurance, the ability to persist. As you know, stronger fast twitch fibers fatigue more readily. Thus endurance and strength are not necessarily related, except when a very heavy load is used in an endurance test.

> I emphasize the term muscular endurance to differentiate it from other uses of the term endurance. It is possible to develop considerable endurance in small muscles, such as the finger flexors used by a pianist or barber, without having any noticeable effect on the heart or respiratory systems. My barber has great endurance in his hands, but his aerobic fitness is poor.

Endurance and Strength.   Endurance and strength are really quite different in physiological terms. Endurance is achieved by repetitive contractions of muscle fibers. Repetitive contractions require a continuous supply of energy, and muscle fibers with aerobic capabilities (slow oxidative or fast oxidative glycolytic) are suited to the job. The repetitive contractions enhance the aerobic enzymes, mitochondria, and fuel and oxygen supplies needed for even more endurance.

Strength comes from lifting heavy loads a few times, and the effects of strength training are most noticeable in fast twitch fibers. Training effects include increases in contractile proteins (actin and myosin) and tougher connective tissue. The increased strength comes from greater cross-sectional area, with more protein filaments and cross bridges to exert force. So the training and the effects of endurance and strength training are quite different. Keep that in mind as you develop your own program. Endurance is important for practice, training, and performance. Repetition leads to skill and repetition requires endurance, so endurance is often the key to success in sport.

Diet and Endurance. Although training is certainly the best way to enhance endurance, there is something else you can do, something as simple as selecting the right foods. The fuel for muscular contractions depends on the intensity of exercise; muscle glycogen is the fuel used for high-intensity effort. But the supply of glycogen, the storage form of glucose, is limited in muscle, and when the supply is gone the muscle's performance drops to a level compatible with fat metabolism. That means long-duration, high-intensity endurance efforts such as a long hard run or bike ride will be enhanced if you have more glycogen stored in the working muscles. The food you eat can directly influence muscle glycogen levels and endurance performance.

In 1939 Scandinavian researchers (Christensen & Hansen, 1939) reported remarkable improvements in endurance for subjects fed a high-carbohydrate diet. That study virtually went unnoticed for years as coaches and trainers continued to order high-protein meals for athletes. More recently, the muscle biopsy technique has been used to study the influence of exercise and diet on endurance performance, and a series of studies has led to several firm conclusions: The best endurance performances are always attained on the high-carbohydrate diet, average performances on a typical mixed diet, and worst performances on the low-carbohydrate (high-fat and high-protein) diet.

Smart athletes follow the high-carbohydrate (high-performance) diet, which is good for fitness, performance, and health. It includes

25% of calories from fat,

15% from protein, and

60% from carbohydrate.

Compare that with the average American diet of 40%, 15%, and 45% from fat, protein, and carbohydrate, respectively. The carbohydrate we advocate is called complex carbohydrate, in contrast to the simple carbohydrate (e.g., refined sugar) found in junk food. Complex carbohydrates include corn, rice, beans, potatoes, and whole grain products (cereals, breads, and pasta). They are a good source of energy and, unlike refined sugar, they include other nutrients and fiber. I will show you the easy way to carbohydrate load in chapter 10.

Flexibility

Flexibility is the range of motion through which the limbs are able to move. Skin, connective tissue, and conditions within joints restrict the range of motion, as does excessive body fat. Injuries occur when a limb is forced beyond its normal range, so improved flexibility reduces this potential.

The range of motion increases when joints and muscles are warmed. Stretching exercises are most successful after some warm-up but before vigorous effort. Stretching after exercise, during the cool-down period, may help reduce muscle soreness. Flexibility exercises are important when training for strength or endurance, because they help you to maintain the range of motion that might otherwise be reduced. Most runners turn to stretching to make their running more enjoyable. Calf, hamstring, groin, and back muscles can become tight and sore, even after years of participation. Daily stretching means the difference between enjoyment and discomfort.

Yoga has gained popularity as a way to achieve relaxation and meditative states. Years ago, yoga positions were viewed as painful contortions, torturous exaggerations on the lunatic fringe of exercise. But today, often stripped of its more mystical elements, yoga has emerged as a safe, enjoyable, and relaxing flexibility program. The greatest benefits are in flexibility, with some potential for improvements in strength and balance, although little evidence supports claims of improved aerobic fitness or significant gains in strength or endurance.

Flexibility contributes to success in work and sport. Lack of flexibility is implicated in the development of acute and chronic injuries and low back problems. All of us profit from regular stretching exercises, and older folks have a special need because connective tissue becomes less elastic with age.

Other Components of Muscular Fitness

In addition to strength, endurance, and flexibility, muscular fitness also includes speed, power, agility, balance, and coordination or skill. Although these components are often important to success in sport or work, they are not believed to be health-related components of muscular fitness.

Speed and Power

These are important and related components of most sports. Both are somewhat related to muscular strength and both can be improved.

Speed may be the most exciting ingredient in sport. Total speed of movement includes reaction time and movement time. Reaction time (the time from the stimulus—such as a starting gun—until the beginning of the movement) is a function of the nervous system. We can't change the speed of nerve impulse transmission along a neuron. Thus any significant improvement in reaction time must be achieved by increasing awareness of appropriate stimuli and by repetition of appropriate responses, which reduce central nervous system processing time. In football, coaches use special drills to improve reaction time.

Movement time, the interval from the beginning to the end of the movement, may often improve (decrease) with appropriate strength training. The key to success lies in the principle of specificity: The movement must be specific to the sport. If you want to throw a baseball with greater velocity, train with light weights at a fast speed. If you are a shot putter, throw heavier weights as fast as possible. Specificity applies to the rate of movement and the resistance employed, which means that the training should simulate the action as closely as possible.

How much can you improve? Remember what I've said about fast twitch fibers; you'll need a high percentage to move fast. If you don't have over 50% fast fibers, don't despair. You may never be as fast as those who do have a high percentage, but you can improve your movement time by following the principles presented in the next chapter. But don't conclude that continued improvements in strength will always lead to improvements in movement time. Strength is more related to speed when the movement is resisted (as in football or shot put). And remember that speed, like strength, is extremely task specific. The speed of arm movement is not necessarily related to the speed of leg movement. Some may be quick with their hands but, because of lack of training, lack of skill, or excess fat, may be slow of foot. Improved skill and strength training reduce the time it takes to complete a movement.

Power is something football coaches often talk about. A lineman needs explosive power to move his opponent. But power is important in other sports, such as cycling and cross-country skiing. Power is defined as work divided by time, or the rate of doing work. Work is defined as force multiplied by distance.

$$\text{Power} = \frac{\text{Work}}{\text{Time}} = F \times \frac{D}{T} = \text{Force} \times \text{Velocity (because Velocity} = D/T)$$

Power combines strength (force) and velocity (distance/time). One who is able to do more work in the same unit of time has more power. If you move 100 kilograms a distance of 1 meter (m) in 1 second (s), you've done 100 kilogram meters (kg/m) of work per second. If you move the same load 2 m in 1 s or 1 m in 1/2 s, you've exhibited twice as much power. Thus power is related to movement time; improve movement time and you'll increase power, or vice versa.

Power is important in a number of sports, but it is seldom required of non-athletic adults. If you want to increase your power for cycling, skiing, basketball, or some other sport, remember the principle of specificity. Even runners can increase power by running uphill, by running against resistance, or by using high-speed repetitions in weight training. I'll provide a power prescription in chapter 6, and tests of power and other components of muscular fitness in Appendix C.

Agility

Agility is the capacity to change position and direction rapidly with precision and without loss of balance. Agility depends on strength, speed, balance, and coordination. Agility is undeniably important in the world of sport, but it is also useful to avoid embarrassment or injury in recreational activities and in potentially dangerous work situations. Because agility is associated with specific skills, no one test predicts agility for all situations. Agility can be improved with practice and experience. Excess weight hinders agility for obvious reasons. Extreme strength isn't a prerequisite, nor is aerobic fitness. However, because agility deteriorates with fatigue, aerobic and muscular fitness should help maintain agility for extended periods, such as a long tennis match.

Balance

Dynamic balance is the ability to maintain equilibrium during vigorous movements. Balance depends on the ability to integrate visual input with information from the semicircular canals in the inner ear and from muscle receptors. It is difficult to measure and predict how dynamic balance contributes to or detracts from sport performance. Evidence indicates that balance can be improved through participation in sports and a variety of movement experiences, especially during childhood. Because it is likely that balance is also task specific, practice of the specific activity should be the best way to improve balance and performance.

Having football or basketball players engage in aerobic dance or ballet classes is likely to result in a profound cultural experience, for both the players and the teacher, and it is sure to make the athletes better dancers. Whether or not it will improve their performance on the field or court has yet to be demonstrated. It is safe to say that few, if any, of the top basketball professionals developed their moves around an arabesque, entrechat, or glissade. And none I've seen shoot fouls in the fifth position!

Coordination or Skill

Coordination implies a harmonious relationship, a smooth union or flow of movement in the execution of a task. In striking the tennis serve, one develops force sequentially. As momentum from body twist approaches its peak, the arm extends at the elbow, and maximum racket speed is finally achieved with the snap of the wrist. If the forces are added in the wrong sequence, the movement appears uncoordinated.

Coordination or skill is achieved with hours of practice. Repetitions lead to changes in the nervous system that make the movement automatic. But every skill is specific; therefore, each must be learned individually. Ability in tennis doesn't assure success in badminton, squash, or racquetball; skill doesn't transfer as readily as was once thought. Another feature of coordination or skill will become apparent as you train for fitness. Skilled individuals work efficiently; they don't waste movement or energy. A skilled runner uses less energy at a given speed, and a skilled worker often can outproduce a stronger or more fit co-worker. We can learn skill, coordination, and technique; with proper skill we make best use of leverage and large muscle groups, thereby avoiding injury and fatigue of smaller muscles.

CHAPTER

5

MUSCULAR FITNESS: THE TRAINING EFFECT

This chapter will help you

understand the effects of training on the components of muscular fitness,

differentiate between the specific effects of strength and endurance training, and

select the type of muscular fitness training most suited to your needs.

How does a session of training lead to changes in the muscles? How does the muscle fiber know the difference between strength and endurance training? Part of the answer to these questions is related to the training stimulus, the characteristic of training related to adaptations.

The Training Stimulus: Strength and Endurance

Strength seems to improve when sufficient tension is applied to the muscles' contractile system. The tension required seems to be above two thirds of the muscles' maximal force. If you do contractions that require less tension you won't gain much strength. Contraction time or the total number of contractions also seems to influence the development of strength. Do more contractions and obtain better results, up to a point. The number of contractions probably depends on level of training, nutrition, hereditary endowment, and other factors. You will receive benefits from any form of strength training, as long as you exert enough tension for a sufficient period of time or number of repetitions.

Overload

In training we often speak of the **overload principle.**

> ### THE OVERLOAD PRINCIPLE
> **For improvements to take place, work loads have to impose a demand (over-load) on the body system (about two thirds of maximal force for strength).**
>
> **As adaptation to loading takes place, more load must be added.**
>
> **Improvements are related to the intensity (tension for strength), duration (time or repetitions), and frequency of training.**

Specificity

Overload training leads to adaptations in the muscles according to the type of training. Here again, the principle of specificity applies, just as it did with aerobic training. The adaptations to *strength* training include increased size, due to increases in contractile protein (actin and myosin) and tougher connective tissue. These changes allow the muscle to exert more force.

The adaptations to *endurance* training include improved aerobic enzyme systems, larger and more numerous mitochondria (increased mitochondrial density), and more capillaries. All these changes promote oxygen delivery and utilization within the muscle fiber, thereby improving endurance (Jackson & Dickinson, 1988). Fatiguing *repetitions* somehow stimulate the muscle fiber to become better adapted to use oxygen and aerobic enzymes for the production of energy (ATP) to sustain contractions. Do more repetitions and you will become better able to use fat as a source of energy.

Table 5.1 reviews the effects of each type of training and suggests that questions remain regarding the effects of training with medium resistance and medium repetitions. In chapter 6 you will learn how to select resistance and repetitions to achieve your goals.

Just how the strength or endurance training stimuli bring about the appropriate changes is not entirely known. But from what is known about how cells work, it is likely that the training stimulus somehow signals the nucleus to make a particular messenger (**messenger RNA** or **mRNA**). This messenger is shaped by the DNA, the cell's blueprint, and sent into the muscle fiber to order the production of more protein (contractile protein for strength training, enzyme protein for endurance). Structures in the muscle fiber, called **ribosomes**, receive the message and begin to produce the protein needed to adapt to the training stimulus. Another RNA (**transfer RNA** or **tRNA**) is used to gather up the amino acids needed to construct the protein, bring them to the ribosome, and place them in the growing chain of amino acids that will become a protein. Because both forms of RNA are formed by the DNA, the training stimulus

Table 5.1 The Strength-Endurance Continuum

	Strength	Short-term (anaerobic) endurance	Intermediate endurance	Long-term endurance
Train with	High resistance Low repetitions		Medium resistance Medium repetitions	Low resistance High repetitions
Training effect	More contractile proteins (actin and myosin) Increased short-term energy (ATP and CP) Stronger connective tissue Reduced inhibitions		?	Aerobic enzymes and mitochondria Improved oxygen intake and fat utilizations Increased capillaries

ATP = adenosine triphosphate

CP = creatine phosphate

must somehow influence the nucleus. We don't know if the nucleus is signaled by tension, electrolytes, waste products, or hormones, so we are unable to trick the muscle into getting stronger or building endurance without training. So you'll have to pursue the prescriptions in chapter 6 to improve your muscular strength or endurance.

Strength Training.   Strength training, which involves high resistance and low repetitions, leads to the following adaptations:

- increased contractile protein (actin and myosin),
- tougher connective tissue,
- contractile efficiency and reduced inhibitions, and
- possibly an increase in number of muscle fibers.

Contractile Protein.   Some years ago, Gordon (1967) compared the effects of strength and endurance training on muscle proteins. His results have since been corroborated in labs throughout the world: Strength training adds to the portion of the muscle that generates tension, the contractile proteins, and endurance training enhances the energy supply system, the aerobic enzymes (all enzymes are constructed of proteins). But the most surprising outcome of his study was the observations that strength training brings about a decline in endurance enzyme protein and that endurance training leads to a decline in contractile protein. Thus if you train for only strength or only endurance, you could lose a bit of the other. This aspect of specificity shouldn't be so surprising; the size and strength of thigh muscles increase during cycling or ski seasons but decline when you return to distance running.

Connective Tissue.   Connective tissue and tendons grow in size and toughness when they are placed under tension. This increased toughness in tendons may help quiet the inhibitory influence of the muscle receptor known as the tendon organ. The increase in thickness contributes a bit to the overall growth or hypertrophy of the muscle.

Nervous System.   Some of the effects of strength training occur in the nervous system. Experienced athletes seem to have fewer inhibitions, both in the central nervous system and from muscle receptors. Practice (repetition) allows us to be more efficient, more skilled in the application of force. Thus, practice alone accounts for some of the improvements in the early stages of training. This may explain why involuntary contractions brought on by an electrical stimulator do not equal the results obtained with voluntary contractions. Involuntary contractions may elicit changes in the muscle, but they don't teach the nervous system how to contract (Massey, Nelson, Sharkey, & Comden, 1965).

Muscle Fibers.   The ability to look at samples of human muscle before and after training has led to some fascinating questions. Can strength training lead to the formation of additional muscle fibers?

For years we believed that the number of muscle fibers was set at birth and was not subject to change. Then Van Linge (1962), using laboratory rats, transplanted the tendon of a small muscle into a position where it would have to assume a tremendous work load. After a period of heavy training, he studied the muscle and found the transplanted muscle doubled its weight and tripled its strength. Furthermore, the heavy work load stimulated the development of new muscle fibers.

Studies on human muscle suggest that we may be able to increase the number of muscle fibers, which happens when overloaded fibers split to form new fibers. However, this finding is still the subject of scientific debate, and I don't suggest that you will form new fibers as the result of ordinary strength training. But for those athletes who spend hours each day lifting weights, or for those who use anabolic steroids to promote unnatural growth, increased fibers may be a possibility.

The available evidence does suggest some differences between the high-resistance, low-volume training of power lifters and the medium-resistance, high-volume training of body builders. The high-resistance, low-volume training seems to increase the size (hypertrophy) of fast twitch fibers, whereas the medium-resistance, high-volume training causes selective hypertrophy of slow twitch fibers (Tesch, Thorsson, & Kaiser, 1984). Here again the response seems to be specific to the type of training.

Endurance Training. Endurance training, which involves low resistance and high repetitions, leads to the following adaptations:

- increased aerobic enzymes and mitochondria,
- increased capillaries, and
- more efficient contractions.

I've already mentioned the effects of endurance training on mitochondria, on capillaries, and on aerobic enzymes, particularly those involved in fat metabolism. More efficient aerobic pathways are able to provide more energy from fat, thereby conserving muscle glycogen as well as blood glucose, which is needed by the nervous system. As a result, muscles that once fatigued in minutes become able to endure for hours. Some of the effects of endurance training take place in the nervous system. Skilled, more efficient movements conserve energy, thereby contributing to endurance. But the most documented effects of muscular endurance training seem to focus on the muscle fibers.

Fiber Type Transformation. Recent evidence suggests that the aerobic enzyme changes noted in endurance training may be a stage in the eventual transformation of fast twitch to slow twitch fibers.

Pette (1984) reported metabolic (enzyme) and structural changes in muscle following prolonged endurance training (electrical stimulation). Studies of rat and rabbit muscles show that fast twitch fibers first take on the oxidative capabilities and eventually assume the contractile properties of slow twitch fibers (Pette, 1984). We do not yet know if these fiber type changes occur in humans.

Successful distance runners have as much as 80% slow twitch fibers. Is that due to fiber type changes or to heredity? At present it appears that endurance training can improve the aerobic or oxidative capabilities of all fibers as well as the ability of fast twitch fibers to utilize oxygen. These studies do show that muscle is extremely adaptable and able to adjust to the demands imposed upon it.

Short Versus Long Muscles. Did you ever hear that running gives you short muscles and swimming gives you long ones? The length of a muscle is fixed by its bony attachments. Running on the toes can develop the size of the calf muscle, but it isn't likely to shorten the muscle itself. Similarly, the long muscle belly seen in the calf of the swimmer could be a product of specific swim training. But it is also possible that the difference existed before training and had something to do with the athlete's success in the sport.

Methods of Training

What is the best way to train for strength or endurance: isometric, isotonic, or isokinetic methods? The answer depends on the goal of your training. If you just want to get stronger, almost any method will work. If you want to gain strength to improve performance in work or sport, the training should be specific to your goal. In one study, college women trained with weights (isotonic), isokinetic devices, or calisthenics. The isotonic group did best on lifting tests, and the calisthenic group scored best on calisthenic tests. The isokinetic group, which gained strength on the isokinetic devices, came in third on the other two tests (Sharkey, Wilson, Whiddon, & Miller, 1978). This study showed how important it is to train in the manner in which the strength will eventually be used.

Isometric Training

Also called **static contractions**, isometrics were the rage of the early 1960s. Professional athletes used the technique, which promised dramatic results with just 6 s of exercise a day. Based on an early study conducted in Germany (Hettinger & Mueller, 1953), the technique was popular until subsequent research put isometrics in the proper perspective. When studies compared isometrics with traditional weight lifting, isometrics came in second. Isometric contractions don't provide knowledge of results, they elevate blood pressure, and they are usually not specific to the training goal. Isometrics do have some uses: in rehabilitation when patients can't perform any other kind of exercise, for work at the sticking point of a lift, and in activities that require static strength or endurance (e.g., archery). More recently, athletes have used isometrics in conjunction with weight lifting to get better results. The weight is lifted and held against an immovable object for several counts in a technique known as **functional isometrics**.

Isotonic Training

Isotonic contractions (weight lifting) have been achieving results since the 1940s, when DeLorme and Watkins (1951) outlined a formula for success. Simply stated, the formula called for high-resistance, low-repetition exercise; minor variations of that formula are used today to develop dynamic strength. Because the resistance is high only at one point of the lift (usually the start), some have questioned the value of the technique. Isotonic programs compare well with isokinetic training, especially when tested on isotonic tests. Free weights and weight machines are readily available in most health clubs, and weight lifting with free weights remains the method of choice for most serious athletes. Although fitness buffs usually lift 3 days per week, serious athletes increase the strength training stimulus by doing multiple sets of each exercise (five or more) and training 5 or 6 days per week.

Isokinetic Training

Isokinetic exercises combine the best features of isometric (near maximal force) and isotonic (full range of motion) training. With the appropriate device it is possible to overload the muscles with a near-maximal contraction throughout the range of motion and control the speed of contraction. Theoretically, this method should lead to strength throughout the range of motion. The problem, if there is one, seems to be the lack of specific devices for many sports skills. But as more devices are developed for specific sports, isokinetic training will become more popular.

Best Method?

No one method is best for strength or endurance training. Free weights are inexpensive and versatile but require more supervision for safety and to prevent theft. Expensive isokinetic devices are effective but limited in application. Isokinetic variations (such as variable resistance or accommodating resistance) are popular in health clubs and they are useful for fitness and sport because of one special advantage; unlike weight lifting, isokinetic training doesn't cause as much muscle soreness. Thus it can be done in conjunction with other activities without adversely affecting performance.

Let me add a note of caution before we go on: Be sure the training program you adopt is appropriate to your level of fitness and ability. What is best for beginners doesn't work for trained athletes, and vice versa. Psychologists base many theories on research conducted on college freshmen and on rats. In exercise physiology, numerous studies have been conducted on "gym rats," college students enrolled in activity classes. Comparisons show that various forms of strength training undertaken by gym rats all seem to yield similar results; in other words, anything works with beginners. But that doesn't predict how the methods will work on athletes or others with higher levels of strength. And it doesn't prove that increased strength will improve performance. We know how to improve strength; now we need to find out how much is needed to improve performance and how best to train to get results. I'll provide partial answers to these questions in later chapters.

Flexibility

To consider the effect of training on range of motion, first we must consider the limits of flexibility. Muscles are covered with tough connective tissue, which is a major restriction to the range of motion, as are the joint capsule and tendons. Thus training must concentrate on altering these limits. Flexibility decreases with age and inactivity. Some injuries may be more likely as flexibility decreases; low back problems are associated with poor flexibility of back muscles and hamstrings and weak abdominal muscles. On the other hand, enhanced flexibility may enhance performance in some sports, especially those with obvious flexibility components (e.g., gymnastics, diving, and wrestling).

Increased muscle and joint temperatures increase flexibility, as do specific stretching exercises. Stretching gradually leads to minor distensions in connective tissue, and the summation of these small changes can dramatically improve range of motion.

How to Stretch

In the past, flexibility exercises conjured up images of vigorous bobbing and jerking movements, but times have changed. Today we engage in static stretching or, at most, light bobbing movements. The reason for the change is the stretch reflex. Rapid stretching invokes a stretch reflex, which calls forth a vigorous contraction of the stretched muscle. Because a vigorous contraction is the opposite of what we seek, we must forget this **ballistic stretching** and learn the gentle art and science of static stretching.

Static stretching involves using slow movements to reach a point of stretch, holding the position 5 to 10 s, and relaxing. The stretch may be repeated, and very light bobbing may be employed. A variation of the static stretch is the **contract-relax** technique. Do a static stretch, relax, contract the muscle briefly, then repeat the static stretch. When done with muscles like those in the calf, the technique seems to help the muscle relax so you can better stretch the tendon. These methods are at least as effective as dynamic stretching, and they provide other advantages such as low risk of injury and reduction of lingering muscle soreness. (See Appendix C for examples of stretching exercises.)

Reducing Soreness

The muscle soreness that becomes evident 24 hr or so after you overdo (delayed onset muscle soreness or DOMS) may be due to slight tears in connective tissue, uncontrolled contractions or spasms of individual muscle fibers, muscle fiber damage, or the lingering effects of metabolic by-products. We are reasonably certain that soreness is not due to leftover lactic acid. That by-product is eliminated within an hour of the cessation of effort. We do know that certain types of exercise lead to soreness that often persists for days and can make subsequent activity less enjoyable. Komi and Buskirk (1972) compared two types of strength training: **concentric** (as in ordinary flexion) and **eccentric** (when the muscle is under high tension as it lets down an overload). Subjects in the eccentric group (the group that lowered the weight) complained of muscle soreness, whereas the other group did not. So if you begin a weight training program, be prepared for some soreness.

Eccentric Training.   You may be surprised to know that the eccentric group in the Komi and Buskirk (1972) study gained a bit more strength, which is a common finding in eccentric training studies, probably because we can let down more weight than we can lift. But before you get excited about eccentric training, remember the rule of specificity: Unless your sport or job calls for letting down heavy loads, the training may not help performance as much as regular weight training or weight machines—and you are certain to get muscle soreness with eccentric contractions.

You can prevent soreness by beginning with light weights, progressing gradually, and avoiding maximal lifting, all-out running, or hard throwing (e.g., serving) at first. Although patience is the best way to prevent soreness, experience shows that we are seldom patient; therefore, we need a way to reduce soreness. Stretching reduces muscle soreness (deVries, 1986), so stretch before and after exercise as well as any other time you feel discomfort. While a recent report casts doubt on postexercise stretching (Buroker & Schwane, 1989), I find it seems to help hours or even days later. If immediate postexercise stretching doesn't reduce soreness, delayed stretching may.

Muscle soreness is correlated with submicroscopic muscle damage and with diminished strength that may persist for up to 2 weeks. The damage may be to older or otherwise susceptible muscle fibers, because recovery is faster and soreness is diminished after successive bouts of exercise. Leakage of the muscle enzyme creatine kinase (CK) suggests membrane damage. Because the soreness peaks 1 to 2 days after the effort, and the enzyme levels peak 2 to 3 days later, the actual cause of the delayed onset muscle soreness is still unclear (Newham, 1988). However, most experts believe that inflammation is involved.

Warm up a bit with light exercise or calisthenics, then do your stretching. Finish the warm-up with more vigorous effort or, if you prefer, begin your run or other exercise at a slow pace. Never substitute skill rehearsal, such as tennis strokes, for stretching. Do your warm-up and stretching before you begin to compete. The results of correct flexibility training are quite persistent; your improved range of motion should remain for at least 8 weeks. But once you have learned to enjoy stretching, you may get hooked on its subtle sensations and move on to esoteric forms such as yoga. If not, just remember to do the stretches you need to avoid soreness and to reduce the risk of injury in the activity.

Speed and Power

Years ago, as I attempted to make some sense of the confusing and sometimes contradictory research on strength and speed, I noticed that strength and speed seemed to be related when heavy loads were used in the test of speed. When little resistance was used, strength and speed were not related. In an effort to generalize the findings to other areas of work and sport I turned to a well-known physiological principle: the force-velocity relationship.

Force-Velocity Relationship

We have long known that velocity of shortening in a contraction is greatest with no load or resistance. As resistance increases, the velocity of shortening decreases (see Figure 5.1). I thought the force-velocity relationship could help simplify basic principles about how and why muscles should be trained for force, speed, or power. From reading the available literature I concluded that strength training would improve heavily loaded movements but would have little effect on the velocity of unloaded movements, and vice versa. Imagine my delight when I happened upon a study that confirmed my hypotheses!

Ikai (1970) demonstrated that training for strength alone led to increased strength and velocity with heavy loads. He also found that training for speed alone improved velocity with light loads but did nothing for strength or velocity under

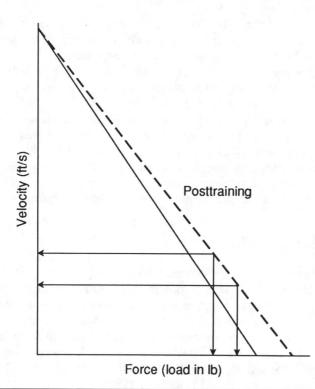

Figure 5.1. Strength training and the force-velocity relationship. The benefits of strength training are more pronounced in events involving loaded or resisted movements. *Note.* From Sharkey (1975).

heavy loads. Most interesting of all was his finding that training with intermediate loads (30 to 60% of maximal strength) at the highest speed possible led to improvements in force, speed, and power.

Japanese researchers (Kanehisa & Miyashita, 1983) confirmed the specificity of velocity in training. They trained three groups at either slow-, medium-, or high-speed contractions. The slow group improved in strength at slow speeds, and subjects in the fast group improved in the force they could exert at fast speeds. But only subjects in the medium-speed group were able to improve at all speeds. It appears that power training (15 to 25 repetitions at 30% to 60% of maximal strength, as fast as possible) may be the way to train when speed or power is desired. Does that negate the concept of specificity?

If you are preparing for the shot put, in which force and speed are both important, you need considerable strength. If high speed is your primary goal, as in pitching a fast ball, you need to train for speed. Power training could help both performances. And the power prescription is ideal for sports like cross-country skiing, a power-endurance sport that requires hundreds of little explosions to power the skier up the hills. The principle of specificity does not imply that you should avoid other types of training, only that training must focus on the movements of the sport if you are to obtain best results.

A final note is in order concerning the use of isotonic and especially isokinetic training for speed, strength, and power development. Both techniques adapt to the advice I've just provided. By reducing the resistance below 30% of maximal force you can increase the velocity of contractions. Increase the resistance above 60% and you'll focus on force development. When power (Force × Velocity) is required, you should contract as fast as possible with weights in the 30 to 60% of maximal range. Although isokinetic contractions seem ideally suited for strength or power development, both can be developed using weight training equipment or even with calisthenics that follow the prescriptions in chapter 6.

Preload–Elastic Recoil

Before we leave the subject of power, I want to acquaint you with one of the secrets of athletic performance. It took me years to realize that a well-known fact of muscle physiology—that a muscle exerts more force if it is stretched just before contraction—describes how muscles should be used. The stretch or preload does several things; it aligns contractile elements for maximal force, takes slack out of the system, and stores elastic energy in the muscle-tendon complex. From studies of the force and efficiency of contraction, this appears to be the way that muscle works most efficiently (Komi, 1986).

Here is how the preload works, for example, in a vertical jump. You sink at the knees to stretch your thigh muscles. Simultaneously you contract the muscles during the stretch and quickly convert the preload into elastic recoil as you jump. To see how effective preload–elastic recoil is, compare that jump with one in which you eliminate the preload. Sink to the starting position, stop for a full second, and then jump. Without preload and elastic recoil the results are inferior. The preload–elastic recoil works whenever you are able to stretch before contraction. It happens in cross-country skiing, in tennis during the serve, and at the ankle and thigh in running. Often it happens automatically, but if it doesn't, see if it can be used to provide more power or the same power with less effort. Done properly, this technique contributes to the efficiency or economy of movement. Chapter 6 describes ways to use this principle to develop power with a training technique called plyometrics.

CHAPTER

6

MUSCULAR FITNESS PRESCRIPTIONS

This chapter will help you

develop a well-rounded program to suit your needs,

select a safe, effective prescription and the most appropriate mode of training,

estimate the rate of progress you may expect, and

maintain the muscular fitness you gain.

By now you have some idea of the values and applications of muscular fitness. First and most important are the health values; all of us need to do flexibility (low back and hamstrings) and abdominal exercises to prevent low back problems. Begin with three sessions per week for 6 to 8 weeks, and then you can maintain with two and occasionally one session weekly. Try to maintain a regular schedule; if you don't you are likely to become one of the millions of Americans whose days are diminished by this preventable problem. Those at risk for osteoporosis should plan a prevention program that consists of moderate weight lifting along with weight-bearing aerobic activity. And middle-aged individuals must understand how muscular fitness contributes to mobility and the quality of life after retirement and that they should begin a program before they retire!

Of course there are many other reasons to improve muscular fitness; many become involved to correct posture, figure, or physique deficiencies (i.e., to look good at the beach). Body shaping and body building motivate many participants. To help decide on a program, you may also want to evaluate your current level of muscular fitness, using the tests in Appendix C. If you are dissatisfied, if you have room for improvement, or if you want to enhance performance in work or sport, use the prescriptions, select your mode of exercise, and get going. Muscular fitness doesn't have to take a lot of time; unless you are seeking high levels of strength or endurance, you should be able to achieve health and other goals in three 15-min weekly sessions. Be sure to begin with a warm-up and end with a cool-down.

Warming up is as important for you as it is for your car. During winter months you can't just jump into the old pickup and expect instant performance; you must start slowly and avoid overloading the engine until it heats up. In the case of the body, muscle is the engine, and increased muscle temperature improves enzyme activity. By slowly increasing heart rate, respiration, and muscle temperature, you avoid wasteful and uncomfortable anaerobic metabolism early in the workout. And by slowly stretching and warming the muscles, you greatly reduce the risk of injury. A 5-min warm-up before and a 5-min cool-down after exercise will enhance your enjoyment of the experience and increase the likelihood that you will be able to participate the next day without soreness. And remember that muscular fitness is only part of total fitness; no program is complete without a well-planned aerobic fitness regimen.

Strength

You may improve your strength with calisthenics, free weights, or weight machines (isometrics work but not as well as the others). You'll get results with hydraulic devices, with accommodating- or variable-resistance equipment, or with old-fashioned free weights. The key is to place the muscle under tension (at least two thirds of maximal strength) for a sufficient period of time or repetitions.

Prescription for Strength

How you intend to use added strength will dictate how you should train. Training is specific in terms of angle, range of motion, and even velocity of contractions; train the muscles and movements you are anxious to improve. Consider the factors described in the following sections on designing a program.

Repetitions. We've known how to prescribe strength training since the early 1950s, when DeLorme and Watkins (1951) published their analysis of progressive resistance exercise. This report and more recent studies confirm the need to use a resistance that can be lifted a maximum of 10 times (repetitions maximum or RM); when more repetitions are possible the load must be increased (hence the term progressive resistance). A recent review of the literature led to the conclusion that there is no one optimal number of repetitions; anything between 2 and 10 RM yields success, so long as each set is in fact the maximal number of repetitions possible (Fleck & Kraemer, 1987).

Sets. In spite of what the manufacturers of some strength training equipment say, research shows that three sets of 2 to 10 RM is about right for newcomers to weight lifting. Later in this chapter I'll point out how more sets are used in advanced weight training. Most programs begin with one set of each exercise, then progress to two and then three as strength develops.

Frequency. One of the early studies to compare different training frequencies (Barham, 1960) found that 3- or 5-day per week formats were superior to 2 days per week, but the 3- and 5-day programs were not significantly different from each other. In their 1987 review, Fleck and Kraemer concluded: "The majority of research indicates that three training sessions per muscle group per week is the minimum frequency which causes maximum gains in strength" (p. 24). Apparently, untrained individuals need 48 hr to recover from a training session and to adapt to the training stimulus.

| **A basic prescription for strength is 3 sets of 2 to 10 RM 3 to 4 times per week (every other day).**

In practice many lifters prefer to vary the program by changing the number of repetitions per set. Some begin at 10 RM, then go to 6 and end at 2; others prefer to begin low and go up (e.g. 2, 6, and 10 RM). Because evidence for either approach is lacking, the choice is yours (6-10 RMs may be safer for newcomers). Just remember to increase the resistance when you are able to do more than 10 repetitions for all three sets. Keep in mind that most of the studies that led to these conclusions were done on gym rats, previously untrained (novice) students in physical education classes, and that the prescription for advanced lifting is more demanding.

The basic prescription can be used with a variety of methods, such as calisthenics, weight training, or isokinetics.

Calisthenics. The least expensive way to train is without equipment. Calisthenics includes a wide range of exercises, such as push-ups, chin-ups, and sit-ups. The strength training prescription calls for high resistance and low repetitions, so you may have to add additional resistance when you are able to do more than 10 repetitions (over 10 repetitions will build short-term, or anaerobic, endurance but not much strength). You can overload the push-up in several ways; have someone place a hand on your back to increase the resistance or put your feet on a chair to place more weight on your arms. You could also do variations, such as fingertip push-ups or power push-ups (push up and clap your hands). Just remember, as the repetitions exceed 10 you shift toward endurance training.

Calisthenics can be used to train for both. See Appendix C for ways to utilize calisthenic exercises.

Weight Training. Use a weight training apparatus (stack weights) or free weights (bar and weights). The machine is somewhat safer and makes it much easier to change resistance as you move from one exercise to another. On the other hand, it restricts you to a set series of lifts and movements, and you don't learn to balance the load as well. But for general training, and especially for groups, the machines have many advantages. Some of the more popular training machines are pictured in Appendix C. Remember, for strength, do three sets of 2 to 10 repetitions, 3 times per week (every other day).

Isokinetics. Isokinetic devices, as well as variable- and accommodating-resistance machines, are becoming available in private health and fitness clubs, in recreation centers, in schools and colleges, and even in private homes. The good ones allow you to exert near-maximum force as the device moves through a full range of motion, and you can vary the speed and resistance to suit specific training needs. Low-cost home devices (e.g., Exergenie, Apollo, and Mini-Gym) can be used in a variety of ways. Least expensive of all is isokinetic exercise with a friend (counterforce). Your partner provides resistance throughout the range of motion; for example, as you attempt forearm flexion your partner provides resistance. You can do fast, medium, or slow isokinetics.

ISOKINETIC TRAINING PRESCRIPTION

Fast: Total movement in 1 s
 15 repetitions
 3 sets

Medium: Total movement in 3 s
 12 repetitions
 3 sets

Slow: Total movement in 5 s
 8 repetitions
 3 sets

Follow the program on an alternate, or every-other-day, schedule. Select the program to suit your needs, not those of your club. If you need medium or fast contractions for your sport, do them regardless of what the instructor may say. Also, if your instructor tells you to do one set, take this advice for the first 4 to 8 weeks; when your strength plateaus, as it will with one set, progress to two and then three sets. Fitness club employees like slow contractions to save wear and tear on the machines, and they often advise one set, not because it is the best way to train, but because it avoids long waits to use the apparatus.

Precautions

If you engage in calisthenics, weight training, or isokinetics, keep the following precautions in mind.

- Ease into the program with light weights and few sets.
- Avoid holding your breath during a lift, because this can cause a marked increase in blood pressure and the work of the heart. It also restricts the return of blood to the heart and the flow of blood in the coronary arteries, which serve the heart muscle. Holding your breath means that just when your heart needs more oxygen, it gets less—a dangerous situation, especially for older, untrained individuals. Breath holding can also increase intra-abdominal pressure and cause a hernia.
- Exhale during the lift and inhale as you lower the weight.
- Always work with a companion or spotter when using free weights.
- Alternate muscle groups during a session; for example, don't do several arm exercises in a row. Allow recovery time between sets of the same exercise.

Suggestions

Keep Records.   Keep records of your progress. Test for maximum strength every few weeks (see Appendix C for a log to keep track of progress). Also record body weight and fat and some dimensions (e.g., chest, waist, and biceps).

Vary the Program.   Experienced athletes use a process called **cycling**, which usually includes four cycles of up to 12 weeks each. For example, Fleck and Kraemer (1987) suggest this program for athletes in high-strength sports. Simply follow each of the following prescriptions for 4 weeks.

> **WEIGHT TRAINING PROGRAM FOR HIGH-STRENGTH SPORTS**
> **Cycle 1: 10 to 20 reps, low resistance—for hypertrophy**
> **Cycle 2: 2 to 6 reps, medium resistance—for strength**
> **Cycle 3: 2 to 3 reps, high resistance—for added strength**
> **Cycle 4: 1 to 3 reps, very high resistance—peaking phase**

Each cycle can be as short as 4 weeks or as long as 12. Because progress begins to plateau after 2 months, I prefer to change my program every 8 weeks. Another approach is to change exercises every 4 to 8 weeks or when you plateau or get bored.

Progress

Although strength doesn't increase rapidly, you can expect the following gains.

- The rate of increase will range from 1 to 3% per week, with the previously untrained individual increasing at a faster rate. With hard training, some people may temporarily achieve a rate of 4 to 5% per week.
- The rate of improvement will decrease or plateau as you approach your potential maximal strength.
- Improvements will take place only in the muscle groups you train.
- Gains will be minimized unless you maintain adequate protein in your diet and increase protein intake if you are on a weight loss diet.

Thus a sedentary individual can expect to increase strength 50% or more in 6 months of training. Hard training could lead to similar gains in less time.

Maintenance

Strength can be maintained with lower volume and frequency of training, as long as intensity (resistance) remains high. One session per week will maintain strength for 6 weeks or more, and two sessions will ensure maintenance for a prolonged period, depending on the level of strength achieved before the maintenance program begins.

Detraining

With normal activity, newly gained strength is largely retained for up to 6 weeks after the cessation of training, and half of the strength you gain will be retained for up to 1 year. When you resume training, you'll return to previous levels with less effort, perhaps because of the learning that took place in earlier training. Studies on older individuals show that strength declines very slowly in muscle groups that are used regularly. Thus an investment in strength could pay dividends later in life. Of course, I recommend that you set aside at least 8 to 12 weeks each year to maintain or improve strength. Find a season when training suits your schedule and follow a program. As the years pass you'll be glad you did.

Advanced Strength Training

Experienced lifters train 6 days per week. When they engage in body building, they do many sets and repetitions. Training for superior strength calls for numerous sets (over 10) with few repetitions and very heavy loads.

Some of these athletes take protein supplements or even drugs to enhance their progress. New research supports the increase of *dietary* protein when the athlete is on a weight loss diet (Butterfield, 1987), but the use of steroid drugs to improve performance, though supported by some research, is dangerous and unhealthy. Anabolic steroids affect glandular function, damage the liver, and lead to early heart disease via an alarming drop in HDL cholesterol. Don't depend on drugs for strength or performance.

For advanced strength training
- **use 5 to 6 sets;**
- **utilize a split program (upper body on M-W-F, trunk and legs on T-Th-Sat);**
- **eat adequate protein, avoid rapid weight loss, and get ample rest.**
- **cut back on endurance training unless you are very fit (best results may occur when serious strength training is conducted separately; Hickson, 1980); and**
- **use training cycles, changing your program every 8 weeks or when progress begins to plateau.**

Strength and Performance

Strength may be related to performance in your work or sport. If so, by all means train to improve your strength. However, don't assume (as many others do) that if some strength training is good, more is better. In most activities performance improves with strength, but only up to a point. Thereafter, you may waste your time or diminish performance with excessive attention to strength. The trick is to know how much is enough. When strength is optimal for the sport, move on to other important phases of training, remembering to maintain the necessary strength with one or two sessions each week.

How much strength is enough? The answer differs according to the sport. For endurance sports, strength is adequate when the force needed in a single contraction (e.g., arm pull in swimming) is below 40% of your maximal ability for that movement. If you exert 20 lb of force in the average arm pull, you need approximately 2.5 × 20 lb, or 50 lb, force in a single maximal pull. More strength will not contribute to performance. So if strength is adequate, move on to endurance training. (Chapter 15 includes more about strength and performance.)

Endurance

I've pointed out how strength and endurance are different and that endurance may be more important than a high level of strength, presuming you have adequate strength. The main difference between training for strength and endurance is the level of tension or resistance, and consequently, the number of repetitions. The lighter weights (less than 66% of maximum strength) don't provide the stimulus for strength development, but if you do enough repetitions, you will develop endurance.

Prescription for Endurance

Years ago we believed that because fewer than 10 repetitions (maximum) developed strength, more than 10 repetitions developed endurance. Recent studies have added to our knowledge of strength and endurance and the territory that lies between them. Studies by Washburn, Sharkey, Narum, and Smith (1983) and Anderson and Kearney (1982b) showed that 15 to 25 repetitions will still develop some strength (1% per week vs. 2 to 3% with 6 to 8 RM strength training) along with short-term or anaerobic endurance. Table 6.1 includes a summary of the effects of various numbers of repetitions and what they are likely to develop. As the number of repetitions increases, less strength and more endurance are developed.

The number of repetitions you need depends on several factors. What are you training for? Is it for anaerobic or for long-term endurance? Training should be specific to the way in which it will be used: Emphasize speed when necessary, or do many repetitions when you need long-term endurance with less resistance. When the activity involves moderate resistance, lift heavier weights and do fewer repetitions. For short (under 2 min) and intense activities, train with 15 to 25 RM to get short-term or anaerobic endurance. If your goals are vague and time is short, use fewer repetitions. A friend once worked up to 400 sit-ups daily, then quit because he became bored. (Incidentally, he didn't get rid of his tummy fat until diet and exercise led to general weight loss.)

> A basic prescription for endurance is
> 3 sets of more than 10 RM 3 days per week.

Follow the same precautions mentioned for strength training. Because the loads are lighter, muscle endurance training is safer than strength training and is probably more related to the activities of the average adult. Be careful, however, to breathe properly, especially as you strain to complete the last few contractions.

Progress

Muscle endurance is very trainable. Whereas it is difficult to go from two to four chin-ups (because that takes strength), it is easy to improve from 20 to 40 push-ups (because that takes endurance). When you have sufficient strength for the task, gains in endurance come with relative ease. Subjects in the Washburn et al. (1983) study improved 10% per week in short-term endurance when they trained with 15 to 25 RM. On a laboratory endurance test, the short-term (anaerobic) endurance training was more effective than strength training, improving

Table 6.1 The Strength-Endurance Continuum

	Strength	Short-term (anaerobic) endurance	Intermediate endurance	Long-term endurance
For	Maximum force	Brief (2-3 min) persistence with heavy load	Persistence with intermediate load	Persistence with lighter load
Prescription	6-8 RM 3 sets	15-25 RM 3 sets	30-50 RM 2 sets	Over 100 RM 1 set
Improves	Contractile protein (actin and myosin) ATP and CP Connective tissue	Some strength and anaerobic metabolism (glycolysis)	Some endurance and anaerobic metabolism Slight improvement in strength (for untrained)	Aerobic enzymes Mitochondria Oxygen and fat utilization
Doesn't improve	Oxygen intake Endurance	Oxygen intake		Strength

ATP = adenosine triphosphate

CP = creatine phosphate

short-term endurance 70% versus 50% for strength training. Most adult activities are enhanced when endurance is improved. Tennis and skiing require hours of practice, and good practice requires endurance. The fatigued student usually practices a sloppy version of the skill.

Of course, your ultimate progress will be dictated by your genetic endowment and your devotion to training. If you have a high percentage of slow twitch muscle fibers, your potential for long-term endurance is excellent. If you do not, don't despair; training improves the endurance capabilities of all fiber types. Although you may not be a world class endurance athlete, you will come closer to your potential.

Diet and Endurance

Best endurance performances take place when muscle fibers are well supplied with muscle glycogen. And glycogen levels are highest when you follow a high-carbohydrate diet. Scandinavian studies show that muscle glycogen stores can be depleted in a full day of alpine skiing. If you dine on steak and salad after skiing, your muscles will not be ready to perform the following day. Do all you can to replace muscle glycogen, and you will be able to ski all day and still have energy for après-ski. More importantly, you will be less likely to fatigue, fall, and get injured. Begin carbohydrate replacement immediately after activity, and continue with a high-carbohydrate diet, which is discussed further in chapter 9.

Speed and Power

As with other types of training, the key is specificity, so you should try to pattern the training after the intended use. To throw a baseball faster, train with a weighted ball or simulate the motion with pulley weights or an isokinetic device. To improve jumping ability, do half squats with weights, jump while wearing a weighted vest, or use an isokinetic device such as the leaper (see Appendix B). For more on speed training consult the newest book on the subject (Dintiman & Ward, 1988).

> For speed (velocity) use high-speed contractions with low resistance.
>
> For power (force × velocity) do three sets of 15 to 25 high-speed contractions with 30 to 60% of maximal resistance.
>
> For strength (force) do three sets of 2 to 10 RM with over 66% of maximal resistance.

A popular technique borrowed from Europe, **plyometrics** consists of explosive movements designed to improve power. Sprinters do one- and two-leg hops to gain power. High jumpers, broad jumpers, volleyball and basketball athletes, and even cross-country skiers use plyometrics to improve performance. Proponents have said that plyometrics trains the capacity for preload–elastic recoil and builds strength and explosive power (Radcliffe & Farentinos, 1985). Unfortunately, the limited research remains inconclusive concerning the value of plyometrics for various sports and for athletes at different levels of development. And excessive use or poor technique leads to painful knee problems. I recommend that you try plyometrics, if only because of the effect of practice on skill and economy. But start with a modest number on a soft surface, and quit at the first sign of discomfort in the knees. Even if you don't gain additional power, you may learn more effective use of the power you possess. (For examples see the exercises for leg strength and power in Appendix C.)

Minimum Muscular Fitness

In the introduction to this section I noted several compelling health reasons for attention to muscular fitness. Even if you decide you don't need muscular fitness for injury prevention, performance, or even body building or shaping, you still need to engage in a minimum program throughout life. The minimum program must address prevention of low back problems and osteoporosis.

The minimum program for prevention of low back problems includes flexibility of back and hamstring muscles and abdominal muscle tone.

Stretch your low back by sitting on the front of a chair with your knees bent and your feet on the floor and comfortably apart. Bend forward and gently stretch the low back region. Stretch hamstring muscles by sitting on the floor with your legs extended. Bend slowly forward and try to touch your toes. Hold the position for a few seconds, then relax. Repeat each stretch several times.

You can achieve abdominal tone with bent knee curl-ups. Recline on your back with your knees flexed at a 90-degree angle and your arms folded across your chest with hands on shoulders. With your chin on your chest, curl up until your arms touch your legs, then return to the starting position. Ten repetitions is minimum, 20 or more is better. Try to do at least 20 curl-ups every other day to maintain the muscle tone you need to counteract the strong muscles of the back. Without abdominal tone the back muscles cause pelvic tilt and excessive curve of the lumbar (lower back) area of the spine. For more low back exercises and a back fitness test see chapter 11 and Appendix E.

Avoidance of osteoporosis requires regular weight-bearing activity, such as walking or jogging, as well as moderate resistance exercises for the upper body. Normal household tasks such as lifting, vacuuming, mowing grass, shoveling snow, and others will help avoid the problem. But research shows that best results are achieved with a combination of weight-bearing and resistance exercises, along with a diet that includes adequate calcium and vitamin D (exposure to sunlight is a natural way to form vitamin D). Excessive endurance training, fat loss, and low calcium intake contribute to osteoporosis in young female athletes, so moderate activity is the sensible approach to prevention. Postmenopausal women may also need to consider hormonal therapy to insure calcium uptake and utilization if they are to avoid crippling fractures of the hip, upper back, and other bones.

PART
III

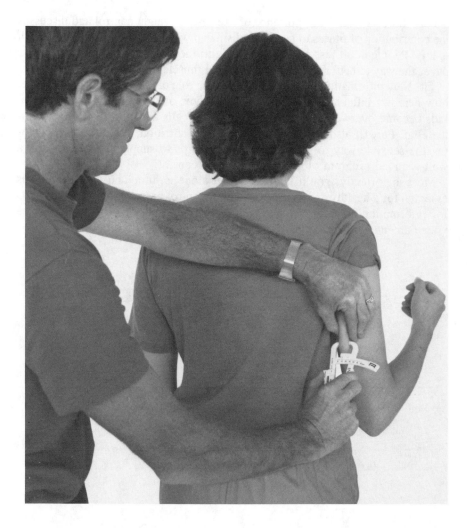

FITNESS AND WEIGHT
CONTROL

For years the importance of exercise in weight control was minimized with statements such as "You have to walk 35 mi to lose 1 lb of fat." You never heard anyone say, "You have to eat three loaves of bread to gain a pound of fat." Both statements are senseless. Fat is gained a few calories or ounces at a time, and this accumulation can be whittled away with a sensible weight control program.

Part III deals with the importance of exercise in weight control and discusses the contribution of fitness to fat metabolism and weight control. The simple truth is this: People don't just want to lose weight; they want to lose fat, and fitness paves the way to better fat control by making muscle cells highly efficient users of fat. New information in Part III includes the role of diet in health and disease, how heredity influences the tendency to become overweight, how overweight kids become overweight adults, and which fat cells are most likely to accumulate fat. Part III also provides information on nutrition, suggestions concerning the sensible way to diet, and behavioral tips to supplement exercise in a well-rounded program of permanent weight control.

Most importantly, you'll learn why diet alone is futile and why exercise is essential for a healthy and successful weight control program. (See Appendix D for information on caloric intake and expenditure and for ways to determine your percentage of body fat.)

CHAPTER

7

ENERGY BALANCE

This chapter will help you

calculate your energy balance (caloric intake vs. expenditure),

estimate your ideal weight and percentage of body fat,

understand the causes and consequences of overweight and obesity, and

establish sensible body weight and body fat goals.

Ages ago, when the food supply was not so predictable and human beings couldn't count on three meals a day plus snacks, they learned how to store energy in the form of fat. Our bodies still store energy, even though the food supply now makes the practice unnecessary for most of us. This ability to store energy, coupled with a plentiful food supply, has created a problem for more than half the population of this country. We put calories in the energy account but seldom draw enough out, so our energy balance grows and grows. This chapter is about energy intake and energy expenditure and what happens when we take in more than we expend.

Energy Intake

Energy is consumed in the forms of carbohydrate, fat, and protein. Once energy is ingested and stored, it remains in our bodies until it is expended.

Carbohydrate

Carbohydrate may be ingested as a complex sugar such as starch in bread or potatoes, as a two-sugar molecule of ordinary table sugar, or as a simple sugar like glucose or fructose. Digestion of complex starch molecules begins in the mouth with the enzyme salivary amylase. Digestion is temporarily halted in the stomach when the enzyme is deactivated by gastric secretions. In the small intestine, starches are further digested with the help of pancreatic amylase. Final breakdown to simple sugar form is completed by enzymes secreted by the wall of the intestine. Glucose and other simple sugar molecules are then absorbed into the bloodstream. The absorption is rather complete; most of the sugar you eat gets into the blood, and complex carbohydrates, like potatoes, can enter the blood as quickly as table sugar (Jenkins, Taylor, & Wolever, 1982).

After a meal, absorbed sugars are taken up by the blood, heart, skeletal muscle, and liver, in that order. When blood sugar levels are restored, heart and skeletal muscle accept glucose. The constantly working heart uses glucose for energy, whereas the skeletal muscle can store glucose as glycogen, for use when energy is needed. The liver takes up the simple sugars from the blood and converts them to glycogen. When sufficient glucose has been stored in the liver (about 80 to 100 g), the excess is converted to fat and stored in adipose tissue for later use. Thus an excess intake of carbohydrate does not become a supply of quick energy; it is stored as fat. The glucose stored in the liver is readily available when needed, but muscle glycogen can only be used directly by the muscle in which it is stored. Blood glucose also can be used by nerves, muscles, or other tissues in need of energy.

Skeletal muscle may convert glucose to lactate, which diffuses from the muscle and travels to the liver for reconversion to glucose or travels to another muscle for use as a source of energy. In other words, lactate is not just a metabolic by-product, but a metabolic intermediate that can shuttle energy from muscle to liver (and then to the blood) or from muscle to muscle (Brooks, 1988).

Fat

During light and moderate work we use mostly fat for energy and switch to carbohydrate during intense effort, only because carbohydrate is more efficient in terms of energy per liter of oxygen. Why do we store excess carbohydrate as fat? Fat is a far more efficient and economical way to store energy; it contains twice as much energy per gram as carbohydrate. Also carbohydrate storage requires a considerable amount of water (about 2 g per gram of glycogen), so it would be a burden to carry much more carbohydrate than we usually do.

Fat digestion is accomplished in the small intestine by pancreatic lipase with the aid of bile salts. The salts break the fat globules into droplets, presenting a large surface area for the action of fat-splitting enzymes. Large fat molecules are thereby broken into fatty acids and glycerol and are absorbed into the lymphatic system. From there the fat passes into the bloodstream, where it may be transported for use as a fuel, deposited as adipose (fat) tissue, or taken to the liver. The liver can use excess carbohydrate or protein to form lipid (fat) molecules. (Chapter 12 includes more about blood lipids, or fats.)

Protein

I will limit the discussion of protein, because its role as a source of energy during exercise is usually small (under 10% of energy; Lemon, 1987). But during periods of dieting, when you restrict caloric intake to lose weight, the body senses starvation and begins a complex survival reaction. Part of that process includes a turn to protein as a way to produce needed blood glucose. Tissue and muscle protein is broken down and converted to glucose in the liver. Hence dieting leads to the loss of *lean tissue*, not just fat. The *only* way to avoid this response is to combine exercise with a moderate diet in a sensible weight loss program (see chapters 8 and 9). Incidentally, if you are losing weight while training or if you are just training hard, you should increase protein intake to insure the benefits of aerobic or muscular fitness training.

In one study, protein requirements increased from less than 1 g per kilogram of body weight to over 2 g/kg when exercise and weight loss were combined (Butterfield, 1987).

Remember that like carbohydrate, excess dietary protein can be converted to sugar and then stored as excess fat. (Nitrogen from protein molecules is split off and spilled out in the urine. The remaining carbon skeleton can be converted to glucose or stored as fat.) So when your energy intake has excess calories, be they carbohydrate, fat, or protein, the excess will remain with you. Energy can neither be created nor destroyed; if you plan to take it in, you better have a use for it. Calories *do* count, and I hope this book helps you learn how to count them.

Energy in Foods

How is the energy or caloric value of food determined? Nutrition researchers use a calorimeter to measure the energy content of foods. A small amount of food is placed in a chamber and burned in the presence of oxygen. The heat liberated in the process indicates the energy content of the food. When a gram of carbohydrate is ignited, the energy yield is 4.1 calories per gram. When fat is tested, more than twice as much energy is released (see Table 7.1).

Table 7.1 Caloric Equivalents of Foods

Food	Energy (cal/g)[a]	Oxygen required (L/g)	Caloric equivalent (cal/L)
Fat	9.3	1.98	4.696
Carbohydrate	4.1	0.81	5.061
Protein	4.3	0.97	4.432

Note. The alcohol in alcoholic beverages has a high caloric value, 7.1 cal/g. The calories are "empty" and provide no nutritional value. Moreover, because alcohol diminishes appetite and interferes with digestion by inflammation of the stomach, pancreas, and intestine, alcohol often leads to malnutrition. Alcohol also interferes with vitamin activation by the liver and causes liver damage (Leiber, 1976). Table from Sharkey (1974).

[a]Cal (kilocalories) refer to the amount of heat energy required to raise the temperature of 1 kg of water 1 °C.

Energy Expenditure

You always expend some energy, even when asleep. If you stay in bed for 24 hr and do nothing at all, you will expend about 1,600 calories (for a 154-lb, or 70-kg, body). This energy is needed by heart and respiratory muscles, for normal cellular metabolism, and for maintaining body temperature. If you do some heavy thinking during that period of rest, the energy expenditure will not increase significantly, but as soon as you begin to move, energy needs increase dramatically. Energy expenditure can go from 1.2 calories per minute during rest to more than 20 calories per minute during vigorous activity. You also need additional energy when you eat, to power the processes of digestion and absorption. But physical activity has the greatest effect on energy expenditure. Walking involves an expenditure of about 5 calories per minute, jogging burns 10 or more, and running can expend more than 15.

Influence of Body Weight

Of course, your caloric expenditure depends on the size of body you carry around. The greater the body weight, the higher the caloric expenditure per minute. The caloric expenditure tables in this book are based on a body weight of about 70 kg (154 lb). If you weigh 7 kg (15 lb) more, add 10%; if you weigh 7 kg less, subtract 10%; and so forth. For example, if you weigh 124 lb and the caloric cost of slow jogging is listed at 10 calories per minute, subtract 20% or 2 calories to find the calories burned when you jog (8 calories per minute).

Exercise for Weight Control

Some types of exercise are better than others for weight control. As you know, we shift from fat to carbohydrate metabolism during vigorous activity. If you desire to burn off excess fat, consider moderate exercise (see Table 7.2). Because extremely vigorous activity cannot be sustained for very long, the total caloric expenditure of heavy exercise may not be great. Also, fat utilization increases over time, with more fat being burned after 30 min of exercise. Moderate activity can be continued for hours without undue fatigue, thereby allowing a significant fat metabolism and caloric expenditure.

Table 7.2   Physical Activity and Caloric Expenditure

Work intensity	Pulse rate	Expenditure (cal/min)	Examples
Light	Below 120	Under 5	Golf, bowling, walking, volleyball, most work
Moderate[a]	120-150	5 to 10	Jogging, tennis, bike riding, aerobic dance, basketball, hiking, racquetball, strenuous work
Heavy	Above 150	Above 10	Running, fast swimming, other brief, intense efforts

Note. From Sharkey (1974).

[a]Preferred for weight control benefits.

Incidentally, the best time to exercise for weight control may be in the morning before you've eaten breakfast. You are more likely to burn fat in the morning, after an overnight fast. So if you are interested in fat metabolism and weight control, try morning exercise. However, if morning exercise doesn't suit your biological clock, don't despair. Exercise always burns calories, so it always contributes to weight control.

Measurement of Energy Expenditure

In the early part of this century, scientists found a way to measure human energy expenditure. They placed subjects in a chamber very much like a calorimeter and then measured heat generated in physical activity, which eventually increased the temperature of the water layer surrounding the chamber. However, this method was far too expensive and cumbersome for the measurement of vigorous activity. Drawing on their knowledge concerning the oxygen requirements of metabolism, researchers developed indirect methods of calorimetry. Because each liter of oxygen consumption was equivalent to about 5 calories, why not just measure the oxygen used during exercise? The **closed-circuit method of indirect calorimetry** is still used in hospitals, usually for resting or basal metabolic studies. The amount of oxygen taken from a large tank is measured directly.

The **open-circuit method** is best suited for vigorous exercise. The subject breathes readily available atmospheric air, and the exhaled air is collected for analysis. The oxygen consumed and carbon dioxide produced during the activity are analyzed along with the total volume of exhaled air. Oxygen consumption per minute is expressed by the following equation.

$$(\text{Atmospheric Oxygen} - \text{Exhaled Oxygen}) \times \text{Volume Exhaled Air}$$
$$(20.93\% - 18.93) \times 50 \text{ L} = 1 \text{ L/min}$$

One liter of oxygen per minute equals 5 calories per minute, the energy cost of a brisk walk.

Energy Balance

Energy balance refers to energy intake, or the calories consumed in the diet, and energy expenditure, or the calories burned in the course of all daily activities (see Figure 7.1). If intake exceeds expenditure, the body stores the excess as fat.

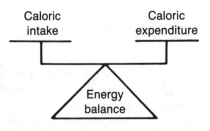

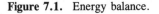
Figure 7.1. Energy balance.

One pound of body fat has the energy equivalent of 3,500 calories. Thus, we must expend (oxidize) about 3,500 calories to remove 1 lb of stored fat. Conversely, 3,500 calories of excess dietary intake will lead to an additional pound of body weight. For example, the daily activity of a young man whose body weight is around 70 kg (154 lb) consists of light office work. He does not engage in any physical activity, so his daily caloric needs approximate 2,400 calories. If he exceeds this number by 200 calories per day (e.g., by eating a 200-calorie cupcake), what will happen to him over the course of a year?

$$200 \text{ cal} \times 5 \text{ d/wk} \times 4 \text{ wk/mo} = 4,000 \text{ cal/mo}$$

Thus, in the few moments it takes to eat the confection, our friend has upset his energy balance to the tune of more than 1 lb per month—more than 12 lb per year! If he keeps the pleasant habit and does nothing about his diet or exercise, he could gain 120 lb in 10 years! Of course the reverse also is true. If he gives up 200 calories each day, he could lose more than 12 lb a year. One purpose of this book is to teach you how you can *have your cake and eat it*—how you can use diet and exercise to control your weight. Use the tables in Appendix D to figure your energy balance.

Overweight and Obesity

In horse racing, the favorite often is "handicapped" with weights to provide a better contest. If a few pounds are added, the favorite may become an also-ran. Excess weight can affect performance in the human race as well; few of us realize how much. Excess weight is a burden physically, socially, psychologically, and economically. It may be the largest health problem shared by the majority of Americans. Yet it is a symptom, not a disease, and it is among the least complicated of all health problems.

What are the medical consequences of overweight and obesity? The death rate is higher than it is among those of normal weight, especially in the younger age groups. The overweight and obese have a higher incidence of atherosclerotic heart disease, hypertension, diabetes, and cirrhosis of the liver. Accidents and surgical complications are more prevalent, as are complications of pregnancy. When the excess weight is removed, these problems are reduced or eliminated.

Overweight

You may say, "I'm not overweight; I weigh the same as I did my senior year of high school." Your *weight* may be the same, but what about your ratio of lean to fat tissue? Isn't it possible that you have lost muscle and gained some fat? Has your waist measurement remained the same? The standard method of determining overweight is by comparison with the *desirable* body weight (see Table 7.3). Desirable weights are those associated with the longest life span for individuals of a certain skeleton size. (Incidentally, because overweight is associated with heart disease, diabetes, and hypertension, insurance companies charge a higher premium for individuals judged to be overweight—10% or more above desirable weight.)

Table 7.3 Desirable Body Weights for Men and Women

Height (in.)	Weight (lb)	
	Men	Women
60		109 ± 9[a]
62		115 ± 9
64	133 ± 11	122 ± 10
66	142 ± 12	129 ± 10
68	151 ± 14	136 ± 10
70	159 ± 14	144 ± 11
72	167 ± 15	152 ± 12
74	175 ± 15	

Note. Heights and weights are without shoes and other clothing. From *Recommended Daily Allowances* (7th ed.) by Food and Nutrition Board, 1968, Washington, DC: National Academy of Sciences, National Research Council.

[a]Desirable weight for a small-framed woman of this height would be approximately 109 lb minus 9 lb, or a total of 100 lb; for an average-framed woman, 109 lb; for a large-framed woman, 118 lb.

Recent attempts to increase the desirable weight standards have been met with skepticism by many health experts. Cigarette smokers and people with chronic diseases often weigh less, making a lower body weight seem less healthy. But lean nonsmokers are as healthy as ever.

Excess pounds of fat *or* muscle can make you overweight, although extra pounds of fat pose more of a burden, because the muscles can do useful work and take less space for equal weight (muscle is denser than fat). But even excess muscle seems unnecessary for the adult, unless it is needed for occupational reasons. Also, there are disturbing suggestions of increased risk of high blood pressure and heart disease among muscular men with excess fat, such as inactive former football players.

Obesity

Obesity is an excessive accumulation of *fat* beyond that considered normal for the age, sex, and body type. Obesity is a case of being *overfat*, not just overweight. It is possible to be *underweight* and still be obese, such as an individual who has excess fat and poorly developed muscles. Obesity is defined as more than 20% fat for men and more than 30% fat for women. These levels are arbitrary and some prefer lower or higher levels, but by this definition a large percentage of the adult population is obese (see Table 7.4).

Table 7.4   Average (Not Desirable or Ideal) Values for Body Fat According to Age or Sex

Age	Men (%)	Women (%)
15	12.0	21.2
18-22	12.5	25.7
23-29	14.0	29.0
30-40	16.5	30.0
40-50	21.0	32.0

Body Fat Measurement

College-aged men average 12.5% fat; college women average about 25%. The standard method for determining percentage of body fat is underwater weighing, with which the nude subject is weighed both in air and while submerged in water. After appropriate adjustments are made for the air in the lungs and gas in the gastrointestinal tract, body density is determined. Because fat is less dense than bone or muscle, it is possible to calculate percentage of body fat.

$$\frac{\text{Weight in Air}}{\text{Weight in Air} - \text{Weight in Water}}$$

As the weight in water goes up the percentage body fat goes down, and vice versa. This is why lean people sink and fat people float; fat weighs less per unit of volume.

A less accurate but serviceable method for the estimation of percentage of body fat utilizes skinfold calipers. The skinfold calculation of body fat is based on the relationship of subcutaneous (under the skin) fat to total body fat. One third of the body's fat may be located just under the skin, so several carefully selected skinfolds provide an estimate of body fat. Appendix D contains charts for this estimation. If skinfold calipers are not available, you can use the pinch test, which involves pinching the skin on the back of the upper arm (midway between shoulder and elbow). If the width of the fold, exclusive of muscle tissue, exceeds 10 mm (more than 3/8 in.), the accumulated fat could indicate a need

Table 7.5 Minimum Thickness of Triceps Indicating Obesity

Age	Male (mm)	Female (mm)
5	12	14
10	16	20
15	16	24
20	16	28
25	20	29
30-50	23	30

Note. Obesity defined as above 20% fat for men; above 30% fat for women. Adapted from "A Simple Criterion of Obesity" by C.C. Seltzer and J. Mayer, 1965, *Postgraduate Medicine*, **38**, p. A101-A106.

for weight control (see Table 7.5). I will talk about the *ideal* percentage body fat later in this chapter.

Other methods can determine body fat, ranging from inexpensive girth or other body measurements to expensive laboratory techniques. Many health clubs use a body impedance analysis technique that estimates fat from water content (and makes large errors when the subject is dehydrated). Scientists also use sophisticated imaging techniques to measure fat. Researchers often compare new methods to hydrostatic weighing to see if they are accurate. However, recent studies have shown that even underwater weighing is subject to errors, especially with younger and older subjects and those at the extremes of leanness and fatness. Age-related differences in body water and bone density can throw off this method, as can dehydration. So studies are underway to improve the equations used to calculate body fat from underwater weighing. Until then, skinfolds or other inexpensive estimates provide enough information to guide your weight control efforts (see Appendix D).

Causes of Overweight and Obesity

Why are 80 million Americans overweight to the point of obesity? Is it merely because their caloric intake exceeds expenditure?

Genetic Versus Environmental Causes

When we see obese parents with obese offspring, we are likely to think the problem "runs in the family." Obesity is more common in offspring whose parents are both obese; such a child has an 80% risk of obesity. Studies of identical twins reared in different environments also indicate that obesity has a genetic root. However, the pattern and extent of that relationship have not been well defined. When one twin is more active the genetic effect seems to be minimized.

Much of the obesity we see in families may be due as much to the environment as to a genetic cause. Overweight people eat more and exercise less; the same may be true of their children. However, in a study of identical and fraternal twins (Stunkard, Foch, & Hrubec, 1986), the authors found a high heritability for weight and body mass index (weight in kilograms divided by height in meters squared) and concluded that body weight, including obesity, is under strong genetic control and that childhood family environment by itself has little effect. Does that mean that energy balance is meaningless? No, it doesn't. In spite of the genetic influence, the basic cause of overweight and obesity remains a positive energy balance due to excess caloric intake, inadequate caloric expenditure, or both. Then what causes this tendency to store fat?

Glandular Causes?

One authority has said, "With the exception of diabetes, glandular disease is associated with obesity in less than one case out of a thousand. Even in the presence of such a disease, the individual is obese because energy acquisition has exceeded energy expenditure" (Gwinup, 1970, p. 20).

Obese individuals have a significantly higher incidence of diabetes than those of normal or desirable weight, but it is not clear whether obesity causes or results from the diabetes. After weight reduction, the diabetes may improve tremendously. In fact, evidence shows that overeating, particularly on a high-fat diet, leads to obesity *and* diabetes.

Diabetes is characterized by a deficiency of the hormone insulin, which is needed to get blood sugar into cells, including fat cells. When sugar doesn't reach the cells, energy is low and the appetite is stimulated. So the overweight individual eats *more*. There is a growing awareness of the possibility that a high-fat diet may inhibit the action of insulin, thereby requiring more insulin to do the same job. After a while, years perhaps, the pancreatic cells responsible for the production of insulin may fatigue, thereby producing a bona fide case of diabetes!

Prior to the discovery of insulin in 1921, diet and exercise were the only treatments available to the diabetic. Now, diabetics use diet and insulin injections to control this metabolic malfunction of insulin production and sugar utilization. Because muscular activity increases the transport of glucose into muscle cells, even in the absence of insulin, and because muscular activity is effective in the reduction of body weight and the risk of heart disease (diabetes and heart disease frequently are associated), it seems logical that attention has turned again to the use of exercise in the treatment and control of diabetes. Moderate physical activity reduces insulin requirements for normal as well as diabetic subjects. Regular participation in aerobic activity often reduces reliance on insulin. When coupled with a low-fat diet and significant weight loss, exercise can further reduce the need for insulin (Leonard, Hofer, & Pritikin, 1974).

Enlarged Fat Cells?

In recent years, researchers have studied the growth and development of fat cells, where excess calories are stored in the form of triglyceride. Some individuals have more fat cells, allowing them to store fat more readily. With the development of methods to determine fat cell size and number, researchers have been able to follow the development of obesity and have found that fat cells are able to increase in size or number and that the increase can be stimulated by overfeeding. Traditionally, a chubby baby has been considered a healthy baby, but overfeeding during the first few years of life will stimulate the development of larger and more numerous fat cells (3 times more). These cells remain for life and may exert an influence on the appetite when they are not filled. This early onset of hypercellularity generally leads to the most severe form of obesity. Although hypercellularity may develop at any age, another period of intense concern comes at or around the time of puberty, when overfeeding can lead to increases in fat cell number and size.

Adult-onset obesity is characterized by enlarged fat cells. But the number of fat cells does not seem subject to significant change. The pattern of obesity is a significant factor in determining health risk. Obesity that begins in childhood and continues into the adult years is a greater risk than adult-onset obesity. The *location* of stored fat also predicts health risk; pot bellies are associated with a higher risk of heart disease, whereas pear shapes are not. Because men accumulate fat in their bellies, that may be a factor in their higher risk of heart disease. Studies are now underway to determine why some cells take in more fat and why that is related to heart disease.

Researchers are beginning to study the waist- to hip-girth ratio (WHR) to determine why one fat storage location carries a greater risk. To calculate your ratio, simply measure your waist at the level of the navel, measure your hips at the greatest circumference of the buttocks, and divide the waist measurement by the hip measurement (measure to the nearest quarter inch). Early results suggest that WHR values above 0.85 to 0.9 for men or 0.75 to 0.8 for women exceed safe limits. One reason may be that abdominal fat, fat stored in and around the viscera, has a direct circulatory route to the liver. Fat cells in that region are likely to send free fatty acids directly to the liver where they can be used to synthesize cholesterol. Whatever the reason for the relationship, we know that exercise is the best way to reduce the amount of metabolically active visceral fat. We also know that smokers have a higher WHR and that those who quit have a lower ratio.

Metabolic Rate?

Studies on obese infants, adolescents, and adults all agree that fat people are more *fuel-efficient*, that is, their bodies burn calories more sparingly than do normal weight subjects. The lower metabolic rate or energy expenditure makes weight loss more difficult, which perhaps helps explain how heredity may influence overweight and obesity. Why is the metabolic rate lower? One line of reasoning points to a lethargic or less active sympathetic nervous system. This portion of the autonomic nervous system secretes epinephrine (adrenaline) to speed up the heart rate and other responses during stress or exercise. Epinephrine also prompts the release of fatty acids from fat cells. Less sympathetic activity means less epinephrine, and less epinephrine means a lower metabolic rate and less fat utilization.

Other lines of research tend to lift some of the blame for excess fat from the shoulders of the obese. However, it is still too early to tell if metabolic problems or overeating cause obesity (Bray, 1983).

Brown Fat Thermogenesis

A form of fat that uses excess food to make heat, brown fat, may be deficient in some obese individuals. Normally brown fat serves to keep extra calories from being stored as fat. Studies on lean and obese humans will shed more light on this potential contributor to obesity.

Lipoprotein Lipase

Lipoprotein lipase (LPL) is an enzyme in adipose tissue and is also found in muscle. Researchers have found that its activity increases in the fat cells of obese individuals who lose weight, leading researchers to wonder if it might be a reason why previously overfat individuals usually regain lost weight. Chapter 8 discusses the effect of exercise on muscle LPL.

Sodium Pump Enzyme

Sodium-potassium ATPase is an enzyme involved in pumping sodium out of cells. Some researchers have found reduced activity in the cells of obese animals and postulate that the deficiency could reduce overall energy expenditure. The findings on obese humans are not conclusive.

If one or several of these lines of research are confirmed on human subjects, we will be better able to understand why so many millions are overweight or obese. Until then, remember the importance of **energy balance**.

> Regardless of genetic, glandular, psychological, or other complications or causes, *overweight and obesity are problems of energy balance.* Too many calories are taken in, too few are expended, or both.

Other Possible Causes

Psychological Causes. Overweight can stem from an underlying emotional problem. Eating may be a defense mechanism, a retreat from reality, or a defiant gesture used to get attention or sympathy. All of us have used food as a crutch when we were bored or lonely, and all of us have eating habits that border on overfeeding, such as doughnuts during coffee break, chips with TV, or late-night snacks. Eating and drinking are complex social behaviors, and failure to participate may be viewed as a social rebuff. The psychological and social causes of overeating are beyond the scope of this book, but eating behaviors are not. I will deal with ways to alter eating behavior in chapter 9.

Although some obese individuals suffer anxiety and depression, it isn't clear if that is a consequence of the excess weight, of social and psychological treatment by others, or of problems related to dieting. In other words, emotional problems associated with obesity may be a cause or a result of excess weight, and some may be a consequence of the treatment—dieting.

Physical Inactivity. Even the most voracious eater would have difficulty gaining weight if he or she ran 10 mi a day. Evidence suggests that overweight children are less active than their thinner counterparts. In one study, trained observers plotted the movements of fat and thin children while they engaged in games such as volleyball. The thin children ranged all over the court, whereas the heavyweights literally held down their positions (Mayer & Bullen, 1974).

You may wonder, "What comes first, inactivity or fat?" The earlier section on fat cells answers part of that question, but we do know that people reduce their activity and range of movement as they become larger, not wishing to call attention to their size. When adult-onset obesity follows an active youth, the individual is likely to be less inhibited and more active. But whatever the case, inactivity leads to weight gain, which leads to further inactivity, which leads to more weight gain, and so on. The problem is to break this vicious cycle and to restore normal levels of activity and food intake.

Dieting! Surprised? How can dieting lead to overweight or obesity? When an animal or human repeatedly loses and gains weight, in a process called **weight cycling,** the body becomes more fuel efficient and metabolic rate declines. Thereafter, more diet or exercise is required to reduce excess weight. Weight loss slows and weight is regained 3 times faster during the second cycle. Eventually, weight is maintained on a reduced caloric intake that inhibits weight loss and promotes regain (Brownell, Greenwood, Stellar, & Shrager, 1986). In other words, the **yoyo** approach to weight control leads to weight *gain,* not loss.

One reason for the yoyo effect is the *loss of lean tissue* with each round of dieting. Lean tissue (mostly muscle) is *metabolically active*; it is the furnace that burns unwanted calories. Remove muscle and you have less ability to burn calories at rest or during exercise. Every time you diet, you lose lean tissue, and hence you must decrease caloric intake to avoid subsequent weight gain. Return to past eating habits and you *increase weight and fat* above previous levels. Exercise is the *only* way to minimize the loss of lean tissue while dieting. In fact, do enough exercise and you can reverse the drop in metabolic rate and also increase lean tissue, thereby easing the problem of weight control.

Ideal Body Composition

Is there such a thing as an ideal body weight or body fat? Should one strive to reduce body fat to the minimum? The minimum amount of fat consistent with good health and nutrition probably is around 5% for young men and 12% for young women. Healthy high school wrestlers and male distance runners sometimes have a bit less than 5%, and female distance runners have had a temporary low of 7%. This does not suggest that all men and women should attempt to achieve these levels. I offer them only to indicate a minimum level consistent with health and performance.

Somewhere between the extremes (5 and 20% for men, 12 and 30% for women) lies a level that is best for you. The level you choose will relate to your current activity and interests. If you are training for a long distance race or bike ride, you'll want to minimize your "handicap." If you've been burdened with a large number of fat cells, you may be doing well to keep the level below 20%. Data indicates that those who weigh less than the desirable body weight for their height and frame live longer than those who weigh more. Because desirable weights are based on average body fat values, it would seem advisable to maintain body weight and fat values at or below desirable weight or average fat levels, respectively. But in the absence of heart disease, hypertension, or diabetes, there is little health difference between the extremes of 5 and 20% fat for men, 12 and 30% for women.

Sex-Specific Fat

Some of the fat differences between males and females are due to sex-specific fat. Female sex hormones dictate different patterns of fat deposition, including breasts, which are largely fat. However, only a portion of the difference shown in Table 7.4, perhaps an extra 6%, is due to sex-specific fat. The rest may be due to lack of activity brought on by outmoded concepts of what is feminine. But that is changing as more women take on the active lifestyle. Active college-age women average 18 to 22% fat, and female endurance athletes are often in the 12 to 17% range (Sharkey, 1984).

Age and Body Fat

With each decade above age 25, the body loses about 4% of its metabolically active cells. If your diet remains relatively unchanged during a 10-year period, you will gain weight, because your total energy expenditure has declined. This means that you should either become more active or eat less in order to maintain a desirable weight. Individuals who can claim that their weight has not changed since college or the day they were married should be congratulated. However, they should also know that the loss of metabolically active cells with age usually means a decline in lean body weight. Therefore, the maintenance of body weight usually indicates an *increase* in the percentage of body fat. *Body weight alone is not sufficient evidence that you are winning the battle of the bulge.*

Seasonal Fluctuation

Body weight and body fat values fluctuate from season to season and year to year. Typically, the lean body weight (body weight minus fat weight, also called the fat-free weight, or FFW) does not change that rapidly. The lean body weight consists mainly of muscles, bones, and organs. Thus, seasonal changes in body weight can be attributed to differences in the amount of fat being stored in adipose tissue. Total body fat storage often is higher during the winter months, when subcutaneous fat serves as insulation against the cold. In the summer, the weight and fat often decline in response to an increase in energy expenditure and a decrease in appetite (stimulated in part by temperature and the increase in daylight).

It seems clear that overweight and obesity can be inherited and that individuals who inherit these tendencies are more metabolically efficient (they use less energy). Thus one can become overweight and yet eat no more than those who remain thin. The reason for this isn't clear at present, although I have presented some hypotheses. What is clear is the importance of physical activity in the battle of the bulge. Exercise is the best medicine for obesity, because it burns fat while preserving lean tissue, something that diet alone cannot do. Chapter 8 will tell you more about exercise, fitness, and weight control.

CHAPTER

8

EXERCISE, FITNESS, AND WEIGHT CONTROL

This chapter will help you

understand why exercise is superior to diet as a means of weight control,

determine the effects of exercise on the appetite, and

understand the extra weight control and fat metabolism benefits associated with improved fitness.

This may be the most important chapter of the book. It discusses the value of exercise in the maintenance of optimal body weight and desirable body fat and shows why exercise is superior to diet for the control of weight and fat. But the best part deals with the *extra* weight control benefits you obtain with fitness, benefits that exceed the effects of exercise alone. This material is only beginning to come to the attention of fitness professionals. In my estimation, it provides the most convincing case for fitness ever compiled.

Exercise and Weight Control

The only way to remove stored fat is to burn it off. By now you know that exercise increases caloric expenditure and that the rate of expenditure is related to both the intensity and duration of activity. As exercise becomes more intense, the duration of participation becomes limited. Although we may be able to expend as many as 125 calories in one all-out mile run, we can jog at a comfortable pace for 3 mi and *triple* caloric expenditure without becoming exhausted. This explains why experts recommend moderate activity instead of high-intensity effort for weight control.

The effects of exercise do not stop when the exercise ceases. Caloric expenditure can remain elevated for 30 min or more after vigorous exercise. Long duration effort such as a distance run will elevate body temperature and call forth hormones to mobilize energy and increase metabolism. When the exercise stops, there is a recovery period when caloric expenditure remains above resting levels. This postexercise increase in energy expenditure is usually neglected when considering the caloric benefits of exercise.

Exercise Versus Diet

Many claim that diet is better than exercise for controlling weight. They point out, quite correctly I might add, that it is easier to reduce the caloric intake by refusing a piece of cake (250 calories) than it is to burn off the cake after it is eaten (by running 2 mi at 120 calories/mi). But let's return to the question, "Is diet a better method of weight control?"

Oscai and Holloszy (1969) compared the effects of diet and exercise on the body composition of laboratory rats. The experiment was controlled so that both groups lost the same amount of weight. After 18 weeks of either food restriction (diet) or swimming (exercise), carcass analysis indicated that the groups lost the following:

Body component	Weight lost (%)	
	Exercise	Diet
Fat	78	62
Protein	5	11
Minerals	1	1
Water	16	26

A control group of sedentary, freely eating animals gained weight during the study. Their weight gain consisted of 87% fat and 10% water. It appears that exercise is a more effective way to lose *fat*. Furthermore, the study provided vivid evidence of the "protein-conserving" effects of exercise. Notice also the amount of water lost through caloric restriction. This water loss is a common occurrence among dieting human beings and accounts for the early success of most fad diets and their eventual failure in reaching the overall goal—fat loss. Can the results of this animal study be generalized to human subjects?

Six months of diet were compared with a similar period of diet and exercise in a study involving 16 obese patients. The exercise group achieved greater fat loss, and the exercise produced other benefits, including a lower resting heart rate and improved heart rate recovery after exercise (Kenrick, Ball, & Canary, 1972). And when 25 women created a 500-calorie/day deficit by diet, exercise, or a combination, the results were the same. All the women lost the same amount of weight, but those in the diet group lost less fat and more lean tissue. The authors of the study, Zuti and Golding (1976), recommended that those interested in losing weight should combine diet and exercise to ensure a greater fat loss and a conservation of lean tissue.

These studies clearly indicate the need for exercise in a program of weight control. Diet or caloric restriction can lead to the loss of weight, but the loss is accompanied by a greater loss of protein (lean tissue) and water. When lean tissue is lost the body becomes less able to burn calories and it eventually gains more fat weight. Weight loss through exercise maximizes the removal of fat and minimizes the loss of protein. Exercise and diet *combine* to provide a positive attack on both causes of overweight—excess caloric intake and inadequate caloric expenditure.

A recent study indicates an added benefit of exercise in relation to weight control and diet. Several weeks of severe caloric restriction imposed by dieting led to the usual loss of lean tissue and a decreased metabolic rate. The drop in metabolic rate makes it difficult for dieters to maintain a lower body weight, because the more efficient body burns 10 to 15% fewer calories daily. However, 2 weeks of *exercise restored the metabolic rate* to pre-diet levels. Moreover, the exercise reduced the loss of protein and increased the utilization of fat as the source of energy (Móle, Stern, Schultz, Bernauer, & Holcomb, 1989).

Exercise and Appetite

In the past, the use of exercise to achieve energy balance and weight control received criticism, with detractors claiming that exercise would increase the appetite as the hunger center, or appestat, attempted to keep pace with energy needs. In fact, the *opposite* is the case. When a person is sedentary, food intake far exceeds energy needs. If a person becomes active, the food intake increases but it doesn't increase above the energy needs. In fact, as the level of activity becomes greater, the caloric intake *falls short* of energy needs. And in time, the appetite returns to normal and remains well below the increased level of caloric expenditure (Mayer & Bullen, 1974).

Exercise and Meals

Years ago, when the American diet was first indicated as a culprit in the heart disease epidemic, researchers roamed the world studying the relationship between diet and the incidence of heart disease. They found that diet alone did not account for the presence or absence of the problem; other factors such as a lack of tension and stress or physical activity confounded the relationship. Since then, several researchers have focused on the effect of *pre- or postmeal exercise* on **postprandial lipemia** (the presence of fat in the blood after eating). Studies conducted at the University of Florida showed that exercise before or after a meal is effective in reducing the magnitude and duration of postprandial lipemia (Zauner, Burt, & Mapes, 1968). Mild exercise proved to be as effective as strenuous effort in this regard.

Lipemia long has been associated with atherosclerosis, reduced myocardial blood flow, inhibition of the fibrinolytic mechanism, and accelerated blood clotting. Thus, anything that reduces the level of fat in the blood seems prudent and advisable. Vigorous premeal exercise can inhibit the appetite and increase the metabolism of fat, even fat ingested after the exercise. The metabolic rate remains somewhat elevated after exercise, and the ingested fat is used quickly to restore energy burned during exercise. Mild postmeal effort such as a walk after dinner also serves to reduce lipemia. Both pre- and postmeal exercise increase caloric expenditure and fat metabolism, lead to improved fitness, and contribute to health and weight control.

And, while we're on the subject of meals and blood lipids, you should know that the *number of meals* you eat has an influence on blood fat levels. Spread the *same* number of calories over more meals (three to six) and your cholesterol level will be lower, presumably because we are able to handle fat better in smaller doses. So if you eat less frequent meals in an effort to lose weight, your metabolic rate will decline and your cholesterol level will climb. And your temporary weight *loss* will be followed by a rapid *gain*.

Fitness and Fat

The effects of exercise on weight control and energy balance are well established. When the exercise is systematic and progressive, it leads to an improvement in aerobic fitness. This section deals with the *extra* benefits associated with improved fitness, benefits that provide dramatic evidence of the role fitness plays in health and the prevention of heart disease. These benefits include

- increased caloric expenditure,
- increased fat mobilization,
- increased fat utilization,
- reduced blood lipids, and
- increased lean body weight (muscle).

Caloric Expenditure

Unfit individuals tire quickly during exercise and are limited in their ability to expend calories. As fitness improves, caloric expenditure increases with the increase in the intensity, duration, and frequency of exercise and because of the inevitable participation in more vigorous activities. The fit individual participates longer without fatiguing, thus, increased fitness undoubtedly enhances energy expenditure and weight control.

One study focused on the effects of training on individuals' perception of effort and fatigue (Docktor & Sharkey, 1971). As fitness improved, the subjects could perform more work at the same heart rate. Work levels once perceived as difficult became less so, and the subjects could manage once-fatiguing exertion with ease. After training, the subjects could accomplish a given task with a lower heart rate as well as a lower level of perceived exertion. Thus, they were able to burn more energy without experiencing a greater sense of fatigue.

We can find further proof of the value of fitness to caloric expenditure in the relationship of caloric expenditure to heart rate. Caloric expenditure is related directly to the heart rate, but the relationship is also influenced by level of fitness. For those in low-fitness categories, a high heart rate does not indicate an extremely high caloric expenditure (see Figure 8.1). For those in high categories, a high heart rate indicates a much higher energy expenditure.

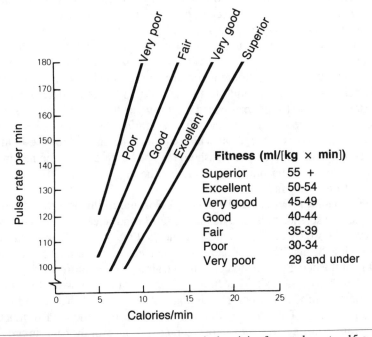

Figure 8.1. Predicting calories burned during physical activity from pulse rate—15-s pulse count taken immediately after exercise (15-s × 4 = rate/min). *Note.* Adapted from Sharkey (1974, 1975).

| **150 HR for very poor fitness level = about 7 cal/min**
| **150 HR for superior fitness level = more than 14 cal/min**

You can use Figure 8.1 to estimate your caloric expenditure in any physical activity. After several minutes of participation, simply stop and immediately take your pulse at wrist, throat (use gentle contact at throat), or temple for 15 s. Multiply by 4 to get your rate per minute. Then use the line corresponding to your fitness level to estimate your caloric expenditure per minute. Also notice how caloric expenditure improves (at the same heart rate) as your fitness improves. This should convince you that fitness provides extra benefits to those who persevere.

Perceived exertion is also related to heart rate. Because training allows you to perform a certain effort, such as jogging at a 10-min/mi pace, at a lower heart rate, your perception of effort will also be lower. I'll say more about perceived exertion and show you how to measure yours in chapter 13.

Fat Mobilization

Fat is stored in fat cells in the form of triglyceride (three molecules of fatty acid and glycerol). This molecule is too large to pass through the wall of the fat cell into the circulation. So when energy is needed, the triglyceride is broken down, and the fatty acid molecules pass into the blood for transport to the working muscles. The hormone epinephrine stimulates the fat cell membrane and leads to the activation of the fat-splitting enzyme lipase. Lipase splits the triglyceride molecule, and the fatty acids are free to circulate (see Figure 2.1 in chapter 2).

As exercise becomes more and more intense, the body begins to produce lactic acid. The point at which lactic acid begins to accumulate in the blood, the lactate threshold (sometimes called the anaerobic threshold), indicates when lactate production exceeds removal and when a significant shift from fat to carbohydrate metabolism takes place. You will recall that the anaerobic threshold is related to activity and fitness. The threshold may be below 50% of the maximal oxygen intake for the unfit and above 80% for the highly trained. But what does that have to do with fat?

Years ago, researchers at Lankanau Hospital in Philadelphia discovered that lactic acid seemed to inhibit the mobilization and release of free fatty acid (FFA) from adipose tissue. The lactic acid blocked the action of epinephrine, thereby reducing the availability of fat for muscle metabolism (Issekutz & Miller, 1962). One of the best documented effects of training is that more work can be accomplished before lactic acid accumulates in the blood. A work load that leads to lactic acid production before training can be accomplished with little increase after training. This may be due to a decrease in lactic acid production or an increase in lactic acid removal (or clearance). Whatever the case, improved aerobic fitness allows more work to be accomplished aerobically; the lactate threshold is raised and *more fat can be mobilized* and made available for use as an energy source.

A recent study of trained subjects illustrated that FFA mobilization and utilization are not affected by moderate levels of lactic acid (Vega deJesus & Siconolfi, 1988). The fit subjects were able to mobilize fat at the lactate threshold (4 mmol lactic acid), which defines the highest level of exercise intensity that can be sustained during prolonged exertion. These findings help to explain the tremendous increase in endurance associated with training. Fat is the most abundant energy source (50 times more abundant than carbohydrate), and improved fitness allows greater access to that immense storehouse of energy.

Lactic acid is produced when the breakdown of muscle glycogen to pyruvic acid exceeds the ability of the mitochondria to process this metabolite. So the pyruvic acid picks up hydrogen, changes to lactic acid, and begins to accumulate in the muscle and the blood. Lactate can be used by the heart and skeletal muscles as a source of energy, and it can be oxidized in the liver. However, when the rate of production exceeds the rate of removal, the level in the blood increases. The rising level of acid in the muscle interferes with contraction and reduces the efficiency of aerobic enzymes. Also, the lactate in the blood blocks the action of epinephrine and inhibits the mobilization of fat. Therefore, less fat can be oxidized by working muscles.

Fat Utilization

The mobilization of FFA does not ensure its metabolism. How does training influence the utilization of FFA as a source of energy for muscular contractions? Studies show that trained animals and humans are capable of extracting a greater percentage of their energy from FFA during submaximal exercise. How does fitness influence fat utilization?

Lipoprotein Lipase. Earlier I talked about LPL in adipose tissue. In muscle the LPL helps grab circulating fat from the blood and use it for energy. Muscle LPL activity increases with endurance training and enhances the muscle's ability to use fat as a fuel (Nikkila, Taskinen, Rehunen, & Harkonen, 1978).

Fat Oxidation. Móle, Oscai, and Holloszy (1971) provided convincing proof of the effect of training on FFA utilization. They found that the ability of the rat gastrocnemius muscle to oxidize the fatty acid palmitate was doubled following 12 weeks of treadmill training. The authors suggested that the shift to fat metabolism was a key factor in the development of endurance fitness and an important mechanism serving to spare carbohydrate stores and prevent low blood sugar during prolonged exertion. Thus, the physically fit individual is able to derive a greater percentage of energy requirements from fat than is the unfit subject. At a given work load, the fit subject may obtain as much as 90% of his or her energy from fat. Our bodies use FFA during all forms of muscular activity, except all-out bursts of effort such as the 100-yd dash. Training even seems to improve the ability of the heart muscle to oxidize fat (Keul, 1971).

Improved fitness, then, leads to improved availability of fat via mobilization of FFA as well as an increase in enzyme activity. Both contribute to the rate of FFA *utilization*. Muscle burns fat, and fitness increases the ratio of lean to fat tissue.

Exercise, Fitness, and Blood Lipids

The blood lipids, cholesterol and triglyceride, have been implicated in or associated with the incidence and severity of coronary heart disease. Both seem to be related to other risk factors, including diet, body weight, and exercise. Recent findings suggest that the lipids are also influenced by fitness training.

Triglycerides

Dietary fat intake shows up in the blood as **chylomicrons**, large clumps of triglycerides. Most of the triglycerides are removed from the plasma in the capillaries adjacent to muscle and adipose tissue, and any remains are cleared from the circulation by the liver.

Chylomicrons are responsible for the milky appearance of blood plasma following a meal (postprandial lipemia). In addition to 80 to 95% triglyceride, chylomicrons contain 2 to 7% cholesterol, 3 to 6% phospholipid, and 1 to 2% protein.

Proper diet or participation in regular physical exercise consistently reduce fasting serum triglyceride levels. The reduction due to exercise occurs several hours afterward and lasts for about 2 days. With regular exercise, further reductions occur until triglyceride levels reach a plateau consistent with the exercise, diet, and other factors, such as inherited blood lipid patterns.

Earlier in this chapter I established the influence of exercise on postmeal fat in blood. Research supports the hypothesis that regular exercise enhances the muscle cells' removal and utilization of triglycerides, rather than allowing their deposit in adipose tissue or removal by the liver.

One researcher trained sedentary rats for 12 weeks on a treadmill. Following the training, the researcher analyzed the rats' muscles for the activity of lipoprotein lipase (LPL), the enzyme responsible for the uptake of plasma triglyceride fatty acids (TGFA) from plasma chylomicrons and other sources in the blood. The researcher reasoned that any increase in the uptake of TGFA by skeletal muscle during exercise would be accompanied by an increase in LPL activity, and the results of the study confirmed this hypothesis. Regular endurance training led to a twofold to fourfold increase in the LPL activity, indicating that training increases the capacity of the muscle fibers to take up and oxidize fatty acids originating in plasma triglycerides (Borensztajn, 1975).

Because the muscle fibers use fat before it can be deposited in adipose tissue, these findings have tremendous significance in the area of weight control. However, the implications for cardiovascular health are even more exciting, as is the realization that these benefits are associated with an entirely natural, enjoyable, and satisfying experience—aerobic fitness training.

Cholesterol

Cholesterol ingested in the diet is absorbed in the small intestine, finds its way into the lymph system, and then is dumped into the blood. There it joins with cholesterol produced in the body in the chylomicrons and in particles of very low-density lipoprotein (VLDL). Once in the plasma, the VLDL is attacked by the same enzymes that act on the chylomicrons, and these enzymes remove much of the triglyceride (within 2 to 6 hr). The VLDL is degraded to low-density lipoprotein (LDL), which the liver removes over a period of 2 to 5 days.

Because of the smaller size of the LDL particle and its high concentration of cholesterol, the LDL particle seems to be involved directly in the development of coronary artery disease. The LDL particles find their way into coronary arteries and contribute to the growth of atherosclerotic plaques. Thus, LDL is believed to be a major culprit in the development of coronary artery disease.

Until the mid-1970s, researchers believed that diet, weight loss, and drugs were the major weapons in the fight against cholesterol. Studies on the effect of exercise on cholesterol typically reported a modest reduction, but only when the exercise was vigorous and of long duration (3 mi or more per day). But cholesterol is transported in the blood in several ways, and a single measure of serum cholesterol does not indicate how the cholesterol is distributed among the several lipoproteins, nor does it indicate the effects of exercise on cholesterol levels.

Dr. Wood (1975) of the Stanford Heart Disease Prevention Program compared the lipoprotein patterns of sedentary and active middle-aged men (35 to 59 years old). The active group consisted of joggers who averaged at least 15 mi per week for the preceding year. As expected, the triglycerides were "strikingly" lower for the active group, whereas total cholesterol was only "modestly" reduced. However, analysis of the lipoprotein pattern showed that the joggers exhibited a significantly lower level of dangerous LDL and an elevated level of high-density lipoprotein (HDL). These findings are astounding, because there is a direct relationship between LDL and heart disease and an inverse relationship between HDL and heart disease (as HDL goes up, the incidence of heart disease goes down; see Table 8.1). HDL seems to carry cholesterol away from the tissues for removal by the liver. (Chapter 12 provides more information on HDL.) Dr. Wood noted that the lipoprotein pattern could be mistaken for that of the typical young woman, who has the lowest risk of heart disease in the entire adult population.

Table 8.1 HDL and Heart Disease Risk

HDL (mg)	Heart disease risk
75	Longevity syndrome (no CAD)
45 (men)	Standard risk (55 for women)
25	High risk

Researchers are currently investigating subfractions of HDL, which may provide more accurate estimates of CAD risk and of the effects of exercise, diet, and weight loss.

I want you to realize the inadequacy of *total cholesterol* as an indicator of the effects of exercise and fitness on blood lipids and health. As a final gesture to the skeptics and those who doubt the validity of cross-sectional studies such as that noted earlier in this section, I offer the following. Researchers at the Louisiana State University School of Medicine studied the effects of 7 weeks of training on the serum lipids and lipoproteins in 13 young medical students (Lopez, Vial, Balart, & Arroyave, 1974). As expected, training reduced triglycerides from 110 to 80 mg—a total reduction of 30 mg. Furthermore, the researchers found a marked reduction of beta lipoprotein cholesterol (cholesterol in LDL and VLDL), a concomitant increase in alpha lipoprotein cholesterol (HDL), and no changes in body weight to confuse the results. Results of this and other studies (Sharkey et al., 1980) agree with those reported by Dr. Wood and many others. These studies clearly indicate how training helps shift cholesterol from the dangerous LDL to the favorable HDL, why total cholesterol fails to indicate all the effects of exercise, and how exercise and fitness training may prevent the development or progression of atherosclerosis and heart disease.

How's that for an extra benefit of fitness? Not only does fitness allow increased caloric expenditure and enhanced fat mobilization and utilization, but it also allows you to have a direct effect on your blood lipids and reduce your risk of heart disease. I feel that this may be the most important benefit of exercise and fitness.

One final word: A growing number of researchers believe that it may be possible to lower serum cholesterol levels enough to actually reverse the process of atherosclerosis, to remove fatty buildup from the lining of the coronary arteries.

If this proves to be true, and if diet, exercise, or even drug therapy can accomplish this reversal, we will be able to cure—instead of just treat—heart disease, the nation's number one killer. (I'll say much more about cholesterol and how to reduce it in chapter 12.)

CHAPTER

9

WEIGHT CONTROL PROGRAMS

This chapter will help you

implement the weight control program most suited to your needs,

understand the essentials of good nutrition, and

lose or gain weight.

This chapter outlines exercise, diet, and behavior therapy programs to provide a three-pronged attack on the problems of overweight and obesity. Any one of the three will help you lose weight, but if you are interested in long-term weight loss, if your weight control problem is significant, and if you want to gain complete and lasting control of the problem, consider the combined benefits of all three. Incidentally, you'll find additional information about weight control in Appendix D.

Exercise: A Positive Approach

I begin with exercise because it represents a positive approach to the problem. When you decide to do something about your weight problem, you commit yourself to a course of action. No other method of weight control is so physiologically sound, so definite, or so enjoyable as exercise. Dieting carries a negative connotation of avoidance, deprivation, and punishment. And dieting, by itself, often leads to increases in weight and fat. Exercise provides a positive approach: It is more psychologically rewarding to *do* something than it is to *avoid* something. When you walk a mile after dinner you relax, improve your digestion, enhance your vitality, and, incidentally, burn calories. After the walk you feel better both physically and emotionally. Problems loom large when you sit and brood, but how quickly they shrink when you undertake a plan of action!

Beginning

If you want to approach weight control systematically, you should determine your energy balance (caloric intake vs. caloric expenditure).

Caloric Expenditure. For the next few days, keep an inventory of your activity. Simply list your activity (exercise, work, and household chores) and the time spent for each (see Table 9.1). Don't omit anything, even sleeping. Then estimate the caloric expenditure of these activities by referring to the tables in Appendix D. This exercise is most educational; it shows you when calories are burned and provides insight about how you can increase caloric expenditures in your normal routine.

Energy expenditure values are based on the oxygen and caloric expenditure of the various activities. These values sometimes underestimate the actual caloric expenditure. For example, if a study of the energy cost of running is conducted on a laboratory treadmill using highly trained endurance runners as subjects, the values obtained underestimate your cost of running because

- the treadmill is perfectly flat (unlike the road or trail you use),
- the air in the lab is still (even on a calm day the moving body must overcome some wind resistance when outdoors),
- trained runners are up to 10% more efficient than untrained, and
- the lab values don't consider the postexercise period, when energy is used to replace stores of energy used during the run. Postexercise oxygen consumption may be elevated for up to an hour after a long, hard run.

These widely used values for the energy cost of running may be over 10% too low for many joggers. Over a period of weeks, an error of that size renders a serious disservice to exercise and its role in weight control.

Caloric Intake. Figure your caloric intake by keeping records of all the food you eat, including snacks (see Table 9.2). Then figure the calories per serving, per meal, per day from the calorie tables (see Appendix D). Estimate portions when necessary, but don't overlook any source of calories, including the sugar in your coffee.

Table 9.1 Energy Expenditure Log

(Use energy expenditure tables in Appendix D)

Activity	Time (min)	Expenditure rate (cal/min)	Total expenditure (cal)
Sleep	_____	_____	_____
Nonwork and household			
_____	_____	_____	_____
_____	_____	_____	_____
_____	_____	_____	_____
Work			
_____	_____	_____	_____
_____	_____	_____	_____
_____	_____	_____	_____
Recreation and sport			
_____	_____	_____	_____
_____	_____	_____	_____
_____	_____	_____	_____
	24 hr	Day's total =	_____

Examples	Time (min)	Expenditure rate (cal/min)	Total expenditure (cal)
Sleep	480	1.2	576
Nonwork			
Personal toilet	10	2.0	20
Cook breakfast	10	1.5	15
Cook dinner	60	1.5	90
Work			
Walk to work and return	20	5.0	100
Work (standard activity)	400	2.6	1,040
Rest breaks	80	1.5	120
Lunch	30	1.5	45
Jogging	30	10.0	300
		Total	2,306

Table 9.2 Caloric Intake

(Use calorie tables in Appendix D)

Date _____ Weight _____

	Food	Portion	Intake (cal)
Breakfast			
Lunch			
Dinner			
Desserts			
Snacks			
Drinks			
Other			

Total caloric intake _____

Total caloric expenditure (Table 9.1) _____

Energy balance (+ or −) _____

Cal/day

Energy Balance. Now figure your energy balance (subtract intake from expenditure). If intake exceeds expenditure on a regular basis you will gain weight. A *mere 100 calories of extra intake daily will lead to more than 10 pounds of extra weight in one year* (100 calories × 364 days = 36,400 ÷ 3,500 calories per pound of fat = 10.4 lb).

Caloric Deficit. When expenditure exceeds intake, you have a deficit. The caloric deficit determines the rate of weight loss. If the deficit is 100 calories per day, you will lose 1 lb every 35 days. If the deficit is 500 calories per day, you'll lose 1 lb each week. *The deficit should never regularly exceed 1,000 calories per day.* A deficit of 1,000 calories leads to a weight loss of 2 lb per week. It is neither necessary nor prudent to exceed this rate of weight loss. In fact, if the deficit regularly exceeds 1,000 calories, fatigue, listlessness, and reduced resistance to infection may occur.

Formulating an Exercise Prescription

The exercise prescription for weight loss or weight control must *maximize caloric expenditure* at the expense of exercise intensity. Exercise *duration* is extended to increase caloric expenditure. Both the duration and frequency of exercise should be increased to achieve the maximal benefit of exercise. Thus, if your fitness prescription suggests 100 to 200 calories of exercise several days per week, you should try to work at the low edge of your training zone (intensity) and increase the caloric expenditure (duration). Also, increase the frequency to daily or twice daily if possible.

Supplemental Activities.   There are many ways to increase caloric expenditure aside from your daily exercise session. Walk to work, to lunch, during coffee break, and after dinner. Be as active as possible while at work, and take an exercise break during the day. Climb stairs, jump rope, do calisthenics. Do *anything* that increases caloric expenditure. If you expend 200 calories in your training session and another 100 walking or climbing stairs, you will accelerate your exercise weight loss by 50%. When you are more fit and are capable of burning 500 calories daily through exercise, you will be able to lose *1 lb per week* (3,500 calories) through exercise alone.

Change of Lifestyle.   The best way to achieve permanent weight loss is to make a change in lifestyle. The change could be to return to old ways of doing things. Avoid unnecessary labor-saving devices (like electric can openers or snow throwers). Seek out and employ energy-*using* devices like the snow shovel, the bicycle, and your own two feet. The best advice is to never use a machine when you can do the job yourself. You will be doing yourself a favor and saving energy (electric, gas, oil, and coal) at the same time.

Perhaps the best idea is to find an active hobby or sport and make it an essential part of your lifestyle. Try woodworking, racquetball, or dancing. Get a bicycle or cross-country skis, or start a garden. Dig out the tennis racket and give it a try. Go ice skating in the winter or roller skating any time of year. You'll enrich your life and lower your weight at the same time.

Dieting for Weight Control

If you're searching for one of those fad diets that regularly come and go, don't look here. When I say diet I mean reduced caloric intake, usually accomplished by reducing high-calorie fat in the diet. As I said in chapter 7, each gram of fat contains 9.3 calories, versus only 4.1 and 4.3 for carbohydrate and protein, respectively. Forty percent of the calories in the average diet come from fat. If you've been eating 2,000 calories daily, 800 may come from fat, so you have plenty of room to cut back. I'll explain the low-fat diet later in this chapter, but first I'll explain what I *don't* mean by dieting.

When you restrict calories, your daily caloric deficit shouldn't exceed 1,000 calories regularly. Of course, it is entirely possible to restrict caloric intake far below energy needs. However, if you do that for more than a few days you'll be on a starvation diet; you won't receive the essential nutrients, your energy level will sag, and you will lower your resistance to infection. Furthermore, your body will interpret the starvation diet as a signal to reduce caloric expenditure, you'll begin to lose lean tissue, and you will be on your way to increased weight loss problems.

Fasting is the ultimate form of caloric restriction. It is guaranteed to bring about a dramatic weight loss, as much as a pound a day—for a while. However, the risks of fasting are many, especially if continued for an extended period. If you are grossly overweight and eager to fast, check into a hospital and proceed; otherwise, avoid extended periods of fasting.

Any diet must consider nutritional needs, so we'll review those requirements as a foundation for advice on dieting for energy balance and weight control.

Nutrition

The requirements of good nutrition are relatively simple and include adequate amounts of energy (calories), protein, fat, carbohydrates (including fiber), and essential vitamins, minerals, and water. In the typical diet, the carbohydrate, fat, and, protein proportions average about 45, 40, and 15% of daily energy intake, respectively.

Fat.   There is a growing consensus regarding the health implications of excess fat in the diet. In discussing the role of fat in heart disease, some argue for a selective reduction of saturated fats and cholesterol, with less concern for polyunsaturated fats. Certain oils, including the tropical oils (palm and coconut), are believed to be more atherogenic (more likely to cause atherosclerosis), whereas others, including safflower, peanut, and olive oil, are thought to be less risky, unless they are hydrogenated to keep them solid at room temperatures (as in some peanut butters). Chapter 12 discusses the influence of fat on heart disease. But in this chapter, weight loss is the issue, and fat is a high-calorie food to avoid if you want to lose weight.

Protein.   The amino acids of the protein we ingest are used to build cell walls, muscles, hormones, enzymes, and a variety of other molecules. Studies show that adult protein needs do not increase markedly during physical activity. In fact, it appears that daily requirements may be met with 0.8 g of protein per kilogram of body weight. Thus, a 70-kg (154-lb) man requires about 56 g, and a 58-kg (128-lb) woman requires 46 g of high-quality protein daily.

High-quality protein describes food sources that are rich in the essential amino acids. Examples include meat, eggs, and dairy products; unfortunately, these food sources also include fat. Low-fat protein sources, such as corn, beans, and grains, don't contain all the essential amino acids. However, these amino acids can be provided by eating a variety of foods including some meat, eggs, or dairy products or by carefully combining vegetable protein sources (e.g., corn and beans, rice and soy).

Excess protein cannot be stored; it is stripped of its nitrogen molecules and the remaining carbon skeleton is converted to glucose or fat. The nitrogenous portion is eliminated through the urine. Small wonder the urine of some over-fed Americans is so rich in nitrogen that municipal sewer facilities convert human waste to nitrogen-rich fertilizer!

Earlier I said that protein needs do not change markedly during exercise. When calories and nutrition are adequate, protein supplementation beyond that needed to maintain nitrogen balance has not proven beneficial to human performance. However, when total protein needs are *not* met or when the essential amino acids are missing from the diet, physical activity could result in a loss of muscle mass. One effect of starvation and most diets is that the body uses muscle protein as a source of energy. When caloric intake is below expenditure, the body has an increased need for protein during vigorous exercise and during training programs that lead to increased contractile protein synthesis (e.g., strength training) or enzyme protein synthesis (e.g., endurance training; Lemon, 1987). An increase to 2 g per 1 kg of body weight will provide a margin of safety for most training programs and will meet the growth and development needs of the young athlete. The increase is *especially important* when *weight loss* accompanies the training. Excessive protein ingestion has no detrimental effect so long as the diet includes an appropriate balance of carbohydrate and fat; but when training or weight loss stop, the protein supplementation should stop. Excess protein isn't necessary on a balanced diet (Butterfield, 1987).

If a 70-kg (154-lb) athlete eats 2,000 calories/day with 15% of the calories from protein, he gets 300 calories of protein ÷ 4.3 c/g = 70 g of protein, or 1 g per 1 kg of body weight. To supply additional protein he can increase food intake to meet the increased energy expenditure of training. If he is *losing weight* while training, he should eat extra protein to supply up to 2 g per kg of body weight (up to 140 g/day).

Some athletes select diets high in protein, probably due to the misconception of the role of protein in vigorous physical activity. More important than the quantity of protein in the diet is the quality, because certain amino acids cannot be synthesized in the body. Thus these *essential* amino acids must be provided in the diet. Failure to supply one of the essential amino acids will put a halt to the synthesis of proteins containing that building block. When planning your diet, include a variety of foods from the four food groups (as shown in Table 9.3) to ensure a *balanced*, nutritious diet.

How much protein is available in common foods?

Food	Portion	Protein (g)
Beans	1/2 cup	6-8
Beef	1/4 lb	20-28
Cheese	1 ounce	7
Chicken	3-1/2 ounces	24-30
Chili	1 cup	20
Corn	1/2 cup	3
Fish	4 ounces	25-30
Hamburger	1/4 lb	20
Milk	1 cup	9
Peanut butter	1 tablespoon	4
Pizza	1 slice	10

Table 9.3 Four Food Groups

Food group	Value in diet	Recommended daily intake
Milk group (milk, cheese, cottage cheese)	Protein, calcium, other minerals, and vitamins	3 or more servings (preferably low-fat)
Meat group (also includes fish, fowl, nuts, peas, beans)	Protein, iron, other minerals, and B vitamins	2 or more servings (consider more fish and beans, and less meat)
Vegetables and fruits (includes potatoes)	Minerals, vitamins, and fiber	4 or more servings
Breads and cerals (includes rice and pasta)	Carbohydrate energy, protein, iron, and B vitamins, fiber	4 or more servings

Carbohydrate. Carbohydrate is the major source of energy throughout the world. In countries where carbohydrates provide a high percentage of dietary energy, the risk of heart disease is low. Simple carbohydrates, such as table sugar and honey, are relatively low in nutrients. But complex carbohydrates (starches), such as potatoes, corn, beans, rice, and whole grain products, provide energy and nutrients. Fresh fruits provide energy, nutrition, and an added plus: Although most carbohydrates stimulate the flow of insulin that hurries sugar out of the bloodstream, fruit sugar (fructose) does not. So fruit is an excellent snack that avoids the eventual drop in blood sugar and energy. For energy, nutrition, a reduced risk of heart disease, and even for good performance, I recommend a diet that contains at least 60% of the calories from carbohydrate. I call this diet the *high-performance diet* and will say more about it later in the chapter.

Vitamins and Minerals. Certain **B vitamins** serve as cofactors on enzymes involved in carbohydrate metabolism. (The cofactor is the active portion of the enzyme.) Thus, it is not surprising that vitamin needs increase with physical activity. Because caloric intake *usually* rises to provide energy for increased activity, the increase in an already sound diet may meet the vitamin needs. If you plan to combine exercise and caloric restriction (as you must to lose weight sensibly), you may want to consider a daily vitamin supplement.

Various vitamin supplements have been tested to determine their effect on athletic performance. A few studies report improved performances, but it is likely that the effect is due to the improvement of previously inadequate nutrition. No type of vitamin supplementation will improve any type of performance for an individual whose nutrition is already adequate.

Excessive vitamin supplementation may carry some undesirable side effects. Those who take huge doses of **vitamin C** in hopes of avoiding the common cold could be doing more harm than good. The recommended allowance for vitamin C is 60 mg for an adult man. Doses of 2 to 3 g (2,000 to 3,000 mg) far exceed human needs. Because vitamin C is ascorbic acid, the large doses could irritate the gastric lining; other possible complications include gout, kidney complications, and leaching of calcium from bones. Because the huge doses do not seem to prevent the common cold or markedly increase resistance to stress, the high doses seem unnecessary. Take modest supplements if you like.

A simple and inexpensive approach is to take a vitamin that meets the recommended dietary allowances (RDA) established by the National Research Council. Select one that provides 100% of the RDA for vitamins (and minerals if necessary). However, the National Research Council discourages the use of vitamin and mineral supplements and argues instead for a low-fat, low-salt, low-alcohol diet that includes fresh fruit, vegetables, adequate protein, and increased calories from complex carbohydrate—the diet I have urged since the first edition of this book.

Excessive doses of **water-soluble vitamins (B and C)** are passed in the urine, but **fat-soluble vitamins (A and D)** accumulate. So excessive supplementation can lead to toxic effects such as headache, nausea, diarrhea, or even decalcification of bones (in the case of excess vitamin A).

The need for additional minerals and trace elements may arise with exercise; hard training can accelerate iron loss in sweat and lower the absorption of iron from food. Also, iron from animal sources is easier to absorb than iron in vegetables. Again, you should meet increased mineral needs with an increase of iron-rich foods in the diet. All active females and young males should eat a balanced diet or consider the need to offset potentially low iron intake with a daily iron supplement (consider multivitamin-plus-iron pills). When caloric restriction and exercise are combined, a well-balanced diet is essential, which is why most of the fad diets are dangerous. To make wise decisions in regard to vitamins and minerals you should understand the amount of vitamins and minerals needed by the body, their functions in the body, and good food sources of these elements (see Table 9.4).

Diets to Avoid

Almost every edition of a popular magazine includes an article on diet. Many offer a ''revolutionary'' new diet plan with such promises as ''eat all you want, calories don't count, quick weight loss, super energy.'' You've heard of the water diet, the drinking man's diet, and high-protein, liquid protein, low-carbohydrate, and other diets. Unfortunately, most of these plans reach more readers than do the critical editorials and reports in medical journals.

Be suspicious of any plan that promises rapid results (more than a 2-lb weight loss per week). Certainly you can lose more weight by fasting or by dehydration. Water is heavy, about 2 lb per quart, and you could easily lose 2 lb in an hour; athletes often lose 6 pounds or more in a hard workout. So what? Your body needs the water and replaces it as soon as possible. Question any plan that calls for a low intake of carbohydrate or protein or encourages a high intake of protein or fat.

Low Carbohydrate Intake.
One fad diet plan advocates the near-exclusion of carbohydrate. The author states that the average overweight man should lose about 7 lb in the first week of the diet! (Remember, carbohydrate is stored with water.) The diet allows a liberal intake of fat and all the protein you want—reasons enough to question the plan. Low-carbohydrate diets are questionable for another reason: When blood sugar levels are low, the fatty acid molecules from adipose tissue are shipped to the liver where they are converted to ketone bodies to provide energy for the manufacture of glucose. Excess ketone bodies spill over into the blood and are carried to the tissues where they are oxidized. During starvation or a low-carbohydrate diet, the production of ketone bodies can exceed the body's ability to remove them metabolically. When this happens, the excess appears in the urine and the expired air. The condition is called **ketosis**, and the main danger is the lowering of the blood pH (acidosis).

Table 9.4 Vitamins and Minerals: Needs, Sources, Functions

	Vitamin	Recommended* daily allowance (men/women)	Some sources	Function
Fat soluble	A	5,000/4,000 (IU)	Liver, milk products	Resistance to infection, light adaptation
	D	200 (IU)	Sunlight, eggs, fish, milk products	Calcium absorption
	E	30/25 (IU)	Vegetable oils, greens	Cell function
	C	60 (mg)	Citrus fruits, tomatoes	Blood vessels, connective tissue, stress
Water soluble	Folacin	400 (μg)	Greens, liver	Red blood cells
	Niacin	18/13 (mg)	Peanuts, grains, greens, poultry, fish	Energy production
	Riboflavin (B$_2$)	1.6/1.2 (mg)	Milk, eggs, fish, meat, greens	Energy production
	Thiamin (B$_1$)	1.4/1.0 (mg)	Meat, grains, milk	Energy production
	B$_6$	2.2/2.0 (mg)	Grains, meat, bananas, lima beans	Energy, protein, hemoglobin
	B$_{12}$	3.0 (μg)	Liver, clams, fish	Red blood cells, energy, nervous system

(Cont.)

Table 9.4 (Continued)

Mineral	Recommended* daily allowance (men/women)	Some sources	Function
Calcium	1,000/1,200 (mg)	Milk products, green leafy vegetables	Bones, muscles, blood
Phosphorous	800 (mg)	Liver, fish, meat, beans, milk	Bones, blood, cells
Iodine	150 (μg)	Seafood, iodized salt	Thyroid hormone
Iron	10/18 (mg)	Liver, meat, beans, dried fruit	Oxygen binding in blood and muscle
Magnesium	350/300 (mg)	Grains, nuts, beans, green leafy vegetables	Enzymes and energy production
Zinc	15 (mg)	Shellfish, grains, meat	Healing growth, blood cell production

Note. Adapted from *Recommended daily allowances* (8th ed.) by the Food and Nutrition Board, 1984, Washington, DC: National Academy of Sciences, National Research Council.

*Designed to maintain good nutrition in healthy people. Covers variations among most normal individuals under usual environmental stresses.

Simple sugar *should* be avoided. But complex carbohydrates (potatoes, whole-grain products, corn, rice, and beans) provide energy and nutrition; they are excellent sources of vitamins and minerals and are usually high in fiber as well. In areas of the world where the dietary energy is largely derived from complex carbohydrates, atherosclerosis and heart disease are *virtually nonexistent*!

Low-Protein Diets. Any diet that restricts intake below the recommended dietary allowance is idiotic. Followed during adolescence, such a plan could stunt normal development. It is certain to cause muscle loss at any age, thus making future caloric expenditure more difficult and leading to increased fat and weight.

High-Protein Diets. You don't need excessive protein; the excess is stored as fat. Because dietary protein often is accompanied by fat, as in meat, you are likely to take in *more* calories on a high-protein diet. (Fat has 9.3 cal/g; carbohydrate has 4.1.) Don't be misled into eating more protein than you actually need.

Reduced-Fat Diets

Very Low–Fat Diet. Reducing fat in the diet makes sense, up to a point. Fat is high in calories and has been related to heart disease, which are good reasons for reducing the proportion of fat in your diet. However, some fat is required for good nutrition, especially during early childhood. Essential fatty acids must be included in the diet, partly because fat-soluble vitamins are not absorbed unless fat is present. Also, fats improve the flavor of food and make it more filling. I would never suggest complete removal of fat from the diet, but I do suggest that you begin now to lower the percentage of your daily calories obtained from fat; 40% is common in this country. I also suggest that you begin to reduce your intake of saturated fats by replacing butter with vegetable-oil margarine, whole milk with skimmed milk, and fat meat with lean meat (including fish and fowl). How far should you go to reduce the fat content of your diet? To date, no one is able to say for sure.

The program recommended by the late Nathan Pritikin, a nutritionist, calls for the following daily energy intake (percentage of total calories):

80% carbohydrate (mostly complex)
10% fat
10% protein

Although the research community awaits solid proof of this dietary regime, researchers at the California-based Longevity Research Institute (Leonard et al., 1974) reported dramatic results among patients with heart and circulatory disorders and diabetes who followed this diet; the study showed that the diet is a surefire way to reduce triglycerides and cholesterol. And when it is joined with an exercise program, as it is at the Institute, the diet may slow or even arrest the progress of atherosclerosis (Leonard et al., 1974).

The very low-fat diet has several advantages in addition to its effect on blood lipids and heart disease. Complex carbohydrates are high in fiber, and low-fiber diets are related to cancer of the colon. Plus, the high-carbohydrate diet is an excellent energy diet. (Remember glycogen supercompensation?) When combined with a sensible exercise program, a diet high in carbohydrate will not lead to the accumulation of fat. In fact, because the carbohydrate has only 4 cal/g, you can eat plenty. Finally, because fat seems to inhibit the action of insulin and this diet reduces the level of fat in the blood, the low-fat diet could reduce the severity of diabetes or the reliance on insulin.

But is there enough protein in the very low-fat diet recommended by Pritikin? There may not be enough for normal activity. Let's assume that your weight is 70 kg and your daily caloric intake averages 2,000 cal. If 10% of that energy comes from protein, you will take in 200 cal from protein. Protein averages 4.3 cal/g, so $200 \div 4.3 = 47$ g of protein. This falls below the daily allowance for protein recommended by the National Research Council (0.8 g/kg × 70 kg = 56 g). For this reason I do not recommend this diet plan. Instead I recommend that you get 15% of your calories from good quality protein, including meat and plant sources.

How much fat does the Pritikin diet allow? Ten percent of 2,000 cal is 200; $200 \div 9.3$ cal/g = 22 g of fat, a very small amount. In our culture, this is a difficult diet indeed. Some spill that much food between plate and mouth! The author of the plan has found the need to retrain the palates of his subjects; the drastic reduction of fat makes food seem bland (Pritikin, 1979). And anyone who attempts to apply the diet in a restaurant encounters frustration on every page of the menu.

Recommendation. You do not have to change your eating habits overnight, and you don't have to reduce fat to 10%, but 25% is an attainable goal. Begin now to reduce the fat content of your diet. If the 10% fat diet checks out in research studies and becomes the thing to do, the food industry will respond with alternatives (lean meats, low-calorie dressings, and fake fat). In the meantime, try to make some of the substitutions I mentioned. Begin to experiment with complex carbohydrates; use beans and corn in a Mexican dinner or rice and soy for an Oriental experience. Use potatoes (without butter and sour cream), and make or buy whole grain breads. The proper combination of these low-fat foods provides for energy, protein needs, and other nutrients. Avoid empty calories like table sugar; substitute a carrot, celery, or fruit for your usual snacks. You can easily reduce fat intake to 25% as we await the final word concerning the relationship of dietary fat to health and disease. I'll say more on the health benefits of diet in chapter 10.

Does lowering the fat in the diet work? Several years ago, when I cut back on dietary fat in an effort to reduce my cholesterol level, I lost a pound a week for 6 weeks—even though I wasn't trying to lose weight! I substituted cereals and fruit for snacks, ate a lot, and still lost weight (yes, the cholesterol came down as well).

> **Switch to the High-Performance Diet, which includes the following.**
> **Carbohydrate—60% of calories**
> **Fat—25%**
> **Protein—15%**

Read labels. To lower the amount of fat in your diet, begin by reading the labels on everything you eat. Of course ice cream and potato chips are loaded with fat, but so are peanuts and many snack crackers. If your goal is 25% of calories from fat and your daily intake is 2,000 cal, you can eat 500 cal or about 54 g of fat (500 ÷ 9.3 cal/g = 54). If you want to snack, choose pretzels with 1 g of fat per serving instead of chips with 11 g per serving. And watch out for coconut and palm oils—the tropical oils—and any oil that is hydrogenated. Read labels, you'll see what I mean.

A Diet Program

This program emphasizes the maintenance of a normal diet, including adequate energy intake; appropriate amounts of carbohydrate (60%), fat (25%), and protein (15%); and adequate levels of vitamins, minerals, and water. (I'll say more about water in chapter 14.)

Assessing Caloric Intake. Take a good look at your caloric intake list. If patterns of behavior are not readily apparent, you should continue to count your calories for several days. In addition to what you eat, consider when, where, and why you eat (see Table 9.5). Do you have a doughnut at coffee break just because it's there? Do you have a candy bar at lunch? Do you have a drink now and then? You may be able to eliminate several hundred calories daily by eliminating unnecessary or ritual eating behaviors. Somehow, I developed the habit of eating peanut butter and jelly crackers after I finished work as a reward for the night's effort. When I realized how quickly the calories added up and what was happening to my weight and waistline, I vowed to break the ritual. Sure, I still get the urge and sometimes I am unable to resist, but for the present (one is never cured) I reward myself with a nutritious but low-calorie treat such as an apple or orange. In this way, I've reduced my daily caloric intake by some 200 to 300 cal.

Modifying Meals. Now that you've eliminated the extras, look at the size and content of your meals. Some of you think that dieting means avoiding meals, usually breakfast. That is the worst thing you can do for several reasons. People

Table 9.5 Daily Eating Log

Weight _____ Date _____

Time	Place (if at home, exactly where were you?)	What did you eat or drink and how much?	What were you doing before you ate?	What did you do while you ate?	Who were you with when you ate?	What did you do after you ate?

Note. From Arkava (personal communication, 1977).

work better when they eat breakfast; when you avoid meals, you become weak and hungry. Those susceptible to low blood sugar may even notice poor performance in skill sports or work. Eventually, you sit down to a meal and overeat. Also, when you eat less than three meals a day, the triglyceride and cholesterol levels are higher than when you eat more frequently. By eating more frequent meals, you avoid the feelings of hunger and fatigue often associated with diet, and you reduce blood lipid levels.

The easiest way to reduce mealtime calories is to reduce the size and number of helpings you consume. Use a smaller plate and fill it only once. Refuse second helpings, except for salad or vegetables. And, of course, eliminate high-calorie desserts, toppings, dressings, gravies, and sauces (see Table 9.6 for a six-meal plan). Eat all you want of fruits, low-fat cereals, whole grain breads (without butter), vegtables, and water.

Table 9.6 Low-Calorie Six-Meal Plan (1,300 cal)

Meal	Menu
Breakfast	Egg or cheese Slice whole grain bread Coffee or tea
Midmorning	Fresh or dried fruit Milk (low fat)
Lunch	Meat, fish, or peanut butter sandwich Milk, fruit, or vegetable juice
Midafternoon	Soup and salad
Dinner	Meat, fish, poultry, or cheese Potato, rice, beans, corn, or whole grain cereal product Vegetables, including leafy green Coffee or tea
Bedtime	Fruit and low-fat yogurt

Substituting. The final step in this simple plan is to make substitutions. Substitute low-calorie snacks for high (e.g., pretzels for potato chips or peanuts) and substitute low-fat foods (e.g., skim milk, low-fat meats, no-fat salad dressing, and low-fat cheese) for similar high-fat products. Once you begin to read labels you will be on your way to a low-fat diet. Try to stay below 50 g of fat daily. If labels don't tell how much fat is in the food, the list of ingredients will help. They are listed in order of concentration, from highest to lowest; when fat comes early in the list, you are looking at a high-fat food. And remember to avoid palm, and coconut oils, which are found in many snack foods, coffee creamers, and other processed products.

Using this plan, many of you easily can achieve a caloric deficit of 500 to 1,000 cal daily. Because you will eat at least three meals a day, you won't feel weak and hungry. And when you combine the benefits of diet with those of exercise and fitness, you are bound to be happy with the results.

Exercise and Diet Combined

When you combine exercise and diet, you can eat more and still achieve a 1,000 cal deficit per day (2 lb per week weight loss). Exercise tones muscles (improving your appearance as you lose weight), conserves protein, and increases the removal of fat. The combination of exercise and sensible caloric intake should be a way of life. Let's see how diet and exercise can be combined in a program of weight loss and weight control (see Table 9.7 and the scenario after it).

Table 9.7 Sample Weight Loss Program

20 lb × 3,500 cal/lb = 70,000 cal overweight		Cal	Total cal
Weeks 1 & 2	Exercise = 200 cal/day × 7 days = Diet = 500 cal/day × 14 days =	1,400 7,000 8,400	8,400
Weeks 3 & 4	Exercise = 250 cal/day × 14 days = Diet = 500 cal/day × 14 days =	3,500 7,000 10,500	18,900
Weeks 5 & 6	Exercise = 300 cal/day × 14 days = Diet = 500 cal/day × 14 days =	4,200 7,000 11,200	30,100
Weeks 7 & 8	Exercise = 350 cal/day × 14 days = Diet = 500 cal/day × 14 days =	4,900 7,000 11,900	42,000
Weeks 9 & 10	Exercise = 400 cal/day × 14 days = Diet = 500 cal/day × 14 days =	5,600 7,000 12,600	54,600
Weeks 11 & 12	Exercise = 450 cal/day × 14 days = Diet = 500 cal/day × 14 days =	6,300 7,000 13,300	67,900

After 12 weeks = 67,900 cal lost.

Weeks 13 & 14—forget the diet. Exercise just 150 cal/day (14 days × 150 cal = 2,100 cal).

67,900 + 2,100 = 70,000 cal or 20 lb.

An analysis of body composition and fitness indicates that John is 20 lb overweight and in the poor fitness category. He achieves energy balance when his caloric intake equals his typical daily expenditure, 2,500 cal. How should he proceed? John should reduce his caloric intake by 500 cal per day and begin exercising.

Once that he has achieved his goal, John has several choices. He can

1. continue his exercise habits and eat as he chooses,
2. become sedentary again and restrict caloric intake for life,
3. return to former exercise and diet habits and begin to regain the weight he has lost, or
4. continue both the active lifestyle and the low-fat diet.

If he chooses to remain active (400 cal of exercise daily), he will be able to eat the things he enjoys and to splurge occasionally on high-fat foods. He should still consider a reduction of fat in the diet, but with sufficient exercise (e.g., running 4 to 5 mi daily) he may be able to eat whatever he wishes with no adverse effect on his health *or* his weight. However, only a cholesterol test will confirm that possibility (see chapters 11 and 12).

Behavior Therapy and Diet

If you follow the instructions in the previous sections and achieve a negative energy balance (caloric deficit), you will lose weight. With a deficit of 1,000 cal daily, you will lose 2 lb per week. However, if you are a difficult case and need additional help, this section is for you. Even if you have your weight completely under control, you may learn a lot about yourself and your eating behavior by reading this section. Behavior therapy (sometimes called behavior modification) is the third and last major weapon in the battle of the bulge. (To read about the use of drugs and surgery for weight control, see chapter 10.)

The essentials of behavior therapy are threefold.

1. Identify the behavior you wish to modify, in this case eating behavior. Keep a food diary that indicates the kind and amount of food you eat; record when, where, why, and with whom you eat, what you do while eating, your mood, and your degree of hunger (see Tables 9.5 and 9.8).

2. Analyze your customary eating behavior and plan new eating behaviors (see the section on diet in this chapter). The new behaviors will include caloric restriction, exercise, and dietary substitutions. To reduce cues or reinforcement for the old eating behavior, try the following aids.

- Eat in one room only (dining room or kitchen).
- Wrap your utensils in a napkin, and wait several minutes before you begin.

Table 9.8 Daily Eating Log—Cognitive Supplement to be Used in Conjunction With Daily Eating Log

Date _____

Instructions: For each instance of eating or drinking recorded on your daily eating log, write down your thoughts and feelings prior to eating—that is, what were you thinking of before you ate, while you ate, and afterward. Indicate your mood and degree of hunger.

Time	What were your thoughts or feelings before you ate?	While you ate?	After you ate?

Note. From Arkava (personal communication, 1977).

- Pause between bites, and set your utensils down between bites. Don't prepare another bite until you've swallowed the last one.
- Wait 30 min before having dessert or have a low-calorie beverage (tea or coffee) instead of dessert.
- Concentrate on what you are eating; take time and enjoy each bite. Save one item to eat later on.
- Purchase a new place setting and eat only from that setting; use a smaller plate.
- After the meal, remove all dishes to the kitchen, then brush your teeth—the meal is over.

When you feel hungry, try to decide if it is real (stomach hunger) or merely boredom (mouth hunger). Avoid eating in front of the TV set or while reading. If you must snack be sure the snack is nutritious and low in fat and calories.

3. Plan new reinforcements or rewards to reinforce the new eating behavior. Develop a schedule of reinforcement (see Table 9.9), a plan of frequent rewards for good behavior. Because the new eating behavior will soon show up on the scale or the tape measure, you can use small units of weight loss and small reductions in girth as indicators of adherence to the new eating behavior. Almost any sort of reward is effective (except food)! A tangible, universally accepted reward such as money seems to work for most. Weigh yourself daily, in the morning after your toilet but before breakfast, and provide a monetary reward for each unit of weight lost. A similar plan to reward reduced girth (waist, thigh) provides added incentive. Spend the reward im-

mediately if you wish, or save it for something you really want but might otherwise refuse to buy. If the plan seems silly, remember this: You will spend far more on food and medical bills if you do not lose the weight.

Table 9.9 Weight Loss Reinforcement Schedule

Date	Weight	Reward	Girth	Reward	Total[a]

Note. For example, $1 per lb; $1 per 1/2 in. of waist girth.

[a]Start new total when you spend the reward.

Behavior Therapy and Exercise

The same general principles apply to those who are having trouble starting an exercise program. Plan the new exercise behavior (active lifestyle) and reward yourself each time you jog, play tennis, or walk instead of ride (see Tables 9.10 and 9.11). You may choose a monetary reward or, if you like, a low-calorie favor. I enjoy a tall drink after a long run. It serves as a reward for my good behavior, and any calories consumed fall far short of those expended in the activity.

Weight Gain

This section is intended to help underweight individuals achieve sensible nonfat weight gain. It is not meant to provide support for the practice of bulking up for sports like football. When normal-weight individuals bulk up they assume a health risk that cannot be ignored. Coaches who encourage such procedures should be responsible for conducting weight loss programs when the sport season or career is over.

Table 9.10 Daily Activity Log

Date _____

Time	Place	Exercise	Intensity	Duration	What were you doing and thinking before exercise?	What were your thoughts during exercise?	What were you doing and thinking after exercise?

Note. Include all forms of physical activity, including work, walking, and household chores.

Score	Intensity	Score	Duration
5	Sustained heavy breathing and perspiration	4	Over 30 min
4	Intermittent heavy breathing and perspiration—as in tennis	3	20 to 30 min
3	Moderately heavy—as in recreational sports and cycling	2	10 to 20 min
2	Moderate—as in volleyball, softball	1	Under 10 min
1	Light—as in fishing, walking		

Table 9.11 Activity Reinforcement Schedule

Date	Activity	Distance of time	Reward[a]	Total
		——		——
		——		——
		——		——
Total for month		——		——

Note. Daily reward—for meeting activity goal (e.g., 2 mi); weekly reward—for meeting activity goal (e.g., 12 mi); monthly reward—for meeting activity goal (e.g., 50 mi; improved fitness score). Adjust goals as fitness improves.

[a]Rewards: daily—a small monetary award (e.g., 25 cents) or a cool drink; weekly—a larger monetary reward (e.g., $1) or a special favor (e.g., movie); monthly—a substantial monetary reward (e.g., $5) or a very special favor (e.g., concert, dinner out). Rewards can be saved for a special purpose (e.g, new warm-up outfit, tennis racket).

As with weight loss, the weight gain program includes exercise, diet, and behavior therapy.

Exercise: Include a strength-training program to build lean body weight and *reduce* calorie-burning activities (e.g., aerobic exercise and sports) to allow a positive caloric balance.

Diet: Include an overall increase in calories, with an extra 750 calories on strength training days and 250 extra on nontraining days. The extra calories should be largely from low-fat, protein-rich foods (e.g., lean meats, low-fat dairy products). A low-fat protein supplement can be used to provide an extra 20 g of protein daily.

Behavior Therapy: Develop a reinforcement schedule to reward gains. Determine a desirable weight and make steady progress toward that goal.

This program should lead to an extra pound of weight each week. If you attempt to gain weight too fast, much of the gain will be fat. So determine current eating behavior and plan needed modifications (such as more meals and nutritious snacks). Start strength training and watch the scale go up. And remember, return to aerobic exercise and weight control when you achieve the desired body weight.

CHAPTER
10

WEIGHT CONTROL:
FALLACIES AND FACTS

This chapter will debunk fallacies and present facts concerning

appetite and hunger,

dehydration and weight loss,

spot reduction,

changing muscle to fat,

drugs, surgery, and weight loss,

eating disorders,

weight control devices,

health clubs and diet centers,

fitness from food,

diet and health, and

exercise and weight loss.

Popular Misconceptions

Although the entire fitness and health field has its share of quacks and is loaded with fallacies, no area has more misconceptions than the area of weight control. Let's replace some of these fallacies with facts.

Appetite Means Hunger

Never assume that the desire for food signifies a real need for nourishment. Appetite is a psychological desire for food that is influenced by several factors.

The control center for food intake, the **appestat**, is located in the hypothalamus of the brain and functions like a thermostat that turns on eating behavior and then turns it off when the desire or hunger has been satisfied. Unfortunately, it takes many minutes for the food you eat to reach the bloodstream, where the appestat can see you've satisfied the need. It is possible to tuck away several hundred extra calories before the appestat says STOP.

Physiological factors like low blood sugar, cold temperatures, hunger pangs from an empty stomach, and unfilled fat cells stimulate the appestat. Exercise can stimulate eating behavior also, but the increase serves only to maintain body weight. Sedentary individuals take in more calories than they need. More exercise means more food intake, but the appetite doesn't keep pace with energy output. Regular activity seems to help the appestat adjust caloric intake to energy needs. The appestat is rather imprecise at a low level of energy expenditure, but for regularly active individuals, appetite control is much more related to energy needs. And at the high end of the activity scale, where endurance athletes burn 4,000 to 6,000 cal daily in running, cycling, and cross-country skiing, the appetite usually underestimates energy needs.

Psychological factors such as the smell, sight, or taste of food can evoke the desire to eat. Habit and emotional factors condition eating behavior. We eat to celebrate, to prolong feelings of excitement. Appetite is a complex phenomenon, subject to many influences and reflecting more than nutritional needs.

The appestat frequently overestimates energy and nutritional needs. Weight control becomes possible when you realize that your eyes are bigger than your stomach, and your potential for energy intake is usually greater than your regular energy expenditure. For example, Table 10.1 shows the amount of running (at about 120 cal/mi) needed to burn off the calories consumed in some common snacks.

Table 10.1 Effort Required to Burn Off Calories

Snack	Running
Highball	1-1/3 mi
Beer (12 ounces)	1-1/2 mi
Potato chips (15)	1-1/2 mi
Peanuts (handful)	2 mi
Peanut butter and jelly (1 tablespoon of each on crackers)	2-1/2 mi

Lose Weight by Losing Water

Water constitutes 55 to 60% of the adult body weight. Thirst, activated by excess sodium or water loss, serves to maintain body fluid levels. Several hormones assist in the maintenance of fluid and electrolyte (sodium, potassium, calcium, and chloride) levels. The kidneys take care of excess fluid intake; in short, the body knows how much water it needs. You should not attempt to take control of the mechanism as a means of weight loss.

Sure, each liter of body fluid weighs about 2 lb and dehydration can lead to impressive weight loss, but the loss is water, not fat! You need the water, and your body will get it back if it can. Water and electrolyte loss from cells affects coordination and strength, and water lost from the blood reduces endurance. So if you lose 4 lb during a vigorous workout in the heat, drink it back (2 quarts). You need it.

Exercise in rubber suits, steam rooms, and saunas should be avoided. The sweat mechanism is a safety valve for heat dissipation. Sweat must be allowed to evaporate, for only when it evaporates is heat taken from the body. Without evaporation you risk serious heat disorders (see chapter 14).

Dehydration weight loss has been attacked by every responsible authority and organization, yet it is still practiced by wrestlers and boxers. Their coaches think it is safe so long as the athlete is able to restore fluids before competition. However, because thirst underestimates water loss, the athlete may be competing with less than normal strength and endurance and flirting with more dangerous consequences.

Dehydration eliminates water, not fat, and the weight loss is temporary. It carries no health or cosmetic benefit and makes you feel and look tired. Don't do it.

Lose Inches, Not Pounds

"Lose inches, not pounds" is the come-on of figure salons that try to appeal to those who don't want to exercise to achieve real fat loss. Of course it is possible to improve one's appearance with exercises that tone muscles and improve posture. But while you are shaping the body you are ignoring the engine and other important parts and missing out on the health benefits associated with body weight and fat loss. Often the inches are not lost at all; a slightly tighter pull on the measuring tape as weeks progress gives the impression of progress. Just remember that fitness and health, like beauty, are more than skin deep.

Spot Reducing

Little evidence shows that fat can be removed from specific areas of the body by localized exercises. Avid tennis players have about the same skinfold measures on both arms. Research studies show little effect of localized exercise, unless there is a significant weight loss due to diet and exercise. One study showed a mere 1 mm of spot reduction after 6 weeks of localized exercise. And my bothersome tummy roll doesn't respond to sit-ups and other abdominal exercises—it only goes away when I lose enough weight.

Each of us has a genetically determined pattern of fat deposition. I gain first around the waist, and that is the very last to go. Why don't sit-ups help? The fat in any region is, in terms of the circulation, quite distant from the adjacent muscles. The fat enters the circulation through capillaries located in the fat depot, then travels through the veins to the heart where the fat can then be pumped to the muscles. The muscles don't really care where the energy comes from. The sympathetic nervous system and its fat mobilizing hormone—epinephrine— have a generalized effect, so when the call goes out for fat, it may come from any of the fat storage deposits. Frank Katch and his colleagues at the University of Massachusetts collected fat biopsies from several fat deposits before and after a 4-week training program consisting entirely of sit-ups. Posttraining analysis of fat cells revealed that the fat loss came from all of the fat storage areas measured, not just the abdomen (Katch & McCardle, 1983).

So don't be misled by promises of spot reduction. The best advice is to forget the spots and the inches and attend to a sound program. Burn off sufficient calories, and the spots and inches will take care of themselves.

Change Fat to Muscle

Does muscle turn to fat, or vice versa? Consider your own abdominal muscles and their overlying layer of subcutaneous fat. Your fingers will tell you that one is separate from the other. Ah yes, you say, but what of the fat within choice cuts of beef? Good point. Some fat is found adjacent to animal or human muscle. But each tissue is so completely different that change from one to the other is highly unlikely.

Adipose tissue is composed of spherical fat cells, which are uniquely designed for fat storage. Long thin muscle fibers are even more specialized, consisting of contractile proteins (actin and myosin) that slide back and forth to produce movement. When muscles are no longer used as much as before, they begin to atrophy (get smaller), and some contractile protein is lost. If you eat too much, some fat will be deposited adjacent to the muscles, but the muscles don't *change* to fat. They just lie dormant, waiting for you to return to an active lifestyle.

While on the subject of fat I want to comment on **cellulite**, that special form of fat supposedly laced with wastes and water. A once-popular book would have you believe that this "orange peel" fat requires special techniques for its removal (the term *cellulite* doesn't appear in the scientific literature on fat). Occasionally you may still see advertisements that describe what must be done to remove this "special" fat. But remember, fat is fat, and chapter 9 tells you how to remove it.

Take Drugs to Lose Weight

Laxatives and diuretics remove only water (thus causing dehydration). So-called weight control specialists prescribe amphetamines to suppress the appetite, in spite of the fact that no conclusive evidence of the long-term effectiveness of such methods exists. Amphetamines stimulate the nervous system and, when taken indiscriminately, lead to dependency. Many continue to use them because of the "high" induced by the drug. Users may not lose weight, but they find a way to avoid confronting overweight and other problems they face.

When users complain that they can't sleep, the doctor may prescribe barbiturates, leading to a roller-coaster drug problem. Reputable physicians do prescribe anorectic agents (appetite suppressants), but only as part of a total program including diet, exercise, and behavior therapy.

Surgery Is a Good Way to Lose Weight

Lipectomy and liposuction are sometimes used to remove fat. Lipectomy involves surgical removal of adipose tissue, and although it certainly removes fat and reduces weight, animal studies suggest that the fat may be regenerated. Liposuction is often used in cosmetic surgery to remove subcutaneous fat deposits. A tube is inserted in an incision and fat is literally vacuumed out of the body. Although this method works, it carries the risk of regeneration and sometimes leads to complications, even death. No surgery is without risk, and no proof exists that surgical removal of superficial fat will change heart disease or other health risks.

Some forms of surgery are used only for the treatment of morbid obesity (over 100 lb above desirable weight). One operation involves bypass of a portion of the small intestine, thereby reducing the absorptive surface area. A less complicated approach literally staples part of the stomach to form a smaller pouch. Surgery is only undertaken when other treatments fail, and in view of the complications commonly associated with operations, I hope you heed my earlier advice and never come close to morbid obesity.

Eating Disorders

Excessive attention to a trim youthful figure has led to the use of dangerous eating behaviors in an effort to become slim. When being thin becomes an obsession, when self-worth is associated with slimness, the stage is set for eating disorders. **Bulimia** is a disorder characterized by a binge-purge cycle. Mild cases purge (vomit) occasionally to avoid weight gain, whereas others may binge and purge regularly. More serious cases combine bingeing and purging with laxatives or diuretics. Serious metabolic and psychological problems can accompany severe cases.

Anorexia nervosa is a serious psychological problem characterized by a distorted body image and a refusal to eat. Sometimes the behavior is associated with the use of drugs and with excessive exercise. If not treated, the individual may experience medical complications or may even die. These disorders are more common among women who seek to please others, who try to be perfect. Fortunately, psychological therapy and medical treatments are available to help victims of eating disorders.

Facts on Fads

Hardly a year goes by without the appearance of a device that is said to remove unsightly fat. In years past, massage, pounding, and vibrating have been promoted for spot reduction and fat removal.

Weight- or Fat-Control Devices

Massage and pounding by human hands or wooden rollers does not break up fat and allow it to be removed from the body. Vibrating belts do not create sufficient heat to burn off fat from hips or thighs. Fat is burned when it is mobilized from adipose tissue, transported to *active* muscle, and used as a source of energy. You wouldn't want extra fat floating around in your circulation unless you planned to burn it off in vigorous exercise. If it were you could suffer blood clots leading to a stroke or heart attack! In spite of the humorous examples from the past, we seem destined to face a never-ending array of fat-loss devices.

Sauna belts, shorts, and body wraps are said to remove fat from the area encased by massage, heat, and who knows what else. Do they really "massage away fatty tissue with the slightest movement of your body"? Of course not; they may temporarily *compress* the tissue and lead you to believe that fat has disappeared, but it will return.

Exercise Devices

Numerous exercise devices are on the market. Most ads carefully avoid statements that are *completely* false, yet they give the impression that the device will lead to significant weight loss. The fact is, the energy cost for most devices averages less than 5 cal per minute. So for caloric expenditure and weight control, exercise devices are far less effective than moderate activities such as walking, jogging, cycling, and swimming.

I call one group the "exer-this and exer-thats," the cylinders with adjustable ropes that provide a variable resistance. With 5 min of "almost effortless" exercise a day, makers of such devices say you can get a firm, healthy, athletic body. These devices *do* provide resistance for strength or muscular endurance training, but they are much less adaptable for aerobic fitness training and can guarantee you nothing for 5 min of almost effortless exercise a day, whether it be for fitness or weight control. And if you are the 79-lb weakling one company refers to in its advertisements (made believable by the endorsement and presence of a famous pro athlete), I doubt that your genetic endowment ever will allow the "splendid physique" promised. Most of these devices end up on a dusty shelf in the basement or garage.

Recently, electrical stimulators have been advertised as an alternative to active exercise. Forty-five minutes of these electrical twitches are said to be equal to 900 sit-ups or 12 mi of running! What is even more preposterous is the comment of one user who says he doesn't have time to exercise, so he uses the stimulator—for 45 min! That many minutes of real exercise would do him some good. Be advised that medical authorities are concerned about the effects of electrical currents on the normal action of the heart, and use your time for real exercise.

A more recent device to come on the exercise market is the passive exercise device. With these wondrous machines you simply lie back while the device moves your body parts. For just a few dollars a day you can move without effort. Do they work? What do you think? What is so surprising is the number of people who believe the advertising and pay hard-earned dollars to avoid the one thing they really need—calorie-burning activity.

Many other devices are on the market, and more appear daily. The advertising claims are aimed at gullible and ill-informed consumers. Several government agencies monitor advertising claims as well as the safety and effectiveness of the devices, but because that takes time, a device can be on the market for months or even years before the manufacturer is forced to correct the advertising, improve the product, or remove it from the marketplace.

Advice on Devices

With so many quacks and charlatans operating in the area of fitness and weight control, how can the layperson separate fact from fraud? Here are some characteristics of fraudulent advertising. The sales pitch often promotes a product that has yet to receive widespread acceptance. The product is often touted as a cure-all, for overweight, back problems, constipation, a small bust, or a bad complexion. Testimonials are used instead of controlled experimental results as evidence of product value (a testimonial is merely an opinion, even when it is expressed by a celebrity or pro athlete who has probably never used the device).

The offer usually involves a special gift for fast action. (Fast action is encouraged because the manufacturers know they'll be forced to revise their advertising at any moment.) The location of the advertisement is another tip-off. Reputable companies don't have to resort to the back pages of cheap magazines; they are in business to stay, and their products are listed in reputable sources. Finally, consider the claims themselves. Is it likely that one device can do everything—muscular and aerobic fitness and weight control? Do manufacturers promise quick results? Compare their claims with my prescriptions. If they promise too much for too little, don't buy. The best advice I can give you is to use the money for something that is sure to please: a tennis racket, cross-country skis, or a 10-speed bicycle. In any event, if it sounds too good to be true, it probably is: *Let the buyer beware.*

Health Clubs

In recent years, health clubs and figure salons have experienced steady growth, much of which can be attributed to a new professionalism in the field. Clubs that offer sound programs and get results are likely to keep their customers. Gone, for the most part, are the fast-buck outfits that lured customers with outlandish claims and long-term contracts. Today, more health clubs are being run for long-term results instead of short-term profits.

A persistent problem in the health club industry is the absence of required professional standards for health club personnel. You can still open, direct, or work in a health club without any formal preparation. Although most states have stringent standards for barbers and hair dressers, few have any standards whatsoever for health club personnel. But things are changing; the American College of Sports Medicine (ACSM) has established professional standards for program directors and fitness instructors. As health club personnel move to meet these standards and as states establish and enforce certification requirements, the health club industry will achieve greater respectability.

How can you differentiate between a good health club and a bad one, between an effective program and a sham, or between a qualified staff and a nonprofessional one? One way is to visit the club for a free introductory session. Talk to the patrons; are they on sensible programs? Are they satisfied with their treatment and their progress? Ask the program director about his or her background and that of the staff. Ask for evidence of formal professional preparation; do employees have academic preparation and ACSM certification? Find out if the club is a social club or a serious business that is dedicated to your fitness and health. Does it require evidence of a recent medical examination? Does it have emergency equipment, and does the staff know how to use it? Finally, does the staff seem overly interested in selling long-term contracts? Refuse to be talked into such an agreement until you are absolutely certain that you are able and willing to continue. A good club will want your business and will do all it can to earn your continued patronage.

Diet Centers

Another recent development is the growth in the number of so-called diet centers, which promise significant weight loss without the bother of exercise. Be careful; such centers provide dieting advice and encouragement, but some also sell special vitamins, salad oils, and other products to patrons. Many of their clients *do* lose weight, but often the loss is rapid, indicating significant water and protein loss.

Few laws govern the conduct of these centers. No professional competence or qualifications are required. Anyone can open and operate a diet center. The centers sometimes advise *against* exercise, as well they should, because anyone following their program may be too weak to enjoy vigorous activity. Because vitamin sales bring in money, some centers advocate excess vitamin use. If you want to use the services of a diet center, follow the advice I gave regarding health and fitness clubs. Ask about the academic preparation and qualifications of the staff. Is a registered dietician a regular employee? Is a reputable local physician associated with the center? Does the center provide any service you can't do for yourself?

Although many diet centers provide a useful service, the existence of so many centers suggests that the facts of energy balance and weight control have reached few people and that many individuals lack the information or the will power to take control of their eating and exercise behaviors.

Food and Fitness

Large food companies spend millions annually to convince us that fitness and health can be achieved by eating their products. Although sound nutrition is absolutely essential for health and fitness, nothing you eat will improve your fitness if you already are on an adequate diet. The only way to achieve fitness is via exercise; unfortunately, you can't get there just by eating.

"Lite" Foods

Interest in weight control has led to the development of so-called "lite" foods and beverages. The products are usually low-calorie versions of the original, such as light beer, light or no-calorie soft drinks, light crackers, light meals, and so forth. Although eating these products will not make you lose weight, they can help you consume fewer calories. Unfortunately, it is common to see someone consume empty calories (e.g., a doughnut) and then drink a diet soda, when a better snack choice would be a piece of fruit or fruit juice. Also, the diet foods prove that people will pay more for less—less calories, less sodium, less caffeine. Sometimes these products contain undesirable substitutes such as coconut or palm oil. Use these products if you like, but don't expect them to cause weight loss, and be sure to read the label so you'll know what you are getting (or not getting) for your money.

Another version of the light meal is the diet platter at the restaurant. People select such a meal believing it is more nutritious and lower in calories. However, a salad isn't high in nutritive value, and a salad dressing could make this a high-calorie choice. One tablespoon of dressing contains 100 cal and 8 g of fat, and the ladle used to pour dressing holds far more than 1 tablespoon!

Some restaurants are beginning to label meals with a heart to indicate good choices for those who must be concerned with fat intake. Look for meals that are nutritious but low in fat. Avoid fried foods, those with cream sauces or butter, and high-calorie desserts. Ask for dressings and other sauces on the side. Request a "dry" muffin or toast. Eating out is difficult for the individual on a weight-loss or low-cholesterol diet, but things will improve as restaurant owners realize what the customer wants. We got rid of smoking in public places and airplanes, didn't we?

Health Foods

Other factors have led to the growth of a "health food" industry. The widespread use of hormones, pesticides, and other chemicals by ranchers and farmers and the use of dyes and preservatives in the preparation of food have led some to be concerned about the food they eat; these consumers see natural or organic foods as an alternative source of nutrition. To the extent that hormones, pesticides, dyes, and preservatives may be harmful to health, especially over extended periods, natural food sources should be safer and, therefore, more desirable. However, the *nutritional* value of any food or vitamin is unrelated to the manner of growth. Foods grown with chemical fertilizers are just as nutritious as those grown with organic fertilizers. Experts from the National Academy of Sciences, the American Medical Association, and the Food and Drug Administration agree:

> The body doesn't care if a vitamin is natural or synthesized in the laboratory—a vitamin is a vitamin.

What *does* matter is the active amount of the essential ingredients and the percentage of their recommended daily allowance. So purchase expensive health foods if you are concerned about the effect of additives on your health, but don't expect to get super nutrition for your money.

High-Performance Diet

Earlier we talked about a low-fat diet and how it could reduce the risk of heart disease and cancer. Another advantage to reducing fat calories is that you replace the energy with carbohydrate calories, which improve performance in many fitness activities. The high-performance diet calls for

- 25% of calories from fat,
- 15% from protein, and
- 60% from carbohydrate.

When eaten in conjunction with regular exercise, the diet insures storage of carbohydrate in muscle and provides the energy you need for the active lifestyle. When the carbohydrate comes from potatoes, corn, beans, rice, and whole grain products, along with fresh fruit, you achieve nutrition, fiber, energy, and good health.

Carbohydrate Loading

For extended periods of exercise such as long runs, all-day downhill or cross-country skiing, bicycle tours, distance swims, and so forth, you need additional muscle glycogen. This is achieved by first depleting the muscle glycogen via the exercise you are preparing for and then eating a high-carbohydrate diet to increase storage above the usual 15 to 20 g per kilogram of muscle. This procedure isn't necessary for events that last less than an hour; typical glycogen levels will meet the need for energy. For longer events, deplete glycogen stores with a long effort 4 days before the date, then go on a high-carbohydrate diet, add even extra carbohydrates, and drink lots of water, because glycogen is stored with water (hence the term carbo*hydrate*). On the morning of the event eat a mixed breakfast to insure fat utilization and glycogen conservation in the early minutes of the activity.

Never attempt several days of vigorous effort without adequate carbohydrate replacement. Don't do what Mimi did on her skiing vacation in Sun Valley. In a mistaken effort to lose weight, this expert skier avoided carbohydrates in the early days of her vacation and saw her skiing deteriorate dangerously. After several days she was losing control after only two runs; at $30 a day for a lift ticket that was quite a mistake! Potatoes and bread restored her form and saved the last days of her vacation. So always plan for carbohydrate replacement and make a special effort at altitudes where glycogen depletion occurs more rapidly.

Diet and Health

It is clear that diet is a necessary part of weight control and the active lifestyle. But is diet related to health for other reasons? Diet has been implicated as a major factor in obesity, heart disease, cancer, and diabetes; in digestive problems such as diverticulitis, irritable colon, and gallstones; and in other problems such as dental caries, hernias, and hemorrhoids. Doctors prescribe a low-fat diet for those at risk for heart disease (see chapter 12), but how does diet influence cancer and other problems?

Anticancer Diet

The anticancer diet recently proposed by the National Academy of Sciences endorses these dietary practices.

- Eat less fat, fatty meats, and dairy products.
- Eat little salt-cured, pickled, or smoked foods.
- Eat more whole grain products, including fiber-rich foods.
- Eat more fruits and vegetables, including those in the cabbage family and those high in vitamins A and C.
- Drink alcohol in moderation, if at all.
- Keep caloric intake low.

Remember, fat is a factor in cancer and heart disease, and exercise is the best way to eliminate excess fat from the body.

Dietary Fiber

Fiber, roughage, bulk, and bran all refer to the portion of plants that is indigestible. Why consume an indigestible material? In addition to its long-standing reputation for maintaining regularity, fiber has other advantages. Insoluble fiber (as in wheat bran and beans) holds water, increases bulk, and increases the rate at which stool and cancerous toxins are removed. Soluble fiber (as in oat bran, apples, and citrus fruits) forms a gel that slows absorption of carbohydrate and binds cholesterol for removal from the body. Soluble fiber may also produce a chemical that slows the rate of cholesterol production.

Epidemiologic studies show that those on a low-fiber diet have a higher incidence of heart disease, cancer, and the other problems mentioned earlier. The average American consumes about one third of the 25 to 35 g of fiber recommended by the National Cancer Institute, and the majority don't eat enough fresh fruits and vegetables. If fiber isn't part of your daily regime, begin now to add bran cereals, fruits, vegetables, beans, and whole grain products to your diet. Read labels and try to seek a balance between soluble and insoluble fiber. Finally, consider this: When you combine fiber with a low-fat diet, you'll be able to eat freely with little concern for weight gain.

Facts About Exercise and Weight Loss

From earlier discussions, you know that exercise indeed helps in weight control. Let's review a few of these facts and learn a few new ones.

Exercise Does Help   Some may still think that exercise doesn't help much, that diet is still the answer. Remember, because exercise spares protein during a weight loss diet, exercise is necessary if you are to avoid the loss of muscle tissue. Why is that important? Because fat is burned only by muscle, thus your metabolic rate and energy expenditure depend on the amount of your lean tissue. Lose lean tissue and you will have to diet, probably for the rest of your life. It is far better to include exercise and a moderate diet than to spend your days on a severe low-calorie diet.

Dieting Leads to Weight Cycling   Repeated cycles of diet-induced weight loss and regain, a process called weight cycling, leads to a drop in metabolic rate, the loss of lean tissue, and increased fat and body weight. With each cycle, weight loss becomes more difficult (due to lower metabolic rate and less muscle) and regain occurs more rapidly and to a *higher* level. Hence dieting can lead to ever higher levels of fat and body weight (Brownell et al., 1986).

Timing Probably Isn't Important   I advise people to exercise when it is most convenient and enjoyable for them. However, one recent study found that morning activity burned more fat. Although that sounds good and could convince the early bird that his way is best, at least for weight control, I'm not convinced. When you wake it has been many hours since your last meal, and the fasted body tends to use fat as an energy source. So it isn't surprising that morning exercise burns more fat. However, that doesn't mean that morning activity will necessarily lead to more weight loss than afternoon or evening exercise. Exercise burns calories whenever it is done. Increased morning fat metabolism could be more effective in the lowering of blood lipids, but that has yet to be demonstrated. And until it is I'll stick to my advice and exercise when the time feels right. Morning exercise could be stressful to a night owl, and heart attacks are more frequent in the morning.

Exercise Does Affect Appetite   People fear they'll eat more if they exercise, and they probably will. Eating does lead to increased appetite, but the food intake doesn't keep pace with the energy expenditure, so you won't gain weight. Active people eat more and weigh less, whereas inactive people eat less and weigh more. Some studies show that moderate activity has little effect on appetite or food intake. And some suggest that exercise depresses the appetite. This may be true after exhaustive effort or in the early stages of training. But those of us who exercise a lot admit that one reason for the dedication to activity is that we love to eat. Regular exercise allows us to indulge our passion for food without guilt or the burden of excess weight. When the exercise is combined with the low-fat, high-carbohydrate (high-performance) diet, we are able to consume a large volume of nutritious food. I have a great appetite and hope I never lose it.

PART
IV

FITNESS AND
HEALTH

Health has been called "the first of all liberties." What we call high-level health, optimal health, or wellness implies a vitality or zest for living and is more than the absence of disease. This state provides a reserve capacity that allows the performance of extraordinary feats when necessary. With the growing awareness of psychosomatic illness, our definition of health has come to embrace psychological or emotional health as well. Thus, the healthy person is free from disease, anxiety, and depression; his or her physical condition, nutritional state, and emotional outlook enable him or her to carry out daily tasks with vigor and alertness, without undue fatigue, and with ample energy to enjoy leisure time pursuits and meet unforeseen emergencies.

Health and fitness coexist and correlate. You can be healthy without being fit, but you cannot improve your fitness without acquiring some benefit to your health. The health that most folks know is only one stage that we pass through on the way to achieving our potential. Fitness can lead to a higher level of physical and emotional health; it can enhance the quality and joy of living. By all means, exercise to improve your health, but don't stop there. Extend yourself; flirt with your potential; aim for the peak. If you only achieve the ridge, it will surely be worth the effort. (See Appendix E for more on fitness and health.)

CHAPTER

11

MEDICAL FITNESS

This chapter will help you

> *decide if and when you need a medical examination,*
>
> *understand the value of the graded exercise electrocardiogram or stress test,*
>
> *appreciate the role of physical activity in the prevention and rehabilitation of heart disease, and*
>
> *develop a program to prevent low-back problems.*

Years ago, when the medical profession was less enthusiastic about exercise, doctors tended to make involvement in a fitness program more difficult, urging a medical examination as well as an exercise stress test. But that is changing, along with the view of the annual medical examination.

Medical Examination

In recent years, health professionals have begun to take a different view of the annual medical examination. In the past, many believed that the annual exam would reduce the incidence of illness or mortality. But when researchers compared those who had annual exams with those who did not, the researchers found an equal number of chronic diseases and deaths in both groups. Nowadays, most doctors agree that for the person with no symptoms or chronic disease, the annual medical examination is a waste of time and money. How can this be so?

You've heard of individuals who have an electrocardiogram one day, receive a clean bill of health, and have a heart attack within 24 hr. Many testing and screening procedures lack the sensitivity to provide early detection of problems; the annual chest X ray seldom detects lung cancer early enough to improve the prognosis. Some tests such as the **exercise stress test**, an electrocardiogram administered during exercise on a treadmill, occasionally suggest heart disease when none actually exists. False findings of this sort not only waste time and money, they also create anxiety that only can be removed by resorting to additional testing and expense.

Does this really mean that all medical examinations are a waste of time and money? Of course not. There are many valid reasons for a medical examination. If you have symptoms or are in doubt about the condition of your health, by all means see your physician.

- If you or any member of your family has a history of hypertension and heart disease, have your blood pressure controlled and checked regularly. You can buy a stethoscope and sphygmomanometer at the drugstore; a physician or nurse will show you how to use it.
- If you have elevated blood cholesterol, have your cholesterol level checked annually or more often at a local laboratory and have a copy of the results sent to your physician.
- If your family has a history of diabetes, supplement annual blood-sugar tests with simple home screening procedures.
- If glaucoma runs in your family, see your eye doctor at regular intervals.
- If you are a woman, have a pelvic examination and a Pap smear for uterine cancer at least once a year and examine your breasts regularly to aid early diagnosis and ensure a more positive prognosis for breast cancer.

The National Conference on Preventive Medicine recommends the following schedule of medical examinations as a minimum for adequate preventive health care.

Infancy: at birth plus four more in the 1st year.

Preschool: at about age 2-1/2 and again at 5-1/2.

School age: at about age 8-1/2 and again at 15-1/2.

Young adulthood: at age 18, around 25, and another at 30 (of course, women should be checked before, at the start of, and throughout pregnancy.)

Middle age: Every 5 years between ages 35 and 65.

Later life: Every 2 years beginning at age 65.

The medical examination should include a thorough medical history. A recent innovation in this regard is a computerized medical history form (health risk or health hazard analysis). After you complete the form, the computer generates a life expectancy based on your medical history and your lifestyle. The computer even tells you how to improve your expectancy by altering habits such as smoking, eating, or inactivity (see also Appendix E).

An obvious part of the medical examination is the physical examination, including measures of height, weight, body fat, blood pressure, and other tests suggested by the patient's age and medical history. For young adults these usually include a resting electrocardiogram (ECG), cholesterol and triglycerides, blood glucose, blood count, and hemoglobin tests. Young men and women should be checked for iron deficiency, especially if they participate in a strenuous endurance activity.

Elevated levels of the blood lipids cholesterol and triglycerides are associated with heart disease. In order to know enough about the problem and how diet and exercise can alter blood lipids, the physician needs a blood lipid profile. With new techniques for the separation of blood lipid fractions, the physician has a better tool to assist in the diagnosis and treatment of blood lipid disorders. Because cholesterol is carried in several lipid fractions, it is important to know more than the total serum cholesterol. Exercise training and diet lower LDL cholesterol and raise HDL cholesterol. This important effect of exercise will be impossible to assess without a blood lipid profile (I'll say more about blood lipids in chapter 12).

Preexercise Medical Examination

Your new level of activity is sure to enhance—not threaten—your health

- if you are free of symptoms,
- if you make a gradual transition to a more active lifestyle, and
- if you follow a sensible program or exercise prescription.

On the other hand, *you should consider a medical examination* before undertaking a more active lifestyle if

- you have been sedentary,
- you are concerned about the status of your health,
- you possess one or several primary or secondary coronary risk factors (high blood pressure, high blood lipids, or cigarette use),
- you haven't seen your physician within the last 5 years, or
- you are over 45 years of age.

The American College of Sports Medicine (1986) has this advice for those over 45 years of age: "At or above age 45, it is desirable . . . to have a maximal exercise test before beginning exercise programs. It is also desirable for those who are already exercising once they reach age 45" (p. 2).

Also, if pending work assignments or fitness training represent a *major* increase in your exercise habits, you should see your physician. However, if you already are quite active and free of risk factors and symptoms, a gradual increase in your activity should pose no problem, regardless of your age.

The preexercise examination includes the same components I mentioned earlier, with specific attention to signs and symptoms that may discourage exercise (e.g., heart disease), those that may limit exercise (cardiopulmonary problems or diabetes), and those that require special attention (drugs, use of a pacemaker, or obesity). The exam should focus on bone and joint problems, heart sounds and rhythms, and chronic lung problems. The exam should also include

- 12-lead resting electrocardiogram (ECG),
- resting systolic and diastolic blood pressure,
- blood tests (e.g., fasting glucose, cholesterol, triglycerides, and blood lipid profile if indicated), and
- a progressive ECG-monitored exercise test (stress test) including
  - stepwise increase in work load,
  - continuous multilead ECG,
  - blood pressure measurement at each work load,
  - maximal or near-maximal work load, and
  - continuous ECG-monitored recovery.

The Exercise Stress Test

Many of the symptoms of previously undiagnosed heart disease appear only during vigorous exercise, when myocardial oxygen needs rise along with blood pressure and heart rate. Narrowed coronary arteries may be able to supply the blood you need for sedentary pursuits, but during exercise the oxygen needs of the heart muscle climb, and electrocardiographic abnormalities or physical symptoms such as chest pain may indicate a problem.

The stress test, a progressive ECG-monitored exercise test, is a diagnostic tool used by the physician to locate the problem early enough to initiate effective treatment. In recent years, the stress test has been used to diagnose or verify the presence of heart disease, as a preexercise test to rule out possible heart disease and to set reasonable exercise limits, as a postcoronary test to indicate extent of damage and subsequent progress in therapeutic programs, and as a postcoronary or coronary bypass follow-up to establish extent of recovery as well as work and exercise limits. Although most stress tests are conducted on the treadmill, arm testing (cranking) may be required for individuals returning to jobs that require strenuous use of the arms.

The **coronary bypass** is an operation to repair a narrowed coronary artery. A small section of vein is taken from the leg and used to replace or bypass a section of diseased coronary artery. A recent approach, called **angioplasty**, involves insertion of a balloon on the end of a catheter. When the balloon is positioned in the damaged artery, the balloon is inflated to open the artery and improve blood flow. Neither procedure is always successful, so prevention seems a far more prudent course of action. Lasers are being tested on animals to perfect a new way to clear arteries blocked by atherosclerosis.

Maximal and Near-Maximal Testing

Some symptoms of heart disease show up only when the heart muscle becomes deprived of sufficient oxygen. For individuals with partial narrowing of the coronary arteries, the ECG symptoms may only become obvious at near-maximal work loads. Those opposed to maximal testing prefer to terminate a test when a subject reaches 85 to 90% of the predicted maximal heart rate. They feel that this severity is sufficient to provide a diagnosis and that near-maximal testing is safer. Although the risk in testing symptom-free subjects in maximal or near-maximal tests is quite small, some feel it is unnecessary to utilize maximal testing for an individual who is only being tested as a safety precaution prior to a fitness training program.

One reason for maximal testing is to evaluate the subject's functional capacity, the maximal attainable work level. When evaluating subjects for employment in an arduous occupation, doctors can use the stress test to determine the subjects' work performance as well as their fitness levels, so long as the subject doesn't hold the railing during the test. This lowers the work load and invalidates the prediction of fitness and work capacity.

Test Termination

The stress test should be terminated when the subject cannot continue or has symptoms of exertional intolerance (chest pain or intolerable fatigue) or distress (e.g., staggering, unsteadiness, confusion, pallor, distressed breathing, nausea, or vomiting), when there are electrocardiographic changes, or when blood pressure drops with an increasing work load.

As I have said, some experts recommend termination of the test when the heart rate reaches a "target heart rate," defined as some percentage of the maximal heart rate predicted for the subject's age. One serious drawback to this approach is the variability in maximal heart rate (see Table 11.1). For example, the predicted maximal heart rate for an active individual of 25 years is 195 bpm, with a standard deviation of ± 12 beats. (The standard deviation, *SD*, is a measure of variability: 68% of the cases fall within one *SD* or ± 12 beats, 95% within ± 24 beats, and 99% within 36 beats). Therefore, it is possible that one in 100 people may have a maximal heart rate above 230 or below 160. Use of a 90% target heart rate gives us 175, a rate higher than that attainable by a few and well below the maximal heart rate for the occasional individual with a rate above 230. So reliance on a target heart rate is no guarantee of test severity *or* safety.

The Exercise Electrocardiogram

The electrocardiogram (ECG) is a strip of paper with a record of the electrical activity of the heart. Each complete ECG cycle (see Figure 11.1) represents one beat of the heart. The *P* wave represents the electrical activity that immediately precedes the contraction of the upper chambers or atria. The *QRS* complex

Table 11.1 Age and Fitness Adjusted Maximal Heart Rates

Age	Below average fitness	Predicted maximal heart rates[a] Average fitness	Above average fitness
20	201	201	196
25	195	197	194
30	190	193	191
35	184	190	188
40	179	186	186
45	174	183	183
50	168	179	180
55	163	176	178
60	158	172	175
65	152	169	173
70	147	165	170

Note. Adapted from "Age-Fitness Adjusted Maximal Heart Rates" by K.H. Cooper, J.G. Purdy, S.R. White, M.L. Pollock, and A.C. Linnerud. In *The Role of Exercise in Internal Medicine* (*Medicine and Sport*, Vol. 10) by D. Brunner and E. Jokl (Eds.), 1975. Basil, Switzerland: Karger.

[a]Maximal heart rate (MHR) declines with age. The rate of decline is related to activity and fitness. The decline is slower among active and fit individuals. These age and fitness adjusted MHRs are based on a sample of more than 2,500 men, but are averages. There is considerable variability in this measure (standard deviation $\cong \pm 12$ bpm). Thus, if the MHR predicted for a given age and fitness is 186, 68% of the subjects are between 174 and 198 (± 1 *SD*), 95% between 162 and 210 (± 2 *SD*), and 99% between 150 and 222 (± 3 *SD*). Thus, there is one chance in a hundred that your maximal heart rate could be 36 beats above *or* below the value in the table!

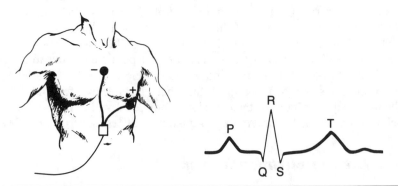

Figure 11.1. The ECG cycle. *P* wave indicates depolarization of atria. *QRS* wave is caused by spread of excitation through ventricles. *T* wave indicates repolarization of ventricles.

represents the electrical discharge of the ventricles, and the *T* wave results when the depolarized ventricles are recharged. Under normal conditions, the heart receives an impulse at the sinoatrial node. The impulse spreads across the atria, causing contractions of the atrial muscle fibers as it goes, and finally arrives at the atrioventricular node. Here, the impulse finds its way to the ventricles.

The electrocardiograph is wired to indicate a positive deflection when the depolarization wave is flowing toward the positive electrode. The *P* wave and *QRS* complex normally yield positive deflections. If the stimulus to contract comes from the wrong direction (e.g., from the ventricles), the *QRS* could deflect downward. Because the recording paper moves at a specified rate (usually 25 mm/s), the width of a wave can provide information about the rate of conduction. For example, if conduction is slow or blocked, the base of the *QRS* will be broad.

The physician, nurse, or technician administering a stress test pays careful attention to the ECG waveform as it travels across the screen of the oscilloscope. Changes of sufficient importance to terminate the test include

- S-T segment depression in excess of 0.2 mv (2 mm below the baseline), an indicator of poor blood flow and myocardial ischemia (lack of blood to the tissue),
- irregular rhythm, particularly when it originates in the ventricles and comes in volleys of 3 or more or as many as 10 per minute, and
- left ventricular conduction disturbances.

Exercise-induced **premature ventricular contractions** may lead to **ventricular tachycardia** (extremely rapid heart rate) and occasionally to **fibrillation**, an uncontrolled and uncoordinated action of heart muscle fibers that is incapable of pumping blood. Fibrillation requires immediate emergency action. The defibrillator provides a strong direct current that depolarizes the entire heart muscle, thereby allowing the normal pattern of stimulation to regain control.

Bruce and Kluge (1971) reported on their early experiences in the testing and training of hundreds of patients with clinically established coronary heart disease. They reported seven cases of exercise-related cardiac fibrillation. Two cases occurred during stress testing and five during the medically supervised training program. All the patients recovered following defibrillation, and six of the seven resumed physical activity within a few weeks. So it is important to provide adequate emergency equipment and a well-trained staff for the testing of patients. Tests conducted on apparently healthy individuals are not considered unsafe, but test administrators should be thoroughly trained in CPR and other emergency techniques.

Test Results

Heart disease is suggested by ECG abnormalities, chest pain, or an abnormal blood pressure response to testing. Stress test findings are verified when they are confirmed with **cardiac catheterization**, an invasive **imaging technique** for the diagnosis of atherosclerosis. With this procedure a catheter is inserted into a blood vessel in the arm and worked into position in the aorta. An opaque fluid (or dye) is injected into each coronary artery to allow detection via X rays of narrowing due to atherosclerosis. Results are considered false when the test reveals evidence of narrowed coronary vessels following a normal stress test or no evidence of narrowing in the case of an abnormal test.

False Negative Results.   False negative results are most disturbing because they indicate failure to diagnose the presence of *abnormal* coronary arteries. A small percentage of cases fall into this category, most of which do not go on for further evaluation, so their first indication of the problem is often their last—a myocardial infarction, or heart attack. The physician cannot rely on the stress test alone but must employ clinical judgment and other diagnostic tools as well. Patient reports of chest pain during other forms of exertion may be useful, because the careful warm-up preceding the stress test may allow some with diseased arteries to adjust to the gradually increased work load.

False Positive Results.   False positive results also are disturbing, because they may cause otherwise healthy individuals to become cardiac neurotics, morbidly concerned with a heart condition that may not exist. Estimates concerning the frequency of false positive results range from more than 50% to as little as 8%. False positive findings seem to occur more frequently in highly active subjects! Furthermore, false positive results are more common among women, perhaps because they may be more likely to hyperventilate during the stress test (for this reason, patients are routinely asked to hyperventilate before the test).

Endurance athletes often exhibit false positive results. A study of 20 top male distance runners revealed that 25% exhibited ECG abnormalities during a stress test (Gibbons, Cooper, Martin, & Pollock, 1977). Because these men were highly successful distance runners, the doctors who administered the test did not worry about the findings. In fact, abnormal ECGs are common among endurance athletes. But consider the plight of the active nonathlete who receives word that the stress test indicates possible coronary artery disease. What does he or she do next?

Until recently, the coronary catheter test was the only way to confirm or deny the existence of coronary artery disease. If a stress test and a subsequent retest indicated possible coronary artery disease, the patient had two choices: Have the catheter test or ignore the stress test and possibly become a cardiac cripple, giving up an active lifestyle for a heart condition that might not exist. Today, the patient has other choices.

Myocardial scintigraphy involves a less invasive assessment of myocardial blood flow during rest and exercise. A radioactive substance is injected into the circulation, and its uptake in cardiac tissue is observed with a scintillation camera. Cold spots indicate areas where blood flow is inadequate during exercise, thereby allowing confirmation of stress test results (Froelicher, 1984). As this and other imaging techniques become available throughout the country, the problem of the false positive test should disappear.

Actually, there may be no such thing as a false positive test. There is the possibility of a coronary artery spasm that occurs only during vigorous effort. Because the catheterization tests are routinely performed at rest, the spasm may not show up. Myocardial scintigraphy during exercise helps solve this problem.

The Risk of Exercise

Several years ago when Jim Fixx, author of a popular book on running, died during a run, millions became concerned about the risks of vigorous exercise. Since then researchers have demonstrated that the risk of heart attack for habitually active individuals rises during exercise to a level above that of sedentary living, but only during the period of exercise. Throughout the rest of the day, the active individual has a much *lower risk* than his sedentary counterpart (Siscovick, LaPorte & Newman, 1985). Chapter 12 provides greater insight into the risk reduction provided by regular moderate activity.

Figure 11.2 provides a graphic view of the relationships between the benefits and risks of activity. The figure shows that benefits increase rapidly at first but eventually plateau with little additional benefit at higher levels of activity. Risks, on the other hand, rise slowly at first then more rapidly at higher levels of activity. Thus it seems prudent to maximize benefits while minimizing risks and

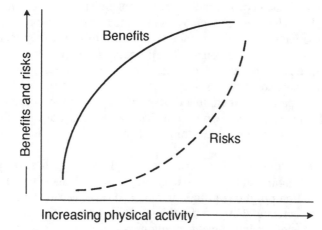

Figure 11.2. Relationships of benefits and risks with level of physical activity. *Note.* From "Workshop on Epidemiologic and Public Health Aspects of Physical Activity and Exercise: A Summary" by K. Powel and R. Paffenbarger, 1985, *Public Health Reports,* **100,** p. 123. Reprinted by permission of the authors.

to engage in a level of activity associated with enhanced health, and relatively low risk. The aerobic fitness prescriptions described in chapter 3 define that level of activity. You will learn more about benefits and risks in subsequent chapters.

"Get Some Exercise"

Doctors have long been cautious about exercise. The medical community has recommended a visit to the physician and even a stress test prior to involvement in strenuous activity. Few Americans receive advice concerning exercise from their physicians, and the advice they get usually consists of the old standby, "Get some exercise." If your doctor tells you to get some exercise, read Part I for the prescription of aerobic exercise.

Cardiac Rehabilitation

In the past, the patient with an acute myocardial infarction, or heart attack, could look forward to a prolonged period of bed rest. Although the rest did reduce the work load demanded of the damaged heart, it also had a severe deconditioning effect. Today, cardiologists advocate early ambulation. Within a few days, the patient is walking the halls of the hospital; within a few weeks, he or she is involved in a progressive reconditioning program. If all goes well, full rehabilitation may be possible within a few months.

Early ambulation and progressive conditioning quickly restore confidence for an individual who has been shaken by an extreme loss of function. After a coronary, many patients question their ability to return to work; they fear exertion of all types, even sexual intercourse. The progressive aerobic conditioning program provides a positive approach to the problem (Pashkow, Pashkow, & Schafer, 1988). As fitness and work capacity grow, so does the confidence needed to face life. Many patients remain in a fitness program after their coronary. Some feel better than they ever have, and some have shown just how complete recovery can be: They have gone on to train for and complete the marathon run, all 26 mi, 385 yd!

Low-intensity, long-duration activity is recognized as the best form of exercise for rehabilitation and continued fitness training. Today, numerous coronary rehabilitation programs utilize running and other aerobic activities as the primary therapeutic modalities. And although programs still avoid heavy lifting and extreme strength training, many programs now utilize moderate weight lifting for muscular endurance and muscle tone. In spite of the fact that one coronary usually leads to another, active participants in these programs seldom experience a serious problem.

Exercise after a coronary is a matter of medical judgment and supervision. The risk and complications can be determined only after a thorough medical examination. Patients often are monitored with cardiac telemetry in the early stages of rehabilitation, and low-level stress tests help define the patient's exercise tolerance and limits. Many hospitals have rehabilitation programs. The YMCA has programs in many cities, and a number of universities have excellent preventive and rehabilitation exercise programs. If your city doesn't have such a program, contact your county medical association or rehabilitation center for advice. Coronary rehabilitation is more than physical; it involves psychological and occupational counseling, nutritional advice, and family counseling. A coronary does not have to be the end of something good; it can be the start of something better. Of course you could decide prevention is the best choice of all.

Low Back Problems

More than 30 million Americans are afflicted with lower back pain, and an estimated 80% (24 million) of these problems are due to improper posture, weak muscles, or inadequate flexibility. Weak abdominal muscles cannot prevent the forward tilt of the pelvis, which displaces the vertebrae and causes pain. Lack of flexibility in back and hamstring muscles also leads to lower back pain. Low back pain has been called a hypokinetic disease, one that results from a lack (hypo) of movement (kinetic). See Appendix E for some simple ways to test flexibility, abdominal tone, and risk of low back problems.

Many cases of lower back pain can be prevented by assuming good posture and adhering to a regular program of flexibility and abdominal exercises. Also keep your body weight low and your waistline trim. To avoid injury to the lower back, use your legs when lifting heavy objects, not your back, and avoid carrying heavy objects above the level of the elbows. Here are some other suggestions for prevention of low back problems.

- Sleep with your knees somewhat flexed; avoid lying flat on your back or stomach. Use a firm mattress or sleep with a piece of plywood under the mattress.
- Sit with one or both knees above your hips; cross your legs or use a foot rest.
- Keep your knees bent while driving. If your car seat doesn't have support for the middle of your back, use a cushion.
- Stand with one foot on a stool, especially while ironing, washing dishes, or working at a counter.

Daily practice of the following exercises will help prevent or improve lower back problems (Williams, 1974).

LYING ON BACK

With knees bent and arms above your head, move one knee as far as possible toward your chest while straightening the other. Return to starting position and repeat, switching leg positions. Relax and repeat (see Figure 11.3).

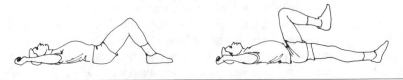

Figure 11.3. Alternately lift each knee to your chest.

Bend knees with feet flat on the floor, arms above head. Tighten the muscles of your lower abdomen and buttocks at the same time, keeping your back flat on the floor. Hold 10 s and relax; repeat (see Figure 11.4).

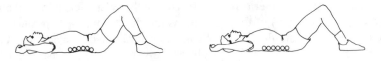

Figure 11.4. Push your lower back into the floor.

Starting in the same position with your arms at your side, draw knees to chest, and clasp hands around knees. Keeping your shoulders flat against the floor, pull knees tightly against chest, hold 10 s and relax; repeat. Repeat and touch your forehead to your knees (see Figure 11.5).

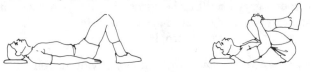

Figure 11.5. Pull both knees to your chest.

Bend your knees with your feet flat on the floor; cross your arms on your chest. Raise your head and shoulders from the floor. With chin to chest and back rounded, curl up to a sitting position. Be sure to pull with the stomach muscles. Lower slowly. Do 5 to 10 repetitions; increase until you can do 20.

ON ALL FOURS

Kneel and place your hands on the floor; Lower your head and contract stomach and buttock muscles; arch your lower back, hold 5 s, and relax.

SITTING IN A CHAIR

With your knees bent, bend forward at the waist to bring your head between your knees; pull your stomach in as you curl forward. Keep your weight back on your hips. Release your stomach muscles and reach to stretch lower back. Come up slowly. Relax, repeat (see Figure 11.6).

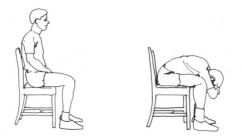

Figure 11.6. Bend from your waist.

HANGING FROM CHIN-UP BAR

Hang from the bar and try to draw your knees up to your chest (see basket hang, in Appendix C).

These exercises are suitable for prevention and rehabilitation; however, you should avoid exercise if pain persists. Your physician may provide additional exercise suggestions.

Abdominal Tone

Because lack of abdominal muscle tone may contribute to low back problems, you should practice preventive exercise. Sit-ups (or curl-ups) exercise the major abdominal muscle, the rectus abdominus. However, because this muscle attaches low on the pelvic girdle, it isn't very effective in counteracting a strong forward tilt of the pelvis. The oblique muscles attach higher up on the pelvis and are better able to counter the forward tilt. So some experts feel that the obliques should be the focus of abdominal training. With practice you can learn to contract the obliques during pelvic tilt exercises. Another approach for the healthy back is to do side sit-ups. Lie on your side, hands behind your head, with feet anchored or held. Come up sideways using the obliques. Then switch sides and repeat. Work up to 20 repetitions on both sides, try the sit-ups while you hold a light weight behind your head.

Flexibility

Because lack of flexibility in the back and hamstrings is another factor in low back problems, you should include stretching in your daily program. Use the static stretch or contract-relax suggestions in chapter 5, and be sure to stretch your lower back and hamstrings.

Stress Reduction

Tense muscles and psychological stress may also contribute to the problem. Try the relaxation techniques described in chapter 13 or sign up for a stress management class.

Fitness

A well-designed program that includes aerobic and muscular fitness training will provide all the elements for prevention of low back problems. You'll get abdominal training and flexibility, and the aerobic exercise will help you reduce or manage stress. See Appendix E for ways to assess your low-back fitness.

Recently specialists in back problems have given attention to new approaches. One makes use of back extension exercises, which maintain back flexibility and strengthen back extensor muscles. Several equipment companies sell sophisticated back testing devices that allow measurements of back flexibility and strength. Back extension training machines are beginning to appear in health clubs.

If you have low back problems, ask your physician about this approach to the prevention, diagnosis, and treatment of low back disorders. If you decide to improve the strength of back extensor muscles, be sure to avoid **hyperextension**, which could lead to low back soreness.

Regardless of the approach utilized, keep one thing in mind: Failure to practice a preventive low back program may leave you vulnerable to a problem that disables millions every year.

CHAPTER

12

EXERCISE, FITNESS, AND CARDIOVASCULAR HEALTH

This chapter will help you

understand the nature and extent of heart disease,

identify heart disease risk factors that are subject to the influence of exercise,

understand the research that links physical inactivity to coronary heart disease, and

understand how physical activity and other lifestyle changes reduce the incidence of heart disease.

The advent of automation, remote control, and robotics and the increased use of other labor-saving devices have led to a reduction in physical activity and the greatest sustained epidemic that mankind has ever experienced—**coronary artery disease** (CAD). Other factors are associated with this hitherto unknown plague, such as increased stress, cigarette smoking, and consumption of fat. CAD is not a simple problem that will yield to a single solution; it is a disease associated with a number of factors.

The greatest single cause of death in the United States and many other highly developed countries—cardiovascular disease (heart attacks, stroke, and other blood vessel diseases)—killed almost one million Americans in 1985, far more than the 636,282 Americans killed in the four major wars of this century! Fifty-five percent die from coronary artery disease, which kills more than 540,000 Americans annually, many by heart attack (or myocardial infarction; American Heart Association, 1988). This sudden death is not so sudden. Coronary arteries are narrowed by **atherosclerosis**, which occurs little by little as cholesterol is deposited beneath the lining of arteries, forming plaques that protrude into the artery. The result is a reduction of blood flow, known as **ischemia**. As the arteries narrow, they restrict the oxygen supply to the heart; its work capacity declines, and the risk of heart attack grows (see Figure 12.1). Death usually results from lethal disturbances in heart rhythms, such as tachycardia or fibrillation, as ischemia leads to electrical instability of the heart tissue.

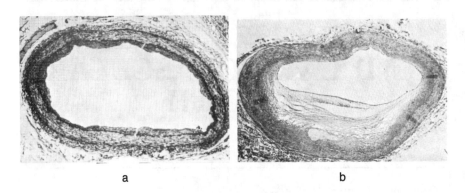

a   b

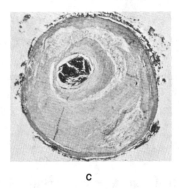

c

Figure 12.1. The coronary artery: (a) a normal coronary artery; (b) cholesterol deposits that narrow the artery; (c) a blood clot completely blocking a severely occluded coronary artery. *Note.* From "Atherosclerosis" by D.M. Spain, 1966, *Scientific American*, **215**.

For every known case of CAD, another case is waiting to be diagnosed. Often the first symptom of CAD is a heart attack. Nearly one million heart attacks occur annually in this country; of those experiencing their first attack, 25% die within 3 hr and another 10% within a week. Those who do survive face the likelihood that death, when it comes, will be by heart attack. What causes this disease, and what can be done about it?

Atherosclerosis

Atherosclerosis begins to develop during childhood. Some risk factors, such as elevated blood lipids (cholesterol), seem to be transmitted as dominant traits. We learn habits and lifestyles, such as overeating, smoking, and inactivity, at an early age. Thus any effort to eliminate, minimize, or control the disease must begin early, before serious damage is done and before dangerous habits are learned.

Atherosclerosis is probably caused by an injury to the arterial wall. The injury may be due to the turbulent flow of blood in the artery. Thereafter, lipoproteins, the carriers of cholesterol in the blood, infiltrate the region. Debris from dead and dying cells joins the growing plaque, and a fibrous cap covers the debris of the plaque as it grows and narrows the arterial passageway (Superko, 1988).

What causes the development of the plaque? A number of factors may contribute to the process, including high blood pressure, which may exacerbate the injury or force cholesterol into the plaque. Cigarette smoke contains substances known to accelerate the process, and LDL cholesterol levels in the blood are highly related to the progress of the disease. Whatever the case, the plaque grows until it blocks flow in the artery or until the artery is clogged by a clot. Then the flow of blood and oxygen to the heart muscle is slowed or stopped, causing a heart attack—and death of cardiac muscle.

Evidence of the early onset and rapid development of the disease comes from postmortem studies of young American soldiers killed in Korea and Vietnam. More than 70% of the autopsied victims had significant evidence of CAD. Thus, it appears that CAD is a disease of early origin that develops rapidly in our society and begins to take its toll among early–middle-aged adults. This means that we must shift our preventive efforts to younger age groups. We cannot ignore the effects of diet, smoking, hypertension, lack of physical activity, and other factors on the development of atherosclerosis.

Several recent surveys identify the presence of CAD risk factors in children of all ages in urban, suburban, and rural settings, and exploratory studies demonstrate that risk factors can be reduced in children. Because the degenerative effects of atherosclerosis eventually become irreversible, and because the disease process has already begun in these children, a program of risk factor identification and reduction for young children is both prudent and advisable.

CAD Risk Factors, Physical Activity, and Fitness

The cause or causes of CAD still are uncertain, but studies identify a number of factors associated with its incidence. Elevated blood lipids (cholesterol and triglycerides), high blood pressure, and cigarette smoking usually rank among the top risk factors (see Table 12.1). An individual who scores high on one of

Table 12.1 CHD Risk Factors

Influenced by physical activity	May be influenced by physical activity	Not influenced by physical activity
Endomesomorphic body type	Carbohydrate intolerance	Family history of heart disease
Overweight	Electrocardiographic abnormalities	
Elevated blood lipids[a]		Sex (male has greater risk until 60s)
High blood pressure or hypertension	Elevated uric acid	
Physical inactivity	Pulmonary function (lung) abnormalities	Cigarette smoking[b]
	Personality or behavior pattern (hard driving, time conscious, aggressive, competitive)	Diet (saturated fats, salt)[b]
	Psychic reactivity (reaction to stress)	

Note. Adapted from Sharkey (1974).

[a]Research continues to identify additional factors associated with heart disease. A subgroup of HDL cholesterol, apolipoprotein, is inversely related to CHD. Estradiol, a female hormone, is highly related to heart disease in men. The fatty substance called cholesterol is the basic chemical structure of estradiol. Some workers feel that body fat, blood lipids, and estradiol are different aspects of the same problem, too much fat.

[b]Diet and cigarette smoking are classified as not influenced by exercise. However, I have seen many individuals become more concerned about their diet as they became involved in a training program, and many have told me they were unable to give up smoking until they started a fitness program.

these factors is said to be **at risk**. A candidate who scores high on two or more factors is a prime candidate for a heart attack and is said to be **coronary prone**. Some of the risk factors are subject to the direct influence of physical activity and some are not.

Many risk factors are interrelated. Psychic reactivity can contribute to hypertension, whereas physical activity seems to reduce stress *and* high blood pressure. Cigarette smokers may reduce, but never eliminate, the influence of cigarettes through vigorous physical activity (see Table 12.2). But those who begin a fitness program are more likely to slow down or stop smoking, if only because vigorous activity leads to a decreased desire to smoke (Pomerleau, 1987).

Several risk factors are related to body fat and fat metabolism. Overweight and obesity and elevated blood lipids are related to heart disease, and exercise can reduce body fat. The appropriate intensity and duration of exercise also can lead to reduced serum triglycerides and cholesterol, particularly LDL cholesterol.

Table 12.2 Exercise, Smoking, and Death Rates[a]

Exercise	Never smoked regularly	Pack or more per day
None	834	1,416
Slight	579	1,347
Moderate	486	1,065
Heavy	474	998

Note. Adapted from "Smoking in Relation to Mortality and Morbidity" by E. Hammond, 1964, *Journal of the National Cancer Institute*, pp. 1161-1170.

[a]Per 100,000 man years.

And because carbohydrate intolerance may be due partly to the effect of fat on insulin, carbohydrate intolerance too can be improved when body fat and blood lipids are reduced, as in a fitness program.

Among those risk factors that physical activity *may* influence, the psychological ones are most intriguing. Psychic reactivity, the reaction to stress and tension, may be improved through participation in some forms of activity and made worse by others; some people crumble under competitive pressure, whereas others find it stimulating. The effect of exercise on the hard-driving, competitive behavior pattern (Type A) that was once associated with CAD has not been well established. But it may be unwise for coronary-prone individuals to carry that competitive behavior into their exercise habits. Proper activity could serve to interrupt the behavior syndrome and help the aggressive personality relax.

Certain risk factors are beyond the influence of activity, or so it seems. Certainly a family history cannot be altered by activity. A family history may indicate inheritance of a blood lipid disorder that predisposes the unfortunate recipient to early heart disease. And one's sex cannot be changed with exercise; being male is a risk factor, and no one can change that. But cigarette smoking and diet are subject to change, and many of those who become active improve their smoking and dietary habits. Thus physical activity helps reduce risks associated with other risk factors.

To say risk factors have been *associated* with CAD means there is a statistically significant relationship but does *not* imply cause and effect. For example, lack of activity may merely allow development of the problem, or it may be related to some other causal factor. Possibly, the lack of physical activity has nothing whatsoever to do with the incidence of CAD, but this seems untenable in view of the many studies that have associated CAD with inactivity.

I have suggested that physical activity directly or indirectly influences several of the coronary risk factors. Most studies loosely describe physical activity as occupational or recreational exercise and seldom specify the amount of regular exercise or describe the fitness of the population measured.

Cooper et al. (1976) at the Institute for Aerobic Research in Dallas set out to determine the relationship of fitness to selected coronary risk factors. They studied approximately 3,000 men (average age 44.6 years) to determine the relationship between fitness and such factors as heart rate, body weight, percentage body fat, glucose, systolic blood pressure, and serum cholesterol and triglycerides. The researchers found a consistent inverse relationship between fitness and the risk factors. This cross-sectional study does not *prove* the effect of fitness training on each risk factor but only proves that the factors are related inversely to fitness in the population studied. However, data do exist to prove the effect of training on many coronary risk factors.

Blair and Kohl (1988) recently reported an update of this ongoing investigation. As before, the data showed a relationship between low fitness and mortality; as fitness improves, the death rate declines for men and women. It is interesting to note that the death rate reaches a plateau at a fitness level of 35 ml/[kg $\times$ min] for men and at 31.5 for women. Thereafter, further increases in fitness are not associated with lower death rates. However, the study did not constitute a random sample; many of the subjects were highly active people who came to the institute's aerobics clinic to test themselves. Those in the low-fitness (and higher risk) categories may have enrolled because they were concerned about their health. These arguments deserve to be noted, but the fact remains that in this sample, those in the low-fitness categories had a higher risk of death. However, among active subjects, the risk of death did not change with improving fitness. Confused? Don't be. Being active probably raises most subjects above the 35 (or 31.5) fitness level. This study suggests that the health benefits of exercise can be achieved at a modest level of fitness (35 is termed low-fitness in chapter 3).

A recent study examined the heart disease risk profiles of 4,351 men and women. Of the 23 factors analyzed, the exercise component accounted for the highest percentage of any factor. In other words, lack of exercise again emerged as a significant predictor of heart disease risk (Collingswood, Bernstein, & Blair, 1987).

In the past 3 decades, many studies have linked physical inactivity with CAD. The following sections represent that literature with a few classic examples. Further elaboration is available in excellent reviews of the literature (Pollock, Wilmore, & Fox, 1984; Wilson, Fardy, & Froelicher, 1981).

Population Studies

One of the first studies to focus on inactivity as a factor in heart disease risk was reported by Morris and Raffle in 1954. They conducted the famous London bus driver study, which compared the incidence of CAD between bus drivers and conductors. The more physically active conductors experienced an incidence rate 30% below that of the drivers. Moreover, the disease appeared earlier among the drivers, and their mortality rate was more than twice as high following the first heart attack. However, subsequent studies indicated the complexity of the problem (Morris, Heady, & Raffle, 1956). The drivers were more likely to be overweight, even before they transferred to the sedentary occupation. The researchers questioned what personality characteristics led some men to be drivers and others to be conductors and acknowledged that piloting a large bus through the busy streets of London may induce significantly more occupational stress than the conductors experienced.

The North Dakota study was reported by Zukel, Lewis, and Enterline in 1959. The researchers tabulated the rate of CAD along with data regarding diet, work history, cigarette smoking, and medical care. When the hours of heavy physical activity were related to the incidence of CAD, the data indicated an impressive argument for physical activity. When compared with those who performed no heavy work, the CAD incidence for those who performed an hour of heavy physical activity daily dropped more than 80% (18.9 per 1,000 per year to 3.5). The researchers found a further decline in those who performed from 2 to 6 hr of work and saw a tendency for an increased CAD rate for the few individuals who performed 7 or more hr of heavy physical activity.

In 1975, Paffenbarger and Hale reported the effects of occupational physical activity on coronary mortality among 6,351 longshoremen, aged 35 to 74. The men were followed for 22 years, to the age of 75, or to death, whichever came first. Their jobs were classified according to high, medium, and low caloric expenditure. The age-adjusted coronary death rate for the highly active workers was 26.9 per 10,000 work years, almost half of that found for the medium and low groups (46.3 and 49.0, respectively). The researchers noted an apparent threshold of protection, which was particularly obvious in the case of sudden death, for which the rate for the highly active was 5.6, compared with 19.9 and 15.7 for the medium and light activity groups. The authors concluded that the repeated bursts of high energy output established a plateau of protection against coronary mortality.

More recently, Paffenbarger et al. (1986) provided further evidence of a threshold of protection provided by vigorous physical activity. In a study of 17,000 Harvard alumni aged 35 to 75, the researchers found fewer heart attacks among those who engaged regularly in strenuous activity for which the energy expenditure exceeded 7.5 cal/min. The protection was evident among those who participated in at least 3 hr of vigorous activity per week, for a total of 2,000 or more cal weekly. Those who totaled 2,000 cal of exercise in light activity (under 7.5 cal/min) were not better off than those who were inactive. The protection afforded by the vigorous activity was independent of other risk factors such as high blood pressure, smoking, overweight, and family history of heart disease. And the protection was a function of current activity, not previous athletic participation or ability.

To summarize these and other studies, *as little as 20 min of walking (about* 100 cal) reduces the risk of CAD by approximately 30% (see Figure 12.2).

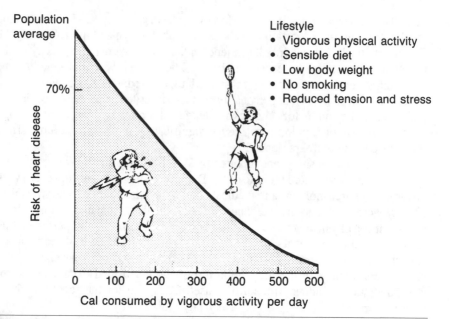

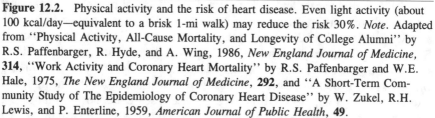

Figure 12.2. Physical activity and the risk of heart disease. Even light activity (about 100 kcal/day—equivalent to a brisk 1-mi walk) may reduce the risk 30%. *Note.* Adapted from "Physical Activity, All-Cause Mortality, and Longevity of College Alumni" by R.S. Paffenbarger, R. Hyde, and A. Wing, 1986, *New England Journal of Medicine,* **314,** "Work Activity and Coronary Heart Mortality" by R.S. Paffenbarger and W.E. Hale, 1975, *The New England Journal of Medicine,* **292,** and "A Short-Term Community Study of The Epidemiology of Coronary Heart Disease" by W. Zukel, R.H. Lewis, and P. Enterline, 1959, *American Journal of Public Health,* **49.**

Increase the daily caloric expenditure, and you reduce the risk further. If you are willing and able to work your way up to 500 to 600 cal of daily activity (the equivalent of 5 to 6 mi of daily running), you will achieve all the protection exercise can offer. Another indicator of cardioprotection is aerobic fitness. The risk seems low for those above 35 ml/[kg × min] and may be even lower for regularly active individuals in the higher categories of fitness.

Although a few population studies fail to show any degree of cardioprotection due to exercise or fitness, the overwhelming tendency is for a 30 to 80% reduction of CAD risk from increased activity. The incidence of myocardial infarction usually is reduced at least 50%, and the physically active individual has less than half the mortality rate of an age-matched but sedentary counterpart.

Recently, Blair and Kohl (1988) attempted to discern if physical activity or fitness was most associated with reduced risk of CAD. They reported on death rates in an 8-year study of 10,223 men. The sedentary men were almost 3 times more likely to die than the active subjects. Among the sedentary subjects, fitness only made a difference at the lowest level. The least fit had twice the risk of other sedentary subjects (5 times the risk for active subjects). Among the active subjects, the death rates were not significantly different, *regardless of the level of fitness*. These findings suggest that for these subjects, *activity conferred most of the benefits of exercise*, and higher levels of fitness didn't provide greater protection from all-cause mortality.

A study of leisure-time physical activity and the risk of coronary heart disease conducted by Dr. Art Leon and associates (Leon, Connett, Jacobs, & Rauramaa, 1987) of the University of Minnesota showed that a small increase in daily activity was associated with reductions in coronary heart disease and overall mortality. These findings have immense implications for those who prescribe exercise for health benefits. If activity is more important than fitness, exercise prescriptions need not emphasize intensity as much as they have in the past.

Autopsy Studies

Autopsy studies analyze tissue for evidence of disease or cause of death. In a postmortem study of 300 American soldiers killed in the Korean conflict, 77% were found to have significant evidence of CAD. Thus, it seems that the pathology of CAD is developed significantly by age 22 (Enos, Beyer, & Holmes, 1955). Morris and Crawford (1958) reported the results of nearly 5,000 autopsies on 45- to 70-year-old men who were classified into light, moderate, and heavy activity groups according to their last recorded occupation. Large fibrous patches were found less frequently in the hearts of those reported to be most active. The incidence of scars, infarcts, and occlusions was reduced 30% or more for the moderately active and even more for those presumed to be heavily active. However, severe coronary atherosclerosis was reduced only 25% for the moderately active and reduced not at all for the most active.

Animal studies suggest that moderate exercise is beneficial, but exhaustive or stressful effort may somehow accelerate the development of atherosclerotic pathology. Rabbits fed a high-cholesterol diet and run to exhaustion daily had more marked pathological changes in the myocardium. (Similar results were reported in a study using dogs.) However, when rabbits were exercised but 10 min a day, the exercised animals had less aortic atherosclerosis (Froelicher, 1972). I should note that exhaustive exercise can be stressful to animals, especially if it is accomplished with the use of electric shock or some other way of forcing the animals to comply. The stress provokes a hormonal response that may accelerate the atherosclerotic process, in animals and in humans.

The pathology associated with ischemic or coronary heart disease develops early in an overfed and inactive society. Regular activity during the elementary and high school years reduces specific CAD risk factors and may reduce this pathological development. There is good evidence that the habitual practice of *moderate* physical activity during the adult years may further retard this development.

Intervention Studies

Researchers are aware that retrospective population and autopsy studies do not *prove* the influence of physical activity on cardiovascular health. Association or relationship studies, or animal studies for that matter, do not prove cause and effect in human beings. Only large, long-term, well-controlled experimental studies in which subjects are assigned randomly to exercise and nonexercise groups will provide the necessary proof. For such a study researchers would have to be able to intervene in the lives of subjects and manipulate their amount of exercise, randomly assigning some subjects to exercise groups and asking the control groups to completely avoid exercise for years. Thus intervention studies are difficult and costly, and in light of what we know about the value of exercise, it may be unethical to ask subjects to live sedentary lives.

No conclusive intervention study has been completed. Due to the large number of dropouts typical in such projects, a well-conceived study must start with thousands of subjects. Various other factors such as diet, stress, occupational physical activity, and body weight must be identified and controlled. For best results, daily exercise has to be documented, and those assigned to the control group must accept the risks associated with lack of activity.

Although such a project seems destined to failure for a multitude of reasons, several pilot studies have been attempted, and each has reported positive effects of exercise on CAD risk. But the large national study needed to provide the final answer to the question has yet to be completed; in fact, our national public health officials gave up trying several years ago. We are left with research data that indicate a strong relationship between physical activity and cardiovascular health. Population studies, autopsy studies, and animal studies support this hypothesis: *The habitual practice of moderate physical activity reduces the risk of developing coronary or ischemic heart disease.*

Most studies link physical activity—*not fitness*—to a lower risk of heart disease. The amount of activity is more related to reduced risk than is the level of fitness. This may be true for several reasons; one is that some aspects of both heart disease risk and fitness are inherited. Thus a high level of fitness doesn't necessarily indicate a high level of activity. Another reason may be that some of the important benefits of physical activity may be associated with fat mobilization and metabolism and the effects of activity on blood lipids (see chapter 8 for discussion). Thus it may be possible to achieve many of the cardioprotective benefits of exercise via participation in moderate activities, such as walking.

The final decision about exercise is yours; it's not up to your doctor or some national scientific or medical organization. You must decide if physical activity and fitness are right for you. In my view, although the effect of exercise may not be *proven*, it certainly seems *prudent* in light of existing evidence.

Cardioprotective Mechanisms

The possible effects of physical activity listed in Table 12.3 may help to reduce the development or severity of CAD. A brief discussion of the more important mechanisms should provide further insight into the nature of cardioprotection and the types of exercise most likely to achieve it. Remember that atherosclerosis results when injury or some other factor leads to changes in the wall of the coronary artery, followed by the entry of LDL cholesterol and the formation of a growing scar or plaque. Reduced oxygen supplies in the artery seem to enhance the rate of cholesterol deposition. Heart attack occurs when the narrowed artery causes ischemia that leads to death of cardiac tissue. Angina pectoris is a chest pain, a signal that occurs when an individual with narrowed coronary arteries attempts vigorous effort.

Table 12.3 Cardioprotective Mechanisms

Physical activity may	
Increase	Decrease
Oxidation of fat	Serum cholesterol and trigylcerides
Number of coronary blood vessels	Glucose intolerance
Vessel size	Obesity, adiposity
Efficiency of heart	Platelet stickiness
Efficiency of peripheral blood distribution and return	Arterial blood pressure
Electron transport capacity	Heart rate
Fibrinolytic (clot-dissolving) capability	Vulnerability to dysrhythmias
Arterial oxygen content	Overreaction to hormones
Red blood cells and blood volume	Psychic stress
Thyroid function	
Growth hormone production	
Tolerance to stress	
Prudent living habits	
Joy of living	

Note. From Sharkey (1974).

Exercise may influence other forms of heart disease. Problems in electrical conduction can lead to failure of the pump, known as heart block. Irregular heart rhythms, or arrhythmia, can reduce blood flow and sometimes lead to fibrillation, an uncoordinated twitching of heart muscle fibers. Because the heart does not pump blood during the fibrillation, it must be stopped quickly to prevent death. Regular moderate activity may diminish these and other problems.

Mechanisms Involving the Heart

Let's consider some mechanisms that have a direct effect on the heart, then move on to mechanisms affecting the vascular system, and conclude with mechanisms related to fat metabolism and blood lipids.

Work Load of the Heart. It is clear that aerobic fitness training reduces the work load of the heart. Changes in trained skeletal muscles, including improved aerobic enzymes, oxygen utilization, and fat metabolism, allow the heart to meet exercise demands with a lower heart rate. The lower heart rate means a lower rate of oxygen utilization in the heart muscle. Although drugs can often achieve the same purpose, exercise and fitness seem to be a more natural approach to the problem.

Efficiency of the Heart. The trained heart uses less oxygen at a given work load. The heart rate is reduced during exercise, and the resting rate often declines from the 70s to the low 50s. Researchers have found hundreds of ski tourers, bicycle riders, and distance runners with rates in the 40s and have recorded several distance athletes in the mid-30s. Part of this decline in heart rate can be attributed to improved contractility of the heart muscle and part to a reduction in secretions of adrenalinelike compounds (or a diminished myocardial reaction to these *oxygen-wasting* hormones).

During exhaustive exercise, a deficient oxygen supply to the untrained muscle may lead to an imbalance of electrolytes (e.g., potassium), electrical instability, and an increased likelihood of arrhythmias, fibrillation, or heart failure (Raab, 1965). Aerobic fitness training greatly reduces this likelihood by correcting electrolyte imbalance, improving oxygen supply, reducing oxygen waste, and improving the efficiency of the heart.

Blood Supply. Studies show that exercise improves the circulation within the heart muscle. One study on rats suggested that regular, moderate activity was more effective than strenuous effort in the development of blood vessels (Stevenson, Felek, Rechnitzer, & Beaton, 1964). Exercise may also increase the development of **coronary collateral circulation** (circulation through the vessels that develop to provide alternative circulatory routes to portions of the ischemic heart muscle). Well-developed collateral circulation, in theory, would minimize the damage caused by a heart attack, reduce the risk of death, and increase the chances for a full recovery. The facts show that physically active individuals are more likely to recover from a heart attack.

Eckstein (1957) demonstrated the development of coronary collaterals in physically active dogs. Collaterals seem to develop where partial occlusion has reduced blood flow in adjacent arteries. Collateralization may serve to relieve ischemic heart tissue, but collaterals do not develop in the absence of exercise unless the circulation is severely impaired. The influence of exercise on the development of collaterals in human subjects remains uncertain. Some who engage in exercise show an increase, but some do not. However, because the pathological symptoms of atherosclerosis develop early, it seems prudent for all of us to exercise while we await final word on this potential benefit.

A fascinating effect of exercise, first suggested after the autopsy on marathon runner Clarance DeMar, is an increase in the size of the coronary arteries themselves. Some scientists hypothesize that this effect, if it occurs, would minimize the effect of plaque formation. Kramsch, Aspen, Abramowitz, Kreimendahl, and Hood (1981) studied the effect of moderate exercise and an atherosclerotic diet on the development of CAD in monkeys. ECG changes and sudden death occurred only in the sedentary animals, whereas the exercise group had larger hearts and *larger diameter* coronary arteries.

Cardiac Hypertrophy. **Cardiac hypertrophy**, an enlarged heart, has long been associated with vigorous exercise. Although the medical community first viewed this condition as a potential problem, we now view it as a normal compensation for increased endurance activity or training. The enlargement is due to an increase in the volume of the left ventricle at rest (left ventricular end diastolic volume). In other words, the trained heart gets bigger mostly because it fills with more blood. Because the healthy heart responds to filling with a vigorous contraction, it can pump more blood with each beat. Therefore this adaptation leads to a more efficient pump. Although some part of this adaptation may be due to changes in cardiac muscle tissue or in the nervous or hormonal activation of the heart, some is also due to increased blood volume with training and with better distribution of blood to working muscles (including the heart).

Vascular Mechanisms

These mechanisms suggest ways that activity may lower the risk of CAD via changes in the vascular system. They include changes in clotting, blood pressure, and blood distribution (or redistribution).

Fibrinolysis. **Fibrinolysis** is a mechanism that retards the formation of clots within the blood vessels. Exercise enhances this mechanism, but the effect lasts only 1 or 2 days. Exhaustive, highly competitive, or unfamiliar activity seems to inhibit this system and allow a more rapid clotting time (Whiddon et al., 1969). This sort of exercise should be avoided, because a clot in an already narrowed coronary vessel could be disastrous. Regular, moderate activity is best suited to enhance the fibrinolytic system (Moxley, Brakman, & Astrup, 1970).

Blood Pressure. High blood pressure, or **hypertension**, increases the work load of the heart by forcing it to contract against a greater resistance. Anything that serves to reduce blood pressure also reduces the work load of the heart.

Studies show that physical activity reduces hypertension among middle-aged (Boyer & Kasch, 1970) or older individuals (Morris & Crawford, 1958). Of course, this change in blood pressure could be a consequence of weight loss or of reduced stress, both of which are known outcomes of regular activity. Lack of physical activity is a risk factor that is associated with other risk factors.

Blood Distribution. One effect of physical training is an improved distribution of blood to the muscles and organs, which reduces the work load of the heart by requiring fewer beats to supply the body's need for blood. Actually this is a redistribution that occurs with training. Blood that might go to the digestive organs is diverted to the muscles during exercise, reducing both the contractile force required (indicated by blood pressure) and the number of beats. Because the oxygen needs of the heart are closely related to the product of Heart Rate × Blood Pressure, the systematic reduction of oxygen needs could help lower the risk of ischemic heart disease.

One study suggests that a moderate increase in red blood cells and blood volume due to training is another cardioprotective mechanism. Both are important components of the oxygen transport system. The importance of blood volume cannot be overstated. When training stops and blood volume declines, other cardiovascular adjustments are also lost (Coyle, Hemmert, & Coggan, 1986).

Fat Metabolism Benefits

Chapter 8 discussed how exercise and fitness influence fat metabolism. In my view, this may be one of the most important benefits of exercise in relation to CAD risk.

Overweight. Even if no relationship exists between overweight and CAD when cases of hypertension and diabetes are excluded, those who maintain their desirable weight enjoy greater protection from this and other diseases. One extremely interesting effect of exercise is a well-proven increase in the ability to mobilize fat from adipose tissue storage and burn it in the exercising muscles. Exercise is more effective than diet alone when it comes to removing fat.

Blood Lipids. Elevated levels of total and LDL cholesterol in the blood are risk factors of considerable importance. Therefore, I shall explore the blood fats and their metabolism in somewhat greater detail.

Triglycerides. Triglycerides consist of three fatty acids and a molecule of glycerol. The fatty acids have an even number of carbon atoms arranged in a straight chain. The fatty acids may be saturated, meaning they have single bonds, such as stearic acid;

```
     H H H H H H H H H H H H H H H H H H
     ' ' ' ' ' ' ' ' ' ' ' ' ' ' ' ' ' '
HC-C-C-C-C-C-C-C-C-C-C-C-C-C-C-C-C-COOH          Stearic Acid
     ' ' ' ' ' ' ' ' ' ' ' ' ' ' ' ' ' '
     H H H H H H H H H H H H H H H H H H
```

they may be monounsaturated, meaning they have one double bond, such as oleic acid;

```
     H H H H H H H H H   H H H H H H H H
     ' ' ' ' ' ' ' ' '   ' ' ' ' ' ' ' '
HC-C-C-C-C-C-C-C-C = C-C-C-C-C-C-C-C-COOH        Oleic Acid
     ' ' ' ' ' ' ' '     ' ' ' ' ' ' '
     H H H H H H H H      H H H H H H H
```

or they may be polyunsaturated, meaning they have two or more double bonds, such as linoleic acid.

```
     H H H H H H   H H H   H H H H H H H H
     ' ' ' ' ' '   ' ' '   ' ' ' ' ' ' ' '
HC-C-C-C-C-C = C-C-C- = C-C-C-C-C-C-C-C-COOH     Linoleic Acid
     ' ' ' ' '       '     ' ' ' ' ' ' '
     H H H H H       H      H H H H H H
```

The double bonds of unsaturated fatty acids may be more susceptible to oxidation. Polyunsaturated fatty acids may reduce cholesterol, and monounsaturated oils may reduce cholesterol without lowering HDL cholesterol. Thus, you can see why nutrition experts advocate the intake of mono- and polyunsaturated fats and a reduction of saturated and hydrogenated fats in the diet. Watch out for the tropical oils, palm and coconut, which are believed to be more atherogenic, especially when they are hydrogenated. Read labels!

Linoleic acid is an essential fatty acid. Because it cannot be formed in the body, we depend on dietary sources to provide for our needs.

Serum triglyceride levels are reduced several hours after exercise, and the effect persists for 1 or 2 days. Several days of exercise lead to a progressive reduction of triglyceride levels. The final plateau attained depends on the diet, body weight loss, and the intensity and duration of exercise. This plateau is also influenced strongly by any genetic tendency toward high serum triglyceride levels. It seems that *regular* activity is needed to achieve and maintain low levels of serum triglycerides.

Cholesterol. In chapter 8, I indicated the effects of exercise on cholesterol and the lipoprotein fractions that contain cholesterol. Training leads to a modest decline in total cholesterol, a significant reduction of LDL cholesterol, and an increase in HDL cholesterol. Because LDL has been implicated as the villain in the development of atherosclerotic plaques, this effect must be considered an important cardioprotective mechanism.

Cholesterol levels in the neighborhood of 240 mg were once considered normal when, in fact, these levels are associated with a significant incidence of heart disease (see Table 12.4). Diet alone can have a considerable effect on cholesterol levels, as well as on the risk of heart disease. Cholesterol is only found in animal products, so substitution of skimmed milk for whole, corn oil margarine for butter, and lean meat, fish, and poultry for fatty meat is a prudent beginning. Add more bran, especially oat bran, as well as apples and carrots to further lower serum cholesterol. Combined with reducing intake of eggs to one or two per week, this program of simple substitutions will lower serum cholesterol. A diet high in saturated fat is probably the biggest problem. Ideally, serum cholesterol should be reduced below 180 mg, the level found in populations where heart disease is virtually nonexistent. These levels are achieved on vegetarianlike diets that are high in complex carbohydrates and low in fat, and the lifestyle typically includes a significant amount of physical activity.

Table 12.4 is based on a study of serum cholesterol and death from CAD in 356,222 men, aged 35 to 57, who were screened for the Multiple Risk Factor Intervention Trial. It is clear from the table that cholesterol and death rate from CAD are highly related and that the risk increases dramatically at higher levels of cholesterol.

Table 12.4 Cholesterol and CAD Death Rate

Cholesterol (mg/100 ml)	Factor of increased risk
Under 181	1.00
182-202	1.29
203-220	1.73
221-244	2.21
Over 245	3.42

Note. Based on the Abell-Kendell Method used by the Centers for Disease Control. Adapted from ''Is Relationship Between Serum Cholesterol and Risk of Premature Death From Coronary Heart Disease Continuous and Graded?'' by J. Stamler, D. Wentworth, and J. Neaton, 1986, *Journal of the American Medical Association*, **256**.

Cholesterol values from 180 to 220 mg should respond to a moderate reduction of dietary fat.

Levels above 220 mg call for a concerted effort to reduce dietary fat and cholesterol. Oat bran, niacin, and other natural foods may also help reduce serum cholesterol.

Values that remain above 240 mg after dietary intervention may require drug therapy if other risk factors exist. Fortunately, several new drugs have successfully reduced cholesterol and the incidence of heart disease. See your physician for details.

LDL Cholesterol. Nobel prize–winning work by Brown and Goldstein (1984) shows why cholesterol contributes to heart disease and provides suggestions concerning what can be done to reduce the risk. The authors identified cellular receptors for LDL cholesterol that control the level of this atherogenic fraction of cholesterol. The story begins when the liver secretes VLDL particles laden with triglycerides. The triglyceride is burned in muscle or stored in adipose tissue, and the remaining portion eventually becomes LDL cholesterol. Cells of the normal liver have LDL receptors that take the dangerous LDL out of the circulation. However, individuals with an inherited error of metabolism (familial hypercholesterolemia) have fewer receptors and twice the normal level of LDL. Those unfortunate to have the severe form of the problem have few if any LDL receptors and LDL levels 6 times higher than normal. These people are likely to have a heart attack before the age of 10. Fortunately this version only affects about 1 in 1,000,000, whereas the milder version affects about 1 in 500.

The most surprising and significant finding of Brown and Goldstein's study was that high dietary fat intake inhibits the formation of LDL receptors. Eat fat and you inhibit the formation of receptors needed to clear the blood of LDL (remember, LDL is the cholesterol that enters the lining of coronary vessels and causes heart attacks). Thus it is very possible that the epidemic of heart disease that has plagued our society for decades is, in part, the result of excessive dietary fat intake. The authors recommend a diet moderately low in animal fat for most people, and for those with a strong family history of CAD, they recommend a diet extremely low in cholesterol and saturated fats.

HDL Cholesterol. The good side of the cholesterol story involves HDL cholesterol. This is a carrier form that is destined for removal by the liver. When HDL levels are elevated the risk of CAD is low, and vice versa. Whereas 45 mg/100 ml is average for adult men (55 for women), CAD risk climbs dramatically when the level drops below 35. On the other hand, an increase from 45 to 55 is associated with a 40% reduction in risk. And when the value reaches 75 the risk is virtually nonexistent (called the longevity syndrome). In the famous Framingham epidemiological study of an entire community, HDL was singled out as the best single indicator of heart disease risk.

Numerous studies show that vigorous exercise can raise HDL values from 5 to 10 mg, conferring a 20 to 40% reduction in risk. The effect is more pronounced when fat weight is lost; weight loss alone, from exercise or diet, leads to an improvement in HDL (Wood et al., 1988). Interestingly, cigarette smoking lowers HDL, whereas alcohol consumption (1 to 2 drinks per day) leads to an increase, although some question if it is the same subfraction of HDL that is inversely associated with heart disease. Of course, inherited differences influence the response of HDL to exercise or other therapies.

Dramatic decreases in HDL have been recorded in subjects using **anabolic steroids** for strength and body building. Values as low as 15 mg/100 ml suggest a severe health risk that could cause steroid-using athletes to experience heart problems in their 30s!

Cholesterol: HDL Ratio.   One of the best predictors of heart disease risk is the ratio formed by dividing cholesterol level by HDL. When the ratio is low (e.g., 180/60 = 3.0) the risk of CAD is low; but when the ratio goes up (e.g., 240/40 = 6) the risk climbs. The ratio holds up as a predictor in spite of the absolute level of cholesterol. In other words, a cholesterol level of 240 is more dangerous when the HDL is low and less dangerous when HDL is high (e.g., 240/75 = 3.2). As the ratio climbs above 4.0 the risk increases, and when it exceeds 6.0 the risk becomes serious. Use a low-fat diet to lower total cholesterol, and exercise and weight loss to raise HDL cholesterol.

Cholesterol Summary.   Serum cholesterol is directly related to heart disease risk; it can be reduced significantly (up to 25%) with a moderate- to low-fat diet. Several years ago, after a good friend had a coronary bypass operation, I embarked on a serious low-fat diet. In 6 weeks I was able to lower my cholesterol more than 20%. Of course I lost body fat during the period, and *weight loss is highly related to improvements in HDL cholesterol.* Although the diet and weight loss probably did the most good, resumption of three or more meals per day probably helped as well, because cholesterol levels are higher with fewer meals. Why do cholesterol levels decline when the same calories are eaten in three or more meals? Probably because the body is better able to handle fat in small doses. Large doses lead to accumulation of fat and inhibition of LDL receptors. Conversely, oat bran, apples, and other foods lower serum cholesterol levels.

Exercise contributes by raising HDL, burning fat, and lowering body weight and the percentage of body fat. More importantly, exercise influences the ratio of HDL to total cholesterol, thereby providing a significant reduction in the risk of atherosclerosis. By combining a prudent low-fat, low-cholesterol diet with moderate exercise, you will achieve a significant reduction in heart disease risk.

Future editions of this book will continue to chronicle the unfolding story of the role of diet and exercise in the reduction of heart disease risk. Future research will document how subfractions of HDL and LDL contribute and how each can be altered. But don't wait for that information. Ample evidence supports the value of the low-fat diet and exercise in the fight against CAD.

Psychological Factors

For years, we have known that stress contributes to heart disease risk. It is possible that CAD may somehow be related to a lifestyle, a behavior pattern becoming ever more prevalent in our society. Friedman and Rosenman (1973) characterized a distinctive personality complex, behavior Type A, which includes extreme competitiveness, ambition, and a profound sense of time urgency. In their studies, men with Type A behavior had a higher serum cholesterol level and a faster clotting time than did their more relaxed counterparts. In spite of similar dietary and exercise habits, the Type A subjects had a sevenfold greater incidence of CAD.

Friedman and Rosenman reported an alarming number of sudden deaths among men diagnosed as Type A. Half of the victims had exercised strenuously within 6 hr of a large meal. The researchers hypothesized that the victims may have carried their competitiveness and time urgency into their leisure activities. Some of the deaths occurred after competitive handball and tennis matches or after jogging. The deaths frequently occurred after a large meal, when serum lipid levels inhibit fibrinolytic activity and when the demands of digestion compromise the blood supply to the heart.

Friedman and Rosenman's data reveal another simple fact: Half of the sudden deaths had *nothing whatsoever* to do with exercise—some deaths occurred in bed, others in the bathroom. Newspapers seem eager to carry stories concerning heart attacks associated with exercise and perhaps exaggerate the risk of sudden death during exercise. Friedman's data may indicate that some Type A individuals are more likely to exercise than non–Type A people and are more likely to exercise within 6 hr of a meal, but the data don't point to the exercise itself as a cause for heart attack.

Although most of us intuitively accept stress as a risk factor, the Framingham study failed to find a link between stress and heart disease risk (Wilson, Castelli, & Kannel, 1987). And there are indications that *anger and repressed hostility* are far more related to heart disease and that Type A behavior in the absence of anger and hostility does not pose a problem. Whatever the case, Glasser (1976) and others suggest that an enjoyable interlude of physical activity may improve our reaction to the stresses of life. If in fact exercise does improve our reaction to psychic stress, reduce tension, and alter the physiologic manifestations associated with CAD, this aspect of exercise may be one of its most important contributions. (See chapter 13 to learn more about stress and the tranquilizing effects of exercise.)

The Future

Since 1968 the cardiovascular death rate has declined more than 20%. Several hundred thousand fewer deaths occur annually than would have been predicted by the grim statistics of 1968. Yet atherosclerosis is still the leading cause of death in the United States. This degenerative disease, called a disease of lifestyle, has responded to the changes people are making in their lives. Although some of the decline may be attributed to improved coronary care and heart surgery, some must also be due to changes in risk factors such as diet, blood pressure, serum cholesterol levels, cigarette smoking, stress, obesity, and physical inactivity.

Business and industry have instituted employee health or wellness programs that analyze individual health risks and encourage improvements. Health and fitness clubs have proliferated, aerobic dance classes overflow, and millions now walk, run, cycle, swim, and cross-country ski. Health articles appear in magazines of all kinds, television shows encourage diet and exercise, and computer programs are available to monitor your diet, exercise, and overall health risk.

Young adults now have the opportunity to avoid the period of inactivity that characterized previous generations. Middle-aged athletes participate in age group competitions, and senior citizens remain active far longer. With all this comes an increase in life expectancy that promises nonsmoking men and women 80 or more full productive years.

And some think that the greatest decline in degenerative diseases is still to come. Continued interest in health and the quality of life could further reduce the risks and costs of degenerative diseases. In light of new approaches to education (e.g., smoking cessation, stress reduction, and behavior therapy) and advances in the prevention and treatment of disease, the future looks good for those who decide to take *personal responsibility* for their health.

A physician cannot keep you from getting sick; that is your responsibility. And pouring more money into treating those who continue to smoke or ignore basic health habits will not reduce the impact of degenerative diseases but will only continue to increase the skyrocketing cost of (so-called) health care. It is time to focus on *prevention*, on *personal responsibility*, and on *cost-effective approaches* to risk reduction. It's also time to focus on the cornerstone of health and wellness—physical activity and fitness. Only you can decide to reduce health risks and costs and to be a contributor instead of a burden to the system.

There is growing awareness that *many of the risk factors associated with CAD originate during childhood* as poor lifestyle or health habits. Many authorities believe that major gains in the war against CAD will be achieved when risk factor modification begins as early as elementary school. In spite of the growing evidence in this area, school fitness and health programs suffer for lack of support. It seems likely that a few dollars spent at this level could save many thousands in future health care costs. Does your school system have a fitness and health program that gets results?

Adults, be they parents, big brothers and sisters, or even grandparents, are role models for kids. If you are concerned about the youth and their health, be a role model for the active lifestyle and all that goes with it (such as a prudent diet, avoidance of smoking, and maintenance of desirable body weight). Plan family outings that involve activity; go on hikes, runs, bike rides, and canoe trips. Involve your kids in your activity and become involved in theirs. Help them establish habits that will insure their health and vitality.

CHAPTER

13

THE PSYCHOLOGY OF FITNESS

This chapter will help you

>*see how mental health can influence physical health,*
>
>*consider ways in which fitness and personality interrelate,*
>
>*understand motivation in physical activity,*
>
>*understand perception of effort, and*
>
>*learn about methods of relaxation.*

Join me for a journey beyond the comfortable landscape of physiology into the fascinating but hazy realm of psychology, where we will seek clues to the relationship of fitness and mental health. I can't promise many answers, but I can assure you that the questions are worth asking.

Mental health may be defined as feeling good about yourself and life in general. A common reply to the question, "Why do you exercise?" is simply that it feels good. Of course a bout of overly strenuous exercise can be uncomfortable, but regular, moderate exercise just feels good. Let's examine some of the reasons why this should be so and why exercise may be good for psychological and physical health.

Stress

The emotional response to events in life is mediated by structures in the brain, including the hypothalmus. When something excites or threatens us, the hypothalmus reacts and tells the anterior pituitary gland to secrete adrenocorticotropic hormones (ACTH), a chemical messenger that travels to the adrenal gland and orders release of hormones called glucocorticoids. These hormones are necessary for the body's response to stressful situations. Without them the body cannot deal with stress, and it collapses and dies.

Stressful situations also elicit a response in the sympathetic nervous system that leads to secretion of other hormones from the adrenal gland, including adrenaline (or epinephrine). These hormones mobilize energy and support the cardiovascular response to the stressor. In terms of exercise, unfamiliar, competitive, and exhaustive events are stressful; that is, they elicit the hormonal response. However, studies show that prior experience with exercise (training) minimizes the stress response (Docktor & Sharkey, 1971). So regular moderate activity is not stressful for humans. In fact, evidence shows that exercise can reduce other forms of stress (e.g., psychosocial) and that improved fitness may minimize the impact of future stressors (Whiddon, 1969).

The stress response is not necessarily unhealthy. It is needed to prepare the body for maximal effort in a race or some other physical challenge. But it can be unhealthy when it occurs in the wrong setting, such as the office. If you become stressed on the job when a natural physical catharsis is impossible or improper, the circulating hormones can be a problem. Some theorize that a bout of exercise (such as running or weight lifting) could minimize problems associated with stress.

Stress has been hard to study because it depends on the individual's response to a situation. One person's stress may be another's excitement. It is likely that the response to stressors is learned and can be unlearned. If a difficult co-worker causes distress, try to find ways to take him or her less seriously. If that doesn't work, try some physical activity.

Stress, tension, and associated personality patterns have been linked with ulcers, hypertension, heart disease, suppression of the immune system, and a variety of other ills that plague modern society. Stress exists when any of a multitude of possible changes either outside or inside the body pose a threat to the body or mind. Selye (1956) found that many possible stressors, including extremes in heat or cold, toxins or infections, trauma, shock, fever, emotional disturbances, and even exhausting physical effort, elicited a fairly consistent series of reactions, which he called the **general adaptation syndrome** and which includes these three phases.

GENERAL ADAPTATION SYNDROME

Alarm stage: The stressor causes initial nervous and circulatory depression, followed by ACTH secretion and the development of resistance to the stressor.

Resistance stage: Full resistance to the stressor is developed as ACTH promotes secretion of hormones from the adrenal cortex. The hormones assist in mobilizing energy and aid the hormones of the adrenal medulla (epinephrine and norepinephrine) in accomplishing their circulatory and metabolic responses to stress.

Exhaustion stage: High levels of adrenal cortical hormones eventually over-tax digestive, circulatory, and immune systems. Ulcers, adrenal hypertrophy, and a reduced resistance to infection indicate imminent exhaustion, shock, and even death.

Selye's theory goes on to suggest that regular exposure to one stressor, such as physical activity, may increase the ability to resist another, such as an emotional problem or even infection. This very appealing theory lacks hard evidence from human subjects, and common sense suggests that vigorous physical training is unlikely to protect one in times of severe emotional unrest (although it certainly seems to help).

The theory is difficult to prove for humans because each of us reacts differently to a stressor. Vigorous exercise may be stressful for the sedentary and relaxing for the fit. A dangerous mountain climb will be stressful for the neophyte and stimulating for the veteran. Exercise can be stressful when it is competitive, unfamiliar, or exhaustive. Fitness training will undoubtedly make exercise more familiar and less exhaustive, and months or years of competition will help us cope with its excitement.

As for the use of fitness training in the protection against infection, the evidence is only beginning to accumulate. It does seem as though fit individuals are less likely to catch the common cold and related infections, and if they do get them they are quick to recover. But little hard evidence exists to support this prejudice. Distance runners may avoid infection because they stay away from crowds, or because they get more rest or a better diet. On the other hand, the exercise may improve resistance to other stressors that lower resistance directly (e.g., infection) or indirectly (e.g., emotional disturbance). Physically fit individuals are less likely to become exhausted, and this reduces the likelihood of infection. And training itself has been shown to reduce the likelihood of infection, even in the presence of fatigue. So there are reasons to support regular physical activity as a means of reducing stress and related problems.

Psychoneuroimmunology

This imposing new field studies links between the brain and nervous system and the immune system, hence the term **psychoneuroimmunology** (PNI). It focuses on how thoughts, emotions, and personality traits interact with the immune system and become manifest in sickness or health. The brain seems to have the capability to influence the immune system; thoughts and emotions can enhance or suppress the immune response. The brain may influence the immune system via neurotransmitters secreted by neurons of the sympathetic nervous system or via hormones released upon command of the brain.

The immune system is immensely complicated, consisting of lymphocytes, T cells, antibodies, immunoglobulins, and more; it serves to protect the body from foreign assaults. When exposed to prolonged stress, the system tends to break down, allowing invading microorganisms to take control. Stress is a reaction to events that leads to increased secretion of hormones. PNI suggests that by altering your perception of the event you can reduce the stress response and spare the immune system. Although you may not be able to will your way to health as some suggest, a positive attitude may indeed reduce the hormonal response that interferes with the function of the immune system.

Studies are now underway to determine the influence of exercise and fitness on the functions of the immune system. Early results suggest an improvement in the body's ability to produce infection-fighting T cells through fitness training. But although it is too early to determine the full effect of activity on the system, we do know that exercise can either cause or reduce stress. Overly strenuous endurance training or competition is a stressor that suppresses some markers of immune response. Stress hormones suppress the immune system, so things that reduce stress may protect the system and allow optimal function. Though the role of exercise is yet to be defined, we do know that regular moderate physical activity helps manage stress.

The commitment to exercise is a positive coping strategy that helps reduce depression, anxiety, hostility, anger, or other negative emotions that release stress hormones that can suppress T cells, immunoglobulins, and other aspects of the immune system. Exercise, imagery, relaxation, and other positive coping strategies help you deal in a rational way with difficult problems, thereby freeing the immune system to function on your behalf.

Personality and Fitness

All of us are amateur psychologists; we feel competent to judge individuals in terms of personality. As with art, we may not know much about the subject, but we know what we like. Personality is a frame of reference used by psychologists in the study of behavior. Personality is more than a mask but less than reality; it is a product of heredity and the environment. Psychologists study personality with paper-and-pencil tests or in-depth interviews, but they have never really defined or measured it. That should not deter scientists in their search. The day may come when we are able to define and measure this elusive concept of personality and thus understand, predict, or even improve behavior and health.

Cattell, who suggested that one's personality indicates what one will do when in a given mood and placed in a given situation, developed the Cattell 16-Personality Factor Questionnaire, a personality test that is used widely by researchers (Cattell, Eber, & Tatsuoka, 1970). The test, typical of the paper-and-pencil approach, presumes to score the subject on each of 16 factors or personality "traits" (see Table 13.1). If we assume that this approach is adequate, we can use it to consider how fitness and personality are related.

Table 13.1 Cattell's Sixteen Personality Factors

Low score description	Personality factors	High score description
Aloof, cold	A	Warm, sociable
Dull, low capacity	B	Bright, intelligent
Emotional, unstable	C	Mature, calm
Submissive, mild	E	Dominant, aggressive
Glum, silent	F	Enthusiastic, talkative
Casual, undependable	G	Conscientious, persistent
Timid, shy	H	Adventurous, "thick-skinned"
Tough, realistic	I	Sensitive, effeminate
Trustful, adaptable	L	Suspecting, jealous
Conventional, practical	M	Bohemian, unconcerned
Simple, awkward	N	Sophisticated, polished
Confident, unshakable	Q	Insecure, anxious
Conservative, accepting	Q_1	Experimenting, critical
Dependent, imitative	Q_2	Self-sufficient, resourceful
Lax, unsure	Q_3	Controlled, exact
Phlegmatic, composed	Q_4	Tense, excitable

Note. From *Handbook for the Sixteen Personality Factor Questionnaire* by R.B. Cattell, H.W. Eber, and M.M. Tatsuoka, 1970, Champaign, IL: Institute for Personality and Ability Testing.

Using the Cattell questionnaire, studies of the personalities of middle-aged men conducted at Purdue University showed that highly fit subjects are more unconventional, composed, secure, easygoing, emotionally stable, adventurous, and higher in intelligence than the low-fitness subjects. The most pronounced personality differences were those related to emotional stability and security. However, the presence of differences between high- and low-fitness groups does not prove that the differences are due to fitness. It could be that in our culture, at this time in history, emotionally stable and secure people are more likely to engage in a fitness program. In fact, when Purdue's researchers studied the effects of a 4-month fitness program on these same subjects, little personality change was noted among the low-fitness subjects, in spite of a conspicuous improvement in fitness. The researchers reasoned that it takes years to become fit or unfit, and that a few months of activity is insufficient to bring about significant personality changes (Ismail & Young, 1977).

Longitudinal studies are necessary to confirm or reject the hypothesis that personality improves with fitness. Meanwhile, we should note that Ismail and Young (1977) found that their subjects did become significantly more conscientious, persistent, and controlled after 4 months of training.

Many studies have attempted to isolate personality traits that differentiate athletes and nonathletes. Does athletic participation influence or alter the personality? The current point of view is that it does not. Rather, those with "acceptable" personality traits are more likely to persist and succeed than those with less acceptable traits. Therefore, the effect of sports and fitness on the quality called personality remains unsettled.

Improving Self-Concept

Your personality undoubtedly has an effect on others, and the way they respond to you influences how you feel about yourself. Does an improvement in fitness influence your self-concept? Before studying the question, we should understand how self-concept is defined and measured. One widely used test of self-concept employs 100 statements and a 5-point answering scale to determine components of self-concept (personal self, physical self, social self, moral and ethical self, and family self). You might not expect improved fitness to alter all the scales, but changes in physical self and personal self seem possible.

I have noted changes in these scales as a result of *significant* improvements in fitness—improvements that took several years to achieve. The most notable change, as expected, is found in the physical self, or body image. When you lose weight and improve your muscular strength, endurance, aerobic fitness, and appearance, you feel better about your body. This new confidence could influence personality traits or other aspects of your self-concept. When middle-aged male subjects in a research study discussed the influence of a fitness program on their personal lives, many volunteered that they had experienced an improvement in their sex lives. As fitness improves, body image is enhanced, and this renewed confidence in the body can be an important step to improved personal relationships.

Possible Influences on Personality

The influence of fitness on the personality is far from established. But for the sake of argument, let's consider some ways in which improved fitness may help you to feel better about yourself and your life.

Anxiety Reduction. The anxious person is troubled, worried, and uneasy because of thoughts and fears about what may happen. Anxiety and worry are forms of negative mental imagery that can influence the immune system. Anxiety dissipates as one takes command of a situation. Regular participation in a fitness program is a positive approach to life. When highly anxious individuals participate regularly, their anxiety is reduced. Those with average or low levels of anxiety do not experience a similar reduction as a result of participation (Morgan & Goldston, 1987). In recent years running has even been used successfully in the treatment of depression.

Tranquilizing Effect.　One study compared a single session of exercise to a tranquilizer to see which was more relaxing. The exercise was more effective in reducing neuromuscular tension. Moreover, the exercise (15 min of walking at a heart rate of 100) produced no undesirable side effects (deVries & Adams, 1972). In view of the tranquilizing effect of exercise, it is distressing to see how often nursing homes, mental health facilities, and other institutions resort to the use of drugs, which impair motor coordination and encourage a passive existence. Exercise improves coordination and function and leads to an active, healthy lifestyle. Moderate exercise even helps people fall asleep.

Blood Sugar.　I have noted how fitness training improves the ability to mobilize and metabolize fat, thereby conserving blood sugar for use by the brain and nervous system. Low levels of blood sugar certainly can affect behavior adversely. On the other hand, fit people have more energy, they accomplish more, and they have a more positive outlook. The conservation of blood sugar may be part of the explanation for the effect of fitness on personality and mental health.

Nerve tissue is almost entirely dependent on the oxidation of blood sugar (glucose) for its energy supply. This means that the brain and nervous system require a constant supply of glucose. Low blood glucose levels (hypoglycemia) adversely affect behavior and performance. Blood glucose rises after a meal and then drops until it reaches a normal resting level (about 80 mg). Thereafter the liver strives to maintain that level, at least until its supply is depleted.

The symptoms of low blood sugar (see Table 13.2) indicate the influence of low blood sugar on behavior. My son used to evidence some of the symptoms when he hadn't eaten for many hours, but a snack always restored his good spirits. And I recall a day when my tennis game went to pieces. I lost my temper, cursed,

Table 13.2　Common Symptoms of Hypoglycemia

Nervousness	Anxiety
Irritability	Confusion
Exhaustion	Rapid pulse
Faintness, dizziness	Muscle pains
Tremor, cold sweat	Indecisiveness
Depression	Lack of coordination
Vertigo	Lack of concentration
Drowsiness	Blurred vision
Headaches	

threw my racket, and became enraged. Eventually, I realized that it was midafternoon, that I had not eaten lunch, and that I had eaten breakfast in the early morning. I apologized to my opponent and rushed off to find some nourishment.

Muscles can use blood sugar as an energy source, so long runs, bike rides, or hikes certainly can lead to hypoglycemia. Fruit, protein, or mixed protein and carbohydrate snacks are recommended to refuel the blood. Sugar snacks such as doughnuts or candy bars lead to a big boost of blood sugar, but they also call forth a large secretion of insulin. The insulin speeds the sugar out of the bloodstream, and within a couple of hours one begins to sag again (reactive hypoglycemia). To avoid the problem simply eat at regular intervals and use nonsugary snacks when necessary to maintain blood sugar levels.

Positive Addiction. In his book *Positive Addiction*, Dr. William Glasser (1976) contrasts positive and negative addictions. Negative additions such as drugs or alcohol relieve pain of failure and provide temporary pleasure but at a terrible cost in terms of family, social, and professional life. Positive addictions lead to psychological strength, imagination, and creativity.

A positive addiction can be any activity you choose, so long as it meets the following criteria:

- **It is noncompetitive.**
- **You do it for approximately an hour each day.**
- **You find it easy to do, and it doesn't take a great deal of mental effort.**
- **You can do it alone or occasionally with others, but you don't rely on others to do it.**
- **You believe that it has some mental, physical, or spiritual value.**
- **You believe that if you persist you will improve at it.**
- **You can do it without criticizing yourself.**

Dr. Glasser suggests that as one participates in meditation, yoga, or running, he or she eventually achieves the state of positive addiction. When this state is achieved, the mind is free to become more imaginative or creative. The mind conceives more options in solving difficult or frustrating problems; it has more strength. Proof of addiction comes when you are forced to neglect your habit, and guilt and anxiety characterize withdrawal from your addiction. In the chapter entitled "Running—The Hardest but Surest Way," Dr. Glasser suggests that running, perhaps because it is our most basic solitary survival activity, produces the non–self-critical state more effectively than any other practice. He recommends running to all, from the weakest to the strongest. He feels that once one can run an hour without fatigue, it is almost certain that the positive addiction state will be achieved on a fairly regular basis. How long this will take depends upon the person, but if competition is avoided and the runner runs alone in a pleasant setting, addiction should occur within the year.

I realized that I was addicted to running long before Dr. Glasser wrote his book; it took far less than a year to achieve. Since I've become a runner, I feel more confident and effective, and I've been more successful. Is all that just a happy coincidence, or is it evidence of the effect of exercise and fitness on my mental health?

Negative Addiction. A sport psychologist and friend of mine, Dr. William Morgan, has mentioned over the years that he worries about runners who become addicted to their sport. He warns that some may devote so much time to running that they begin to neglect family and work. I have seen examples of negative addiction to running, but they were often confounded by other problems, such as recent alcoholism. For my part I'd prefer a negative addiction to running over an addiction to alcohol or drugs. The running may alter family relationships and work performance, but so does drug or alcohol abuse, and running isn't likely to destroy the body and the mind. The obsession with running may be a form of therapy, just as it is for anxiety and depression.

The Psychology of Motivation

Almost half of all adult Americans fail to engage in any form of regular exercise. Among those who do exercise, only a very small percentage do so in such a way as to bring about an improvement in fitness. The rest lack the interest or motivation necessary to ensure regular participation. Let's examine the psychology of motivation in hopes of finding ways to motivate ourselves and our friends. Motivation involves the *arousal* and *direction* of behavior.

Arousal of Behavior

Physiological motives or drives are triggered by basic biological needs such as food, water, elimination, and sex. Safety and health needs—to be safe from threat, to be secure—are next in the hierarchy of human motives or needs. Then come love and belonging, needs involving genuine affection and a place in one's group. Next in the hierarchy are the esteem needs—to be liked and respected and to respect oneself. At the top of the hierarchy is the need for self-actualization, to realize one's potential (Maslow, 1954). Any of these needs may serve to arouse an individual to action.

Direction of Behavior

The direction of behavior, that is, where and how one behaves when aroused, is a complex study involving a multitude of learned behaviors and the interaction of these behaviors with ever-varying situations. Kenyon (1968) attempted to categorize the reasons why individuals engage in physical activity; he identified socializing, health and fitness, vertigo (the thrill of speed and change of direction while remaining in control), aesthetics (the beauty of movement), catharsis (relief from stress and tension), and asceticism (self-denial, discipline, and training). Many forms of activity may satisfy an individual's needs. One could walk, jog, run, swim, or cycle for health and fitness. The direction chosen will depend on the level of arousal, previous exercise experiences, and just a little bit of chance.

Before I moved west over 25 years ago, I had never seen a pair of skis, let alone a real mountain. Somehow I was motivated to give skiing a try, probably because many of the people I knew were skiers. It didn't take long to realize that skiing was for me. Soon I was doing it—not for belonging or esteem but because it felt good and was a way to test myself and find my potential. Now I am hopelessly hooked, positively addicted.

Intrinsic or self-directed goals are more effective in long-term motivation and adherence to exercise. Extrinsic or external sources of motivation may arouse and direct efforts to win a prize, medal, trophy, or scholarship, but the motivation necessary to persist, to ensure lifelong participation in an active lifestyle, must come from within, from the upper reaches of the hierarchy of human needs (self-respect and self-actualization). Consider all the ex-athletes who lose interest in their sport when the glory fades and the medals tarnish. Then look at your habitually active friends, the runners, tennis and racquetball players, and skiers. What keeps them going? Do they seek health, a trophy, or a championship? They most likely go out each day because they must, because they are addicted. They go out to be themselves, and in the process they come closer to their potential. (For more on motivation and exercise adherence see Dishman, 1988.)

Perceived Exertion

Physiologists, coaches, and teachers once ignored comments from subjects or students regarding the difficulty of exertion, reasoning that personal perceptions of effort were too subjective, too prone to error and variation. When subjects said they were pooped, that they couldn't go on, they were told, "Don't be silly, of course you can."

But Swedish psychologist Dr. Gunnar Borg changed all that when he developed his ratings of perceived exertion (see Table 13.3). Borg (1973) realized that the sensory stimuli generated during physical effort are integrated by the brain into a perception of effort; the brain perceives and evaluates respiratory distress, pain, the sensation of a pounding heart, and stimuli from muscles. Subsequent studies have shown that these subjective estimates of effort are highly related to work load, heart rate, oxygen consumption, and even lactic acid and hormones. In other words, our subjective estimate of work intensity provides a rather accurate estimate of the load itself, as well as of the internal factors affected by the work.

Table 13.3 Perceived Exertion

How does the exercise feel?	Rating
	6
Very, very light	7
	8
Very light	9
	10
Fairly light	11
	12
Somewhat hard	13
	14
Hard	15
	16
Very hard	17
	18
Very, very hard	19
	20

Note. Rating × 10 is approximately equal to the heart rate (e.g., "somewhat hard" = 13 × 10 or 130). From "Perceived Exertion: A Note on History and Methods" by G. Borg, 1973, *Medicine and Science in Sports, 5*, p. 91.

Because we are able to accurately judge our effort in an exercise such as cycling or running, and because the heart rate and metabolic cost of the effort are closely related to those ratings, we should be more inclined to "listen to ourselves" during exercise. If the exercise feels too difficult, it probably is. The use of the heart rate training zone in exercise prescription is an attempt to employ important physiological criteria in the determination of a safe and effective dosage of exercise. You may find that running at your training heart rate feels "somewhat hard." Thereafter, you can use that sense of difficulty to guide your exertion. If high temperatures cause your heart rate to rise, your perception of exertion will adjust your pace to a more prudent level.

While I'm on the subject of perceived exertion, I want to spend a moment on the concept of **preferred exertion**. Experienced exercisers seem to require a certain level of exertion to be satisfied. If the exertion is either too easy or too difficult, it diminishes their sense of satisfaction. Training increases the amount of exertion preferred, whereas inactivity lowers it. Those who have been involved in highly competitive sports often seem to prefer a high level of exertion. They have erroneously learned that exercise has to *hurt* to be good, and they believe in the saying, *No pain, no gain* (which is also untrue). Therefore, when they resume activity after a long layoff, they often overdo and end up with severe soreness or an injury.

Preferred exertion is learned; most Americans prefer little more than walking to and from the car. This could be different. If schools and parents demonstrated and encouraged sensible and inexpensive exercise habits, more kids would grow up with a predisposition to exercise. Elementary, high school, and even college students can be encouraged to prepare for and participate in activities like running. If parents become involved, kids will soon make activity a family affair. Communities and organizations like the YMCA sponsor distance runs, bike rides, and ski tours for which participation is the major goal.

Some years ago, one of our local banks decided to sponsor a road race and advertised the upcoming race for weeks to allow people to prepare. Participation was encouraged in several ways: race T-shirts, certificates of participation, prizes, and a postrace lunch with beer, soda pop, and sandwiches. Bank officials were astonished to see more than 400 runners line up for the race. Now, years later, the race has grown to an annual event attracting more than 1,500 runners, who come out to test themselves over the 7-mi course and to share the event with fellow runners.

Perception of Quality

Psychologists and sensory physiologists have long known how to measure the quantity of stimuli (e.g., sound, light, and exertion). It is far more difficult to assess the *quality* of an experience, yet the quality of an exercise experience is likely to bring us back for more. Ask someone to rate the quality of an exercise experience, and he or she will respond with a long-winded evaluation of the conditions—the weather, the companions, personal sensations, and expectations. Many factors are involved in the quality of an exercise experience.

A creek-side distance run on a tree-shaded path amid the beauty of the mountains is an experience to be savored and long remembered. Cover the same distance on a short, crowded running track in a steamy gym and the experience becomes an ordeal, unless, of course, you are with company you enjoy or are glad for the chance to get away from the office.

You can control the factors that enhance the quality of your exercise experiences. If you abhor noisy, crowded public tennis courts and constantly are bothered by players who either don't know or don't practice the etiquette of the sport, build your own court, join a private club, play before the crowds arrive, or encourage the city recreation department to teach court etiquette.

Your exercise experiences will be more enjoyable if you follow these guidelines.

- **Be flexible. Don't depend on one activity, time, or place for satisfaction.**
- **Plan ahead. Plan your participation, your companions, the time of day, and the place. If the afternoon winds diminish the quality of tennis, plan to play in the morning.**

- **Don't set unrealistic goals.** If you set out to run 10 mi on a hot, humid day and don't finish, you may feel you've failed, but you haven't. You've merely set an unrealistic goal.
- **Recognize your moods.** We all get depressed, concerned, and worried. Sometimes exercise can help you calm down when you're too excited or pick you up when you're depressed; but a really foul mood can ruin a friendly game.
- **Be prepared.** Get adequate rest, eat sensibly so you don't become fatigued, bring extra food or drink if it may be needed, keep your equipment in good condition, and have extra parts available.
- **Learn to relax.** (See the next section.)

It is up to you to enhance the quality of your exercise experiences. If your daily activity is satisfying, it may bubble over and affect other phases of life. If it isn't, you may feel cheated, lose interest in the activity, and quit. In that case, you will be the loser.

Relaxation Techniques

Learn to relax. It sounds simple, but that oft-given advice has been terribly difficult to follow until recently. Now, thanks to two very different books, it is easy to learn.

Years ago, Edmund Jacobson (1938) recognized the relationships among anxiety, stress, and neuromuscular tension. He measured the activity of skeletal muscles to determine neuromuscular tension, then he taught subjects to recognize this tension and relax it, thereby achieving reduced anxiety and psychological tension. In classes and through his book *Progressive Relaxation*, Jacobson taught thousands to relax.

The subject of relaxation did not receive a great deal of additional scientific attention until recently. The popularity of Eastern mystics and gurus and the commercial promotion of various meditative techniques prompted a renewed interest in relaxation research. Dr. Herbet Benson (1975) studied meditation and its outcomes and concluded that most systems were essentially similar. In his popular book *The Relaxation Response*, Benson outlined the essence of the method: Sit in a comfortable chair in a quiet room for 20 min and repeat a simple sound (sometimes called a mantra) such as "one" each time you exhale (use the word "easy" and apply the principles of relaxation in your sport). Do this daily or twice daily, and you certainly will become more relaxed. As for the health benefits claimed by the proponents of transcendental meditation, you may experience a reduction in heart rate and an insignificant reduction in blood pressure and metabolic rate (you may burn slightly fewer calories while meditating). More important will be the reduction in tension and stress. Of course, as Glasser (1976) notes, you can achieve similar benefits by running an equivalent amount of time each day, which guarantees the substantial health benefits of exercise as well.

Whereas Jacobson's method involves a physical approach to achieve mental relaxation, Benson's does the opposite. Concentration on the mantra or the breathing rate frees the mind of disturbing thoughts, and the body relaxes. And as one becomes more proficient at the technique, he or she may achieve the state of positive addiction—a transcendent state of relaxation, clear thought, imagery, well-being, and openness. Is meditation a substitute for exercise? Not at all. It is a way to achieve relaxation and, perhaps, positive addiction but will not induce the many physiological changes that result from regular physical activity. For some, activity may be as effective as meditation in the achievement of relaxation and positive addiction. If you are anxious, worried, or tense, exercise— and learn to relax.

Somatopsychic Effect

Everyone is familiar with the concept of psychosomatic illness, which implies physical illness caused or exacerbated by psychological factors. But you seldom hear the term **somatopsychic**, which implies the effect of the body on the mind. This chapter indicates ways in which the right amount of exercise can have a beneficial effect on the mind, or how mental health can be enhanced via physical activity. Research in this area is in its infancy.

Runner's High

Several years ago there was a flurry of interest in the concept of the runner's high, a trancelike state reported by many runners during and after a long run. The interest grew when researchers found increased levels of beta endorphins in the blood of distance runners after a marathon. Runners were quick to speculate that these morphinelike chemicals were responsible for the sensation known as the runner's high. Although blood endorphin levels are elevated during and after an endurance effort, subsequent studies showed that the levels do not correlate with the perceived sensations or moods (Markoff, Ryan, & Young, 1982).

Endorphins

Endorphins are natural opiates (narcotics) that are secreted by nerve cells in the brain. It isn't surprising that blood levels and moods might not correlate, because a blood-brain barrier prevents easy transport between the two. Hence blood levels of endorphins do not tell us what is happening with endorphins in the brain, where moods are formed. The increased levels in the blood are probably a reflection of another function of endorphins, their ability to *kill pain*. Experienced runners report that running feels easier after the first 20 min, which is just about how long endorphin levels take to increase. So if you've tried running and found it uncomfortable, try to last 20 min or more. You may find it becomes easier with the help of your natural painkillers.

Coping Strategies

The underlying theme throughout this chapter is that physical activity can serve as a positive coping strategy. This theme has implications for health and for adherence to health behaviors.

Locus of Control

This concept separates people into **internals**, those who believe they can control outcomes in their lives, and **externals**, who believe their lives are controlled by chance or by others. Internal controllers may be more likely to adhere to healthy behaviors, whereas externals may be less likely. Can the locus of control be influenced or changed to insure adherence to healthy behavior, such as regular activity?

Self-Efficacy

This theory suggests that coping behavior is influenced by the perception of acquiring mastery in that area. Perception of mastery influences performance and, some theorize that experience alters this perception. Thus successful experience may reinforce a coping behavior (such as weight loss or running), leading to continuation of the behavior. Some have even suggested that enhanced self-efficacy in one behavior may generalize to others.

Although research has yet to prove the validity and effect of these theories, they provide a new way to study exercise and other coping strategies. For more information consult Dishman's book *Exercise Adherence* (1988).

In this chapter I've attempted to show how thoughts, feelings, and actions can influence moods and health itself. Thoughts appear to influence hormones just as hormones can influence thoughts. Therefore, the way you think about a person, event, or even yourself will automatically influence physiological responses. Negative thoughts lead to negative feelings and can influence performance and health. Used properly, exercise can be a **positive coping strategy** that puts control back in your own hands. Exercise can reduce anxiety and depression, serve as a tranquilizer, and help you fall asleep. Months of training may improve your body image and self-concept and could improve your personality and the way you view life. Give it a try!

CHAPTER

14

EXERCISE AND THE ENVIRONMENT

This chapter will help you

anticipate the effects of the environment on performance and health,

take appropriate steps to minimize environmental effects, and

understand how fitness enhances your ability to acclimatize and work in difficult situations.

Environmental factors such as temperature, humidity, altitude, and air pollution have profound effects on health and performance. Failure to consider these effects can lead to serious problems, even death. On the other hand, it is entirely possible to adjust to the environment, enabling you to perform well and comfortably under a wide range of conditions. Let's consider the problems caused by extremes of temperature, humidity, altitude, and air pollution to see how fitness and proper planning can minimize their effects.

Heat Stress

At rest, metabolic heat production amounts to about 1.2 calories per minute, or 72 calories per hour. Moderate exercise can elevate heat production to 600 calories or more per hour. You can see that exercise by itself can create considerable heat. Normally, the heat is lost by convection, radiation, or evaporation of sweat, but when exercise is performed in a hot environment or when the humidity is high, metabolic heat cannot be dissipated, and the body temperature rises. **Heat cramps** occur when considerable salt is lost in the sweat. Take lightly salted fluids and use stretching and massage to relieve the cramp. **Heat exhaustion** occurs when the heat stress exceeds the capacity of the temperature-regulating mechanism. The individual with cold, pale skin, a weak pulse, and dizziness should drink fluids and rest in a cool environment. **Heat stroke** means that the temperature-regulating mechanism has given up. The skin is flushed, hot, and dry, sweating stops, and the body temperature may rise above 106 °F. *Heat stroke can lead to permanent damage*, especially to the temperature-regulating center of the brain, or even to death. *Heat stroke is a medical emergency.*

Temperature Regulation

The temperature-regulating mechanism of the body consists of three parts:

1. a regulating center located in the hypothalamus that acts like a thermostat to maintain body temperature at or near 37 °C (98.6 °F),
2. regulators such as muscles that increase body heat by shivering, or vasomotor controls that constrict or dilate arterioles to conserve or lose body heat, and
3. heat and cold receptors located in the skin to sense changes in environmental temperature conditions.

The regulating center responds to the temperature of the blood flowing by the hypothalamus. If the blood cools, the thermostat sends information to conserve heat loss by constriction of blood vessels in the skin. Shivering can also generate some heat.

If the blood temperature rises above the desired level (sometimes called a set point), the regulating center can cause dilation of cutaneous (skin) blood vessels and also stimulate the production of sweat. Consequently, blood is brought from the warmer core of the body to the surface, allowing heat loss by conduction, convection, and radiation, as well as by evaporation of sweat from the surface of the skin. Note that *complete* evaporation of 1 L of sweat leads to a 540-calorie heat loss. However, if the sweat drips off the body, little heat is lost.

Heat and cold receptors in the skin also aid in the maintenance of body temperature. The cold of the ski slopes causes constriction of blood vessels, especially in the hands and feet. The extremities will stay cold until you elevate the body temperature, warm the blood, and reopen the blood vessels. This can best be done by vigorous exercise. You also can put on more clothing or seek relief in the lodge.

The stifling heat of the tennis court causes vasodilation that diverts a significant amount of blood from the muscles to the surface of the skin. The heart rate increases in an effort to maintain blood flow to the working muscles. Sweating eventually reduces blood volume, and unless the water is replaced, your performance will suffer. If you persist in the activity and fail to replace the water loss, you may end up with heat exhaustion or heatstroke. So you are wise to listen to your body's call for rest, shade, and fluid replacement.

Each person responds differently to heat stress because of variations in body fat, number of sweat glands, fitness level, and possibly sex.

Body fat serves as a layer of insulation beneath the surface of the skin. Those with more subcutaneous fat may be better insulated from the cold, but are they less able to lose excess heat to the environment? Probably not, because the body learns to route blood around the fat for cooling purposes. But excess fat is a handicap, because just carrying it around takes energy.

Each of us inherits a certain number and pattern of sweat glands. Because evaporative heat loss is the most important protection against heat stress, a good supply of active sweat glands is important. Like almost everything else, sweat glands respond to use. If you use them a lot, they become more efficient.

Physical fitness seems to enhance our ability to regulate body temperature during work in the heat. Fitness does so by lowering the temperature (set point) at which sweating begins. Thus, fit individuals can work or play with lower heart rates and core temperatures. Acclimatization further lowers the point at which sweating begins; therefore, the physically fit and heat-acclimated individual is even *better* prepared for work in the heat (Nadel, 1977). And recent evidence indicates that fitness *hastens* the process of acclimatization.

Men produce more sweat for a given increase in body temperature, perhaps even too much. Women are more efficient sweaters; their sweat production is more suited to the heat load so they don't waste water. When men and women are compared on the same task, men *seem* better able to work in the heat. However, the difference is due to fitness, not sex. When the fitness level is the same or when the work load is equated (e.g., a given percentage of maximal oxygen intake), women seem quite able to work in the heat. In several recent marathons, the women seemed to tolerate the heat as well as or better than many men, probably because women are more efficient sweaters.

Exercising in the Heat

When exercise begins, the temperature-regulating center increases the thermostatic set point, allowing the body temperature to increase. The rise in temperature depends on the intensity of exercise. In a moderate environment, the temperature will increase about 1 °C at 50% of the maximal oxygen intake and will rise to about 39 °C at the maximal level (above 102 °F). This resetting of the core temperature during exercise can be viewed as an adjustment favorable to the enzyme activity within the muscles, and it also serves to reduce the problem of heat dissipation. Under moderate environmental conditions, the methods of heat dissipation are not employed *until* the elevated set point has been reached.

In hot environments, we are able to maintain temporary thermal balance during exercise by virtue of circulatory adjustments and the evaporation of sweat. In a hot, dry environment the body actually gains heat when the air temperature exceeds the temperature of the skin. Under these conditions, the evaporation of sweat allows the maintenance of thermal equilibrium. However, when the humidity also is high and *evaporation cannot take place*, the body temperature continues to rise, severely impairing performance. Blood is diverted from muscles to the skin, blood volume is reduced via sweating, and water and electrolytes are lost in the sweat. Stroke volume declines, heart rate increases, and lactic acid accumulates. Blood may even begin to pool in the large veins, further reducing venous return and cardiac output. All this sets the stage for **hyperthermia**, an alarming rise in body temperature, and the imminent collapse of the temperature-regulating mechanism.

Sweating

In a normal day, we lose and must replace about 2.5 L of water (Remember, 1 L = 1.057 qt; 1 qt = 0.946 L). Of this amount, about 0.7 L is lost from the lungs and skin (insensible water loss), 1.5 L through the urine, 0.2 L with the feces, and about 0.1 L through perspiration. During heavy exercise in the heat, the water lost through sweating can be increased beyond 2 L *per hour*. Sweat production may amount to as much as 12 L per day. Because work capacity becomes impaired as water loss progresses, the fluid must be replaced. Dehydration in excess of 5% of body weight leads to a marked decline in work capacity, strength, and endurance. Estimate 1 L for each 2-lb weight loss; therefore, if you lost 8 lb, or over 5% of 150 lb, you will be about 4 L low on fluid!

The thirst mechanism always underestimates fluid needs during work in the heat and after the work is over. Therefore, it is wise to take frequent small drinks throughout the work period. If you drink 250 ml (about 1 cup) every 15 min, you can replace 1 L per hour. If the sweat rate is higher, it is extremely difficult to keep up with fluid needs. Marathon runners are wise to drink as much as possible (up to 500 ml) before the event to offset the tremendous water loss and difficulty of replacement. If during prolonged periods of work in the heat (i.e., several days), weight loss exceeds 2% prior to the next day's effort (e.g., 3 lb for a 150-lb individual), the individual should be rehydrated *before* returning to work or exercise.

Sweating rates and evaporative cooling depend on adequate rehydration. Hyperhydration, or excess water intake, allows you to sweat more and work with a lower rectal temperature and heart rate, thus leading to increased work performance in hot industrial or sporting environments.

Salt Loss

Water replacement alone will not compensate for the loss of electrolytes (such as sodium and potassium) in the sweat. For each liter of sweat lost, approximately 1.5 g of salt are lost as well, because the average meal includes 3 to 4 g of salt, three meals will satisfy most salt needs. For long periods of work in the heat (8 hr or more) when considerable water and salt will be lost, workers should salt food liberally (8 hr at 1.5 g of salt per liter = 12 g salt loss). I don't recommend salt tablets for several reasons. They are slow to dissolve and leave the stomach. While in the stomach, the high salt content encourages the movement of water into the digestive tract via osmosis. Salt tablets will not provide aid for hours, and while they are dissolving they take needed water from the bloodstream. Also, excessive salt intake can cause stomach cramps, weakness, high blood pressure, and other problems. Avoid such an intake if you can.

There are several choices for the replacement of water and salt. Solutions containing the necessary electrolytes as well as some glucose can be obtained commercially, but remember that you may have to replace several quarts of fluid, which could become expensive. You can save money by using the saltshaker at mealtime, drinking citrus fruit drinks for potassium, and obtaining the balance of fluid needs in *water*. Or you can prepare your own solution by adding 1/4 teaspoon of salt to each quart of half-strength frozen lemonade. Another approach is to replace some of your fluid needs with tomato juice and the rest with water. When long periods of work in the heat make it absolutely necessary to add salt to water, use commercial replacement drinks or add 1/4 teaspoon of salt to each quart of water and be sure to replace potassium during mealtime with citrus fruits or drinks, bananas, or other potassium-rich foods.

Never use excess salt or glucose in fluid replacement solutions, especially during running. When too much glucose is added to a solution to be used *during* continuous physical effort, the glucose retards gastrointestinal absorption by keeping the solution in the stomach (Costill, Saltin, Soderberg, & Jansson, 1973). In marathon or other long duration races, runners should drink cool (40 °F) electrolyte solutions that are relatively low in glucose (about 25 g per liter). Cyclists and cross-country skiers can tolerate higher glucose concentrations during exercise. After exercise continue to replace fluids, electrolytes, and energy. You may want to use commercially available fluid replacement solutions to insure rehydration and to maintain a healthy thirst after exercise in the heat (Nadel, 1988).

A recent alternative, glucose polymer solutions, quickly replace fluid while providing 3 times more energy in the form of clumps (polymers) of glucose molecules.

Heat Stress Index

As you may have guessed, we cannot predict heat stress on the basis of air temperature alone. Relative humidity is an important factor that determines how effective sweating will be. If the sweat cannot evaporate and merely drips from the body, little heat is lost, and the water loss only adds to the problem. Air movement and radiant heat also are important factors to consider in evaluating the effect of a given environment on human comfort and performance. Even the type and color of clothing have an effect on heat loss. Finally, we must consider the metabolic heat production due to physical activity, because this is the major heat source.

The wet bulb globe temperature (WBGT) provides a simple and accurate indication of the effect of environmental factors on active human beings. The index uses dry and wet bulb thermometers to assess air temperature and relative humidity (see Table 14.1). The black copper globe thermometer indicates radiant heat as well as air movement. The several temperatures are weighted to indicate their relative contribution to the total heat stress. As you can see, relative humidity measured by the wet bulb, is the greatest contributor to heat stress (70% of total).

The U.S. Marine Corps uses the WBGT to determine when physical training activities should be reduced or cancelled, and many high school and college athletic trainers and coaches use it to determine when practice sessions or distance

Table 14.1 WBGT Heat Stress Index

	WBGT heat stress index		Example
Wet bulb	= _____ °F = .7 = _____		80 × .7 = 56
Dry bulb	= _____ °F × .1 = _____		90 × .1 = 9
Black globe	= _____ °F × .2 = _____		120 × .2 = 24
WBGT	= _____ °F		WBGT = 89 °F

Where: The wet bulb indicates humidity, the dry bulb measures the ambient temperature, and the black copper globe measures radiant heat and air movement.

Standards for Work or Exercise
   Above 80 °—utilize discretion
   Above 85 °—avoid strenuous activity
   Above 88 °—cease physical activity[a]

Note. From Sharkey (1974).

[a]Trained individuals who have been acclimated to the heat are allowed to continue limited activity.

runs should be scheduled. The WBGT does not allow an estimate of the effect of clothing or energy expenditure; dark or nonporous clothing can increase radiant heating or reduce evaporation. Also, high levels of energy expenditure can create internal heat problems in rather moderate environments. No simple index tells you everything about heat stress. But for moderate energy expenditures (up to 425 calories per hour) that you undertake while wearing sensible clothing, the WBGT is an excellent indicator of heat stress.

Another approach is to use the heat stress chart (see Figure 14.1).

This chart is based on the shaded air temperature, moderate radiant heat from the sun, a light breeze, and a moderate work rate. Unfit or nonacclimated individuals will suffer at lower levels of heat, humidity, or work than might affect fit people.

Heat stress

When heat and hard work combine to drive the body temperature up, the temperature-regulating mechanism begins to fail and the worker faces serious heat stress disorders. This dangerous—often deadly—combination of circumstances can be avoided by monitoring the environment with simple measurements of temperature and humidity. This chart can help alert individuals to dangerous heat stress conditions.*

Extreme heat stress conditions. Only heat acclimated individuals can work safely for extended periods. Take frequent breaks and replace fluids.

Watch for changing conditions. Heat sensitive and nonacclimated individuals may suffer. Increase rest periods and be sure to replace fluids.

Little danger of heat stress for acclimated individuals. Lack of air movement, high radiant heat (from sun or fire), and hard effort can raise danger.

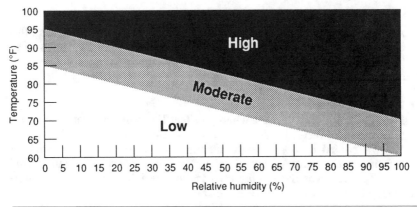

Figure 14.1. Heat stress chart. *Note.* From Sharkey (1979).

Heat Acclimatization

On the first day of vigorous exercise in a hot environment, you may experience a near-maximal heart rate, elevated skin and core temperatures, and severe fatigue.

After just a few days of similar exposure to work in the heat, you can accomplish the same task with a reduced heart rate, made possible by improved blood distribution and increased blood volme. Your skin and core temperatures are lower, because sweating begins at a lower temperature. The loss of water in the urine diminishes, and the salt concentration of the sweat gradually reduces. This increase in circulatory and cooling efficiency is called **heat acclimatization**, and most of the process usually occurs after 4 to 8 days of work in the heat (increases in sweat rate may take longer; Wenger, 1988).

Highly fit individuals become acclimatized within 4 to 5 days, whereas sedentary subjects take twice as long. The best way to achieve acclimatization is to work in the actual temperature and humidity conditions you'll have to endure. However, if you live in a cool climate and don't have a heat chamber to work in, high-intensity training can get you halfway there, probably because of the heat generated during vigorous effort (use a nonrubberized sweat suit to increase the temperature close to the skin). Fit individuals start to sweat at a lower body temperature, and they increase sweat production at a faster rate. Acclimatization helps move the set point for sweating even lower.

Less fit individuals would be wise to acclimatize using periods of light to moderate activity in a hot environment, alternated with rest periods when fluid is replaced. Electrolytes can be replaced with commercial drinks or the saltshaker at meals, plus potassium-rich citrus fruits or bananas. The vitamin C in the citrus drinks may hasten the acclimatization process.

> **In summary, the prescription for exercise in a hot, humid environment includes the following advice.**
>
> - **Wear sensible, porous, light-colored, loose-fitting clothing.**
> - **Acclimatize to the expected environment and work load (i.e., do 50% of your work load the first day, 60% the second, 70% the third, 80% the fourth, 90% the fifth. By the sixth you should be acclimatized and able to do 100% of your work load.**
> - **Always replace water and electrolytes.**
> - **Find a cool place for rest periods.**
> - **Don't be too proud to quit when you feel the symptoms of heat stress (dizziness, confusion, cramps, nausea, and clammy skin).**
> - **Keep a record of body weight during prolonged periods of work or training in the heat. Weigh in before and after exercise to gauge fluid loss. To check for day-to-day rehydration, weigh yourself in the morning, after toilet but before breakfast.**
> - **Maintain a high level of aerobic fitness. You'll work better in the heat, acclimatize faster, and hold your acclimatization longer.**

Exercising in the Cold

Because of the metabolic heat generated during exercise, cold temperatures do not pose a threat similar to that posed by hot, humid conditions. But severe exposure to low temperatures and high winds can lead to frostbite, freezing, hypothermia, and even death. Peripheral vasoconstriction increases the insulating capacity of the skin, but it also markedly reduces the temperature of the extremities. It's as if the body is willing to lose a few fingers or toes to save the more important parts. Protective vasoconstriction often leads to severe discomfort in the fingers and toes. To relieve the pain, it is necessary to warm the affected area or raise the core temperature to allow reflexive return of blood to the extremities. Although shivering may cause some increase in temperature, gross muscular activity is far more effective in restoring heat to the troubled area. Because large-muscle activity takes considerable energy, the cold weather enthusiast is wise to maintain a reserve of energy for use in emergencies. Excessive fatigue is the first step toward hypothermia and possible death.

Windchill

Windchill describes the effect of wind speed on heat loss (see Table 14.2). A 10 °F reading is equivalent to -25 °F when the wind speed is 20 miles per hour. Runners, skiers, and skaters can create their own windchill. Skiing at 20 mph on a 10 °F day is equivalent to -25 °F. And if the skier is moving into a wind, the effect is even worse. When possible, run, ski or skate away from the wind. If you must face into the wind on a cold day, be sure to cover exposed flesh, including earlobes and nose, and be on the lookout for frostbite.

Frostbite

Frostbite is damage to the skin resulting from exposure to extreme cold or windchill. As you can see on the windchill table, there is little danger of frostbite at temperatures above 20 °F. A temperature or windchill of -20 °F seems necessary to produce the condition.

At first, frostbite appears as a patch of pale or white skin, due to the constriction of blood vessels in the area. After mild frostbite, the skin appears red and swollen when the blood returns. In severe frostbite, the skin may appear purple or black after it is warmed. Immersion in warm (not hot) water will hasten the return of blood to the area. *Do not massage the affected part.* Protect the groin and other sensitive areas to avoid the excruciating pain that occurs when circulation returns.

Don't worry about freezing the delicate tissues of the lungs during cold weather exercise. Cold, dry air may make your breathing uncomfortable but poses little danger of damage to the tissue. The respiratory system has a remarkable ability to warm and humidify air. People can tolerate air temperatures well below 0 °F without damage, because the cold air is warmed to above freezing before it reaches the bronchi. However, when the temperature goes below -20 °F, you should modify or curtail your exercise plans. The danger to earlobes, nose, fingers, and toes is great, and at much lower temperatures respiratory tract damage

Table 14.2 Wind Chill Index

Wind speed (mph)	Actual thermometer reading (°F)											
	50	40	30	20	10	0	-10	-20	-30	-40	-50	-60
	Equivalent temperature (°F)											
Calm	50	40	30	20	10	0	-10	-20	-30	-40	-50	-60
5	48	37	27	16	6	-5	-15	-26	-36	-47	-57	-68
10	40	28	16	4	-9	-21	-33	-46	-58	-70	-83	-95
15	36	22	9	-5	-18	-36	-45	-58	-72	-85	-99	-112
20	32	18	4	-10	-25	-39	-53	-67	-82	-96	-110	-124
25	30	16	0	-15	-29	-44	-59	-74	-88	-104	-118	-133
30	28	13	-2	-18	-33	-48	-63	-79	-94	-109	-125	-140
35	27	11	-4	-20	-35	-49	-67	-82	-98	-113	-129	-145
40	26	10	-6	-21	-37	-53	-69	-85	-100	-116	-132	-148

(Wind speeds greater than 40 mph have little additional effect)

LITTLE DANGER (for properly clothed person)

INCREASING DANGER

GREAT DANGER

Danger from freezing of exposed flesh

Note. From Sharkey (1974).

is possible, though unlikely. Very cold air will cause bronchoconstriction and make vigorous effort difficult.

Hypothermia

When your body begins to lose heat faster than it can be produced, you are at risk for hypothermia. Prolonged exertion leads to progressive muscular fatigue, and shivering and vasoconstriction are the body's attempts to preserve heat and the temperature of the vital organs. Neuromuscular impairment and exhaustion of energy stores lead to the virtual termination of activity. As exposure continues you lose additional body heat, and the cold reaches the brain; you lose judgment and the ability to reason. Your speech becomes slow and slurred, you lose control of your hands, your walking becomes clumsy, and you want to lie down and rest. *Don't do it!* You have **hypothermia**. Your core temperature is dropping, and without treatment you will lose consciousness and die.

Surprisingly, most hypothermia cases develop in air temperatures above 30 °F. Cold water, windchill, and fatigue combine to set the stage for hypothermia. Avoid the problem by staying dry. If you become wet, dry off as soon as possible. Be aware of the windchill and how wind refrigerates wet clothing. During a cold weather hike or ski tour, take off layers of clothing before you perspire, and put them back on as you begin to cool. Eat and rest often to maintain your energy level. Make camp when you still have energy; don't wait until rest and heat are critical.

> If someone exhibits the symptoms of hypothermia, transport the victim to a medical facility as quickly as possible. The victim's heart may begin to fibrillate during rewarming, and emergency equipment will be needed. If immediate transport isn't possible, or if the case isn't severe, try the following:
>
> - **Get the victim out of the wind and rain.**
> - **Remove all wet clothing.**
> - **Provide warm drinks, dry clothing, and a warm, dry sleeping bag for a mildly impaired victim.**
> - **If victim is only semiconscious, try to keep him awake, leave him stripped, and put him in a sleeping bag with another person to provide warmth.**
> - **Build a fire to warm the camp.**

Cold Weather Clothing

For extended periods of outdoor exertion when you'll be away from protective shelter and central heating, dress in layers. Layers of clothing provide an insulating barrier of air and can be peeled off as your temperature rises and put back on as it falls. Wool is one of the best fabrics to wear for under and outer garments. It doesn't have the insulating value of dry down, but it is far better when wet.

Physiologists rate the insulating value of clothing in "Clo" units, with one Clo unit being equivalent to the dress that will maintain comfort at a room temperature of 70 °F (roughly equivalent to cotton shirt and slacks). Table 14.3 and Figure 14.2 illustrate how insulating requirements change during vigorous activity such as cross-country skiing or hiking, light work, and rest. That is precisely why it is necessary to dress in layers in cold weather. At a temperature of 0 °F, a light shirt will be adequate during vigorous effort, but you may need 2 in. of insulation to maintain comfort at rest and more for a good night's sleep.

Table 14.3 Comfort Data

Effective temperature °F	Thickness of insulation required for comfort (in.)		
	Sleeping	Light work	Heavy work
40	1.5	.8	.20
20	2.0	1.0	.27
0	2.5	1.3	.35
−20	3.0	1.6	.40
−40	3.5	1.9	.48

Note. These figures are approximate but are a good base for an average healthy person. From various U.S. Government sources.

Because perspiration is a major problem during exercise in the cold, you would be smart to purchase a set of synthetic (polypropylene) undergarments. This amazing fabric wicks perspiration away from the skin so evaporative cooling won't strip heat from the body. Next, wear a wool shirt or sweater for warmth. A wind- and rain-proof slicker should be all the additional clothing you need during exercise. Invest in a "breathable" slicker if you can afford one, but don't expect any garment to handle the tremendous moisture load created during vigorous skiing or running. You can carry a down or pile coat in your pack for use in camp. Modern, light, synthetic fabrics have several advantages over goose down. They are less expensive, easier to care for, and don't mat and lose insulating qualities when wet.

Cold Acclimatization

Are we able to adjust to the cold as we are able to acclimatize to hot environments? If so, what are the physiological mechanisms involved? Specific examples of cold acclimatization do appear in the research literature (Folk, 1974). One mechanism is a metabolic adjustment wherein metabolism increases as much as 35%. The female divers (called Ama) of the Korean Peninsula evidence this

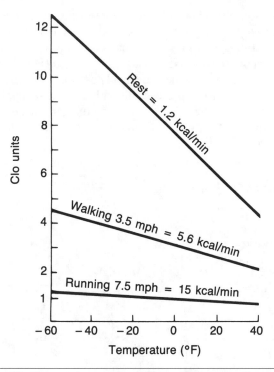

Figure 14.2. Clothing requirements at different energy expenditures in the cold.

adjustment as well as improved tissue insulation during the winter months when the water temperature falls to 50 °F. Australian aborigines adapt to cold conditions with a hypothermic response, that is, a lowering of the core temperature to a more easily maintained level (95 °F). Of course, natural selection and heredity play important roles in the adaptation to cold environments, and a large body mass, short extremities, increased levels of body fat, and a deep routing of venous circulation also help.

It also seems likely that repeated cold exposures can lead to physiological and psychological adjustments that allow one to tolerate and enjoy physical activity in cold environments. I'm sure that my extra eating in the winter and the extra weight I carry are my way of adding an insulating layer of subcutaneous fat. At least that's the excuse I use!

Exercising at Altitudes

More than 40 million people live at altitudes above 10,000 ft, and some live above 17,000 ft in the Andes. However, no permanent habitations are found above 18,000 feet, indicating that such an elevation may be incompatible with adaptation and long-term survival. Elevations below 5,000 ft have little notice-able effect on otherwise healthy individuals. But as you ascend to higher eleva-tions to ski, hike, climb, or even to live, barometric pressure declines along with available levels of atmospheric and alveolar oxygen (PO_2). When this oc-curs, the arterial blood is unable to become highly saturated, less oxygen is trans-ported, and the tissues are forced to operate with a reduced supply (see Table 14.4). Thus, in spite of the heroic efforts of the oxygen intake and transport systems, altitude always leads to a reduction in aerobic fitness and associated endurance performances.

Table 14.4 Altitude and Oxygen

Altitude (ft)	Barometric pressure (mmHg)	PO_2 in air (mmHg)	PO_2 alveoli (mmHg)	Arterial O_2 saturation (%)	Aerobic fitness (% of sea level)
0	760	159	105	97	100
3,200	680	142	94	96	
6,500	600	125	78	94	90
10,000	523	111	62	90	
14,100	450	94	51	86	75
18,400	380	75	42	80	
23,000	305	64	31	63	50
29,141	230	48	19	30	

Note. Adapted from "Variation in Altitude and its Effects on Exercise Performance" by B. Balke, 1968, in *Exercise Physiology* by H.B. Falls (Ed.), 1968, New York: Academic Press; *Environmental Physiology* by G.E. Folk, 1974, Philadelphia: Lea & Febiger; and *Compendium of Human Responses to the Aerospace Environment III* by E.M. Roth (Ed.), 1968, Washington, DC: National Aeronautics and Space Administration.

In this age of rapid transit, it doesn't take long to ascend to a national park or ski resort located above 5,000 ft. When you arrive, you'll have to adjust cardiac output for a given work load. The heart rate is higher, but the stroke volume may be lower because of a diminished oxygen supply to the heart muscle. More air is brought into the lungs each minute, and this hyperventilation leads to in-creased carbon dioxide exhalation and the acid-base disturbances associated with acute mountain sickness. The symptoms—headache, shortness of breath, rapid heartbeat, and loss of appetite—appear at 8,000 ft or above. Needless to say, work capacity declines at this altitude, as does the motivation to perform hard work.

Does a high level of physical fitness provide some advantage to the newcomer? On arrival, the conditioned individual maintains his sea-level advantage over the unfit, but no more. The trained individual will be able to do less than he or she could at sea level and is just as likely to suffer mountain sickness. At very high elevations, some highly trained endurance athletes have been found to be nonresponders whose respiration fails to adjust adequately to the added demands of the altitude (Jackson & Sharkey, 1988).

Acclimatization to Altitude

Profound changes occur soon after you move to a higher elevation. Pulmonary ventilation increases so more air can be moved into the lungs. This increase doesn't take more energy, because the air is less dense at higher elevations. Increases in red blood cells, hemoglobin, and blood volume gradually enhance oxygen transport. Above 15,000 ft the red cells increase from 5 million per cubic millimeter to 6.6 million, and hemoglobin rises from 15 g per 100 ml to above 20. This makes the blood more viscous, but that isn't a problem, because the hypoxia (lower oxygen tension) of altitude serves to vasodilate, or relax, the arterioles. Altitude exposure also may cause an increase in lung and muscle capillaries; likewise myoglobin, the molecule that serves to store oxygen in muscles, increases at higher elevations (Smith & Sharkey, 1984).

Our bodies require about 3 weeks to make a good adjustment to a higher elevation, or about 1 week for each 1,000 ft above 5,000 ft. Once you have acclimatized, your oxygen intake and transport systems will be better able to supply oxygen to the working muscles. These adjustments reduce but never eliminate the effect of altitude on aerobic fitness. Endurance performances always will be reduced at altitude, regardless of your state of acclimatization. Unfortunately, these hard-earned changes (they occur only when you work at a high altitude) are reversible; they return to prealtitude values within weeks after leaving the mountains.

Altitude Training

Because of the reduced oxygen intake ability above 5,000 ft altitude, your usual pace will be more anaerobic than usual. You will have several options: Do your usual distance but go slower, go at your usual pace but for shorter distances, or (my favorite) relax and enjoy the view. Go sightseeing as you exercise and forget about distance or pace. If you are training to compete at a high altitude, you should realize that the slower pace of running may cause your speed to slip a little. Occasional shorter but faster runs should help avoid that problem (athletes sometimes drop to lower elevations for speed work).

For years, coaches and athletes have sought the ultimate training stimulus at altitude. They believe that muscle hypoxia is the stimulus that causes changes in aerobic fitness and that exercise at altitude ensures extreme tissue hypoxia.

So they travel to a training site at 6,000 to 9,000 ft and train for several weeks or months before returning to sea level for a major event like the Olympic Games. Unfortunately, this may not be worth the effort and cost, because arduous effort at sea level also leads to tissue hypoxia. One research study produced a small benefit from altitude training on return from sea level; however, no control group was used. When the study was repeated with a control group, the altitude training was no more effective than equally arduous sea level training. The subjects were highly trained middle-distance runners, 17 to 23 years old, who trained at either sea level or 7,500 ft for 3 weeks (Adams, Bernauer, Dill, & Bornar, 1975).

Casual observers of the sport scene are always quick to conclude that a certain athlete's performance is due to his or her residence at high altitude. Several outstanding African athletes have emerged to perpetuate the practice of altitude training. Of course, the athletes do live above 7,000 ft. What many forget is that these athletes were *born* there and lived most of their lives there as well. Their parents were born there as were their parents' parents. So the benefit that many seek really is a product of natural selection and long-term residence at a higher elevation, not just a few weeks of altitude training.

The benefits of altitude acclimatization do not seem to help all athletes equally. If altitude were the only secret to success, all our great distance athletes would be from high altitude areas, and that certainly is not the case. Some athletes, particularly those with low hemoglobin levels, may profit from altitude training. But others do no better and some do worse, perhaps because altitude training is more stressful or because their already high hemoglobin is raised, becoming more viscous and difficult to pump at sea level (Smith & Sharkey, 1984).

Air Pollution and Exercise

Should you check the local air pollution index before you can safely go outside to exercise? In some cities you should. If you fly over any major city in this country, you can see the pall of pollution that diminishes the quality of our lives. Although some forms of pollution are most dangerous for old or weak individuals and those with respiratory problems, other forms attack physically active individuals. Exercise increases the volume of air taken into the lungs each minute. Because pollution-related respiratory disorders often are related to the degree of exposure, it seems wise to avoid exercise in polluted atmospheres.

On one warm, humid fall afternoon thousands of cars circled the suburban communities outside New York City. A haze created by the action of sunlight on the hydrocarbon emissions hung heavily in the air. As the players of a suburban New Jersey football team practiced, some began to complain of troubled breathing, chest pains, tightness, nausea, and vomiting. The scene was repeated at other area schools where young, healthy athletes engaged in vigorous physical activity were learning firsthand about the growing problem of air pollution. Adults also were affected as they attempted to mow lawns or work in gardens. The urban East was experiencing the choking pall that regularly forces Los Angeles schoolchildren to cancel games or remain indoors for recess when the photochemical smog is particularly bad.

Air pollution comes from many sources, and we are beginning to recognize them as threats to the quality of life and to life itself. Some pollutants are relatively harmless by themselves but in combination with others are capable of exerting potent biological effects.

The biological effects of air pollution include
- **irritation of conducting airways (bronchial tubes),**
- **effect on diffusing surfaces (e.g., alveolar breakdown in emphysema),**
- **reduction in oxygen-transporting capacity (carbon monoxide competes for space on hemoglobin molecule), and**
- **cancer.**

But although many forms of industrial and automotive pollution are nauseating, troublesome, or even fatal, no *single* source of pollution is as deadly as the cigarette, which can cause all the biological effects listed above. It can irritate the bronchial tubes, make the smoker more susceptible to infection, cause emphysema, reduce oxygen transport 10% (thereby reducing aerobic fitness and performance capacity), and cause lung cancer and heart disease.

Carbon Monoxide

Carbon monoxide (CO) is a colorless, odorless gas that results from imperfect combustion. The smoldering cigarette produces high levels of CO, so much so that the average smoker is likely to have at least 5% carboxyhemoglobin (COHb) in the blood (see Table 14.5). COHb occurs when CO unites with hemoglobin, a union that takes precedence over the union of oxygen and hemoglobin. If the air you breathe contains CO, it will find its way into your blood. The level of COHb depends on its concentration in the air and the duration of exposure. Eventually, blood levels reach an equilibrium with the breathing mixture (about 5%

Table 14.5 Levels of COHb Produced by Cigarettes

Cigarettes/day	COHb
10-15	5%
15-25	6.3%
30-40	9.3%

COHb after 8 hr exposure to 35 ppm CO). Although your body requires time to reach this equilibrium, flushing the deadly gas from your system may take just as long.

The effects of carbon monoxide are additive to those of altitude. If your aerobic fitness is down 10% at 6,500 ft, you can lose another 5 to 10% by smoking (e.g., 80% × 45 = 36; altitude and smoking adjusted fitness score).

Though the smoker gets the worse part of the deal, a nearby nonsmoker also is subjected to high levels of CO, especially in a crowded or poorly ventilated room. One study measured levels as high as 166 ppm in an automobile. It wouldn't be long before the nonsmoker felt symptoms of distress, headache, and nausea. (The smoker has become less sensitive.) We should all support efforts to restrict smoking in public places, to assert our right to an unpolluted atmosphere. I agree with the sign that tells smokers, "If you must smoke, please do not exhale." And I agree with the public health goal of making the country smoke-free by the year 2000!

Practical Suggestions

Let us hope that we can clean up the air we breathe, that we need never regulate our activities in accordance with the air pollution index, and that our enjoyment of physical activity need not be compromised by human mistreatment of the environment. In the meantime, avoid exercise in obviously dangerous areas (along expressways, near industrial pollution) and when air pollution warnings are in effect (that doesn't mean you shouldn't exercise, just find a way to avoid the pollution). And be sure to add your voice to the growing fight against pollution and smoking. (For more on the subject of air pollution see McCafferty, 1981.)

PART
V

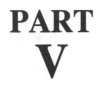

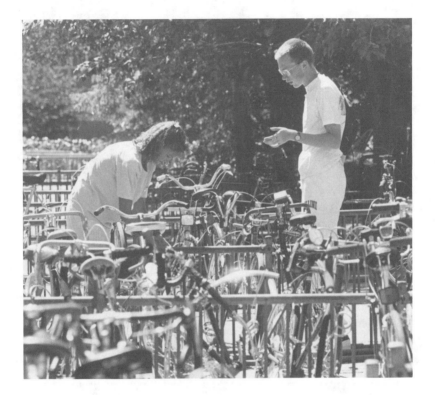

FITNESS AND
LIFESTYLE

The final chapters of this book show how decisions you make influence your health and the quality of your life. You can add excitement to your life as you pursue your potential in athletic competition, and improved fitness can make your workday more enjoyable. Daily habits are part of your lifestyle, and the appropriate lifestyle contributes to health and the quality of life. The suggestions in Part V and Appendix F may help you improve your mental health, achieve success in athletics, lower your medical bills, obtain a raise or a promotion, and, possibly, find the secret to a longer, fuller life. Preposterous, you say? Maybe, and maybe not.

CHAPTER

15

FITNESS FOR
WORK AND SPORT

This chapter will help you

understand the relationship between fitness and work capacity,

improve work performance and job satisfaction,

better integrate your job into your lifestyle,

improve performance in your favorite sport, and

play your best game more often.

Most of us spend about 8 hr in sleep and 8 hr at work. The rest is largely dedicated to preparation for one or the other, or for so-called leisure time pursuits, including physical activity and sport. Improved fitness will enhance work capacity and improve performance in sport.

Fitness and Work

Until recently, the primary source of power for the production of useful work was derived from the contractions of muscles, both human and animal. Of course, people devised ways to augment muscle power with the ingenious use of wind, water, and tools, but it was not until the 18th century that mechanization began to reduce the need for muscular work. Robots, computers, and other devices have replaced the need for human muscle power. Today, when men and women go to *work*, few actually engage in arduous muscular effort.

Much of the credit for the reduction in physical labor must go to the inventors and engineers whose attempts at mechanization and, more recently, automation and robotics have made work relatively effortless. Some credit also is due to specialists in ergonomics, the scientific study of work. Work physiologists, psychologists, and engineers combine to study people in their working environments, with the goal of *adapting the job to the ability of the average worker*. A host of labor-saving devices are eliminating the need for muscular work at home, and the automobile makes the task of getting to and from work physically effortless.

The consequences of these trends are obvious: The average worker is incapable of delivering a full day's effort in a physically demanding job, and degenerative diseases associated with inactivity—such as heart disease, the nation's number one killer—are epidemic. If job requirements are continually lowered to meet the abilities of the average workers, the trend will continue. Perhaps it is time for a change; perhaps we could benefit by working *up* to job requirements, *not down*. Perhaps it is time to adapt the worker to the job rather than to continue adapting the job to the worker.

Certain jobs still require strength and endurance at least some of the time. Workers in heavy industry, construction, agriculture, forestry, and the military often engage in strenuous effort. Without proper conditioning, the stress of arduous work can be unpleasant or worse, so concern for these employees' health and safety has prompted screening procedures to make sure the worker is capable of meeting the job's demands. Many companies have instituted employee fitness programs to help workers meet and maintain required levels of work capacity.

Studies show that the unfit worker can become a safety hazard to himself as well as to co-workers. Fit workers are more productive than their sedentary colleagues, are absent fewer days, and are far less likely to incur job-related disabilities or retire early due to heart or other degenerative diseases. Moreover, physically fit workers have a more positive attitude about work and life in general. For safety, health, production, and morale, fitness is good business.

Work Capacity

Work capacity is the ability to accomplish production goals without undue fatigue and without becoming a hazard to yourself or your co-workers. Work capacity is the product of a number of factors, including natural endowment, skill, nutrition, aerobic fitness, muscular fitness, intelligence, experience, acclimatization, and lean body weight.

Aerobic or muscular fitness, acclimatization to heat or altitude, or even skill and experience do not ensure work output. A worker may rate high in all of these categories but fail to produce adequately due to lack of *motivation*. On the other hand, even the most highly motivated workers will fail if they lack strength or endurance, ignore the need to acclimatize to a hot working environment, or lack the physical skills required for the job.

Aerobic Fitness and Work Capacity. The relationship between aerobic fitness and work capacity is this: The body requires energy to perform work, energy created by burning fat and carbohydrate. This process takes oxygen; the tougher the job the more energy and oxygen are needed. When oxygen and energy needs are light, such as for office duties, work performance isn't strongly related to aerobic fitness; but when oxygen and energy needs are high (over 7.6 calories per minute), production relates directly to the ability to produce energy aerobically (see Table 15.1).

Table 15.1 Occupational Work Classifications

Classification	Energy expenditure (cal/min)	Lifting (lb)	Carrying (lb)
Very light work	Under 2.5	Up to 10	Small objects
Light work	2.6-4.9	Up to 20	Up to 10
Medium work	5.0-7.5	Up to 50	Up to 25
Heavy work	Above 7.6	Up to 100	Up to 50
Very heavy work	Above 7.6	Over 100	Over 50

Note. From *Dictionary of Occupational Titles* (p. 48) by the U.S. Department of Labor, 1968, Washington, DC: U.S. Government Printing Office.

When heavy work is required, individuals with a low level of aerobic fitness are able to work at only 25% of capacity for 8 hr. Those of average fitness can sustain about 33% of their capacity for 8 hr, and those with above average fitness can maintain 40%. Only highly conditioned and motivated individuals can sustain levels as high as 50% of their aerobic fitness level for 8 hr. Those with higher fitness levels have the capacity to outperform less fit individuals (see Figure 15.1; Åstrand & Rodahl, 1977). In some systems better performance is rewarded with better pay; in others it is not. One study found fit workers able to produce 4 to 6 times more than the unfit (Sharkey, Jukkala, Putnam, & Tietz, 1980). Which one would you hire?

Muscular Fitness and Work Capacity. Dynamic muscular strength is clearly related to work capacity for heavy lifting or using heavy tools, but for *repeated* lifting (as in work with hand tools), strength, muscular endurance, and aerobic fitness combine to set the limits of work capacity (see Figure 15.2).

Combinations of work rate and percentage of maximum strength that fall to the right of the line for one's fitness level cannot be sustained for a full working

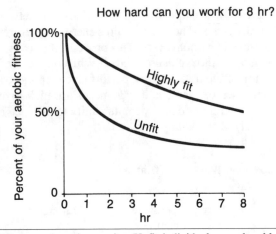

Figure 15.1. Fitness and work capacity. Unfit individuals may be able to work at only 25% of their aerobic fitness level for prolonged periods, whereas the highly fit may work at 50% of their maximum for long periods. The fit worker is able to sustain a higher work rate than the unfit. *Note.* Adapted from *Textbook of Work Physiology: Physiological Bases of Exercise* (2nd ed.) by P.O. Åstrand and K. Rodahl, 1977, New York: McGraw-Hill; from Sharkey (1977).

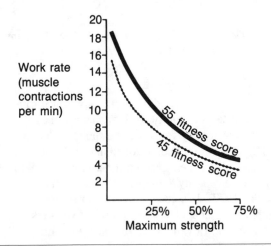

Figure 15.2. Interrelationships of strength, aerobic fitness, and work rate.

day. Highly fit workers (55 ml/[kg × min]) can produce more by working at a higher rate, and stronger individuals can lift more with each contraction. The ideal combination includes levels of aerobic fitness and strength suited to the task.

How much strength is necessary? Generally speaking, the average load in repetitive heavy lifting should not exceed 20% of your maximal strength in that movement. In other words, strength should be 5 times greater than the load lifted on the job (the ratio is different in sports, as explained in the next section). If the job requires daylong work with a shovel that weighs 10 lb when loaded, the worker should possess at least 50 lb of dynamic muscular strength in the arm and shoulder muscles used in the task. Once the worker achieves the minimum strength required, further increases in work capacity can be achieved by increasing muscular endurance and aerobic fitness. If the job involves only occasional lifts of very heavy loads (e.g., 100 lb), the worker can succeed with 100 lb of strength, plus a bit more for safety's sake.

Most work tasks require more endurance than strength; in fact, many individuals mistakenly use the term strength when they really mean endurance. If an individual already has the strength to accomplish a task, physical conditioning should focus on muscular endurance and aerobic fitness. Only those with inadequate strength need engage in strength training.

Of course, skill is also needed to work safely and efficiently, and fitness cannot make up for deficiencies in skill. Skill leads to efficiency, and efficiency allows the worker to conserve energy and avoid fatigue.

Body Fat and Work Capacity. Excess fat certainly limits work capacity. Recently, an additional fact has come to light: When considerable muscular strength is needed on the job, the individual with a high lean body weight (LBW) is more likely to excel (LBW = Body Weight − Fat Weight). The LBW indicates how much muscle is available; body weight alone doesn't tell enough about an individual's body composition. Body fat alone can also be misleading: 20% of body fat sounds high, unless it's on top of 200 lb of LBW. In a study of wildland firefighters, Sharkey et al. (1980) found work capacity is highly related to LBW. When strength is an important job requirement, use skinfold calipers to estimate body fat and lean body weight (see Appendix D).

Body fat has considerable relevance when women apply for heavy work. Because women typically have a greater percentage body fat, men and women of the same weight will not have the same LBW. The female applicant will have to be unusually lean or weigh more than the average man to have a similar LBW.

Fitness Is Good Business

Fit employees are a good investment; thousands of companies spend billions on fitness and recreation programs for their employees. The expenditure is justified on several grounds.

> *Cost Effectiveness:* **Each dollar spent on fitness or wellness in the work place saves several dollars. Fit workers are less likely to smoke, and smoking costs business and industry billions for health costs, cleaning costs, and wasted time. Cost effectiveness is also achieved via increased production and safety and enhanced health and morale.**

Production: Fit employees are more productive in any line of work.

Safety: Fit workers are safe workers; they are far less likely to experience debilitating low back injuries.

Health: Fit workers miss fewer days of work; they are far less likely to suffer from degenerative problems like heart disease. They spend a smaller share of the health care dollar.

Morale: Fitness programs improve morale among employees.

If your company doesn't have a fitness or wellness program, you should *write to the President's Council on Physical Fitness and Sports* in Washington, DC, 20202, for information on how to start such a program.

Flextime.   Recently, many employers have adopted an alternative to the rigid 8:00 a.m. to 5:00 p.m. work schedule. Prompted by congestion in parking lots and highways, congestion in lunch areas, and employee requests for more flexible work schedules, employers have tested and confirmed the feasibility of the flexible work schedule. The typical flextime program calls for 8 to 10 hr of work that may begin as early as 6:00 a.m. and end as late as 6:00 p.m. Employees are required to be at work during a core period so that company business can be carried out. Flextime allows individuals to work during their most productive time and to take longer lunch breaks for shopping, exercise, or family. As a result, production goes up and absenteeism goes down. Flextime allows each worker a freer hand in the creation of his or her own lifestyle.

4-Day Work Week.   Another interesting variation of the traditional work-rest cycle promises even greater individual benefits. The 4-day work week may provide a simple solution to the overwhelming weekend congestion on beaches, tennis courts, golf courses, ski lifts, even wilderness areas. The 4-day (10 hr per day) work week has been tried with considerable success in a number of industries. Schedules can be staggered to provide flexible 3-day rest periods. Some possible work weeks are M-T-W-Th, T-W-Th-F, W-Th-F-S, or even S-M-T-W. Some may even prefer to take their "weekend" during the week. When combined with flextime, the 4-day work week cannot help but further humanize the world of work, thereby providing a greater opportunity for a creative adaptation to life. For more information on the relationship between fitness and work performance, see *Fitness and Work Capacity* (Sharkey, 1977).

Fitness and Sport

In an earlier chapter, I spoke of the stressful side of competition and how competition can be bad for some people's health. This section tells you how to prepare for athletic competition safely and effectively, so you can enjoy the intense pleasure and excitement of sport.

Opportunities for adult (Masters, senior, or veteran) competition include distance running, orienteering, track and field, swimming, alpine and cross-country skiing, tennis, racquetball, handball, golf, softball, volleyball, bowling, judo, karate, and many others. Adults participate in age groups, and it is not unusual to find active athletes of 60, 70, and even 80 years of age. A few, such as the amazing Larry Lewis, continue to participate beyond their 100th birthdays. If you enjoy the thrill of sport, of getting high on your own hormones, this section is for you.

Just remember:

▌ Don't play sports to get in shape; get in shape to play sports!

The physiology of training has received a great deal of attention in recent years. Working together, coaches, athletes, and sports scientists have added to the body of knowledge on training. This section provides an overview of the topic.

Energy Training

In order to tailor a training program suited to your needs, you first must know the energy sources required in the activity. Figure 15.3 illustrates the relative contribution of anaerobic and aerobic energy sources in relation to the distance or duration of running events (use the time scale to determine the energy sources for other activities). Next, you need to know something about your individual capabilities, both anaerobic and aerobic (see tests in Appendix B). If you are eager to prepare for a marathon, for which the energy source is primarily aerobic, you should be as strong as possible in aerobic fitness. If your event is primarily anaerobic, like a 100-m swim, you will need anaerobic capabilities. Once you know the energy sources used in the activity and your own capabilities, you can begin to design your training program.

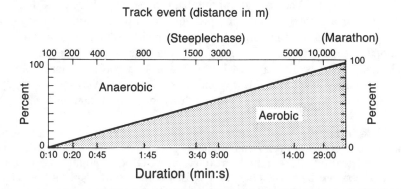

Figure 15.3. Anaerobic and aerobic energy sources in relation to distance and duration of events. Shorter events are primarily anaerobic. For distances over 1500 m (over 4 min) training should concentrate on aerobic fitness. *Note.* From Sharkey (1975).

Year-Round Training

Although you can make significant improvements in aerobic energy sources in as little as 3 months, a year-round program is bound to be safer and more effective (see Figure 15.4). *All* training begins with an aerobic buildup, a period of

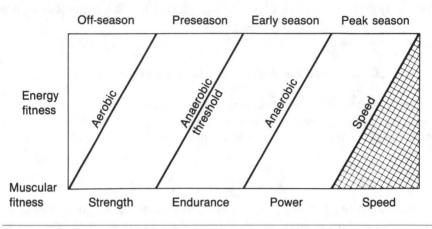

Figure 15.4. Seasonal training goals.

slow distance work. Once you establish a sound aerobic foundation, you are ready to train your anaerobic threshold. This is accomplished by interval training, using long intervals (2 to 5 min). Anaerobic training then follows with shorter and faster efforts (30 to 90 s). Finally, and only if speed is required in the event, sprints can be added to the program (see Table 15.2).

The year-round approach to training provides the strong aerobic foundation needed in all sports, and it minimizes the risk of injury that accompanies anaerobic and speed training. Year-round training leads to a competitive peak that can be sustained for a month or more and provides for a postseason recovery period prior to a renewed training effort. If you are involved in several activities and cannot devote 12 months to any one activity, use the same approach but shorten each phase. Always allow at least 1 month each for aerobic and anaerobic buildup. If necessary, use the first few weeks of the competitive season for any speed training, but don't expect your best performances until later in the season.

Athletes often use heart rate monitors to make sure that they are training at the correct intensity. The best heart rate monitors are those that utilize the electrical signal from the heart (e.g., an ECG). One popular version transmits the signal from the chest to a wrist monitor that displays the rate and stores minute-by-minute heart rates for later analysis.

Table 15.2 Seasonal Training Goals and Methods

Season	Training goals	Training methods
Off-season	Aerobic fitness of slow twitch fibers	Long slow distance, medium distance, Fartlek,* hills
Preseason	Raise anaerobic threshold and aerobic fitness of fast oxidative glycolytic (FOG) fibers	Long intervals (2-5 min), Fartlek, pace work, fast distance
Early season	Anaerobic capability and short-term energy and speed	Medium intervals (60-90 s), short intervals (30-60 s), sprints
Peak season	Maintain training gains and achieve peak performances	Reduce training volume, emphasize quality not quantity

*Fartlek—speed play; a medium distance effort that consists of faster sections followed by slower ones for recovery.

Race-Pace Training

To ensure the specificity of training and the development of needed energy sources, be sure to spend part of your time on race-pace training. If your goal is to ski or run a 35-min 10-km (6.2-mi) race, you'll have to average 3.5 min/km. To provide the physiological and psychological base for the effort, do a number of kilometers at that pace (at least 1 km at race pace for each 20 km of training). If the pace sometimes feels difficult, remember that the excitement of the race and the competition provided by others will elicit hormonal support to help ease the burden. (For more advice on aerobic training, see Part I.)

Anaerobic Threshold Training

To run, ski, swim, or cycle fast, you'll need well-trained fast twitch muscle fibers. Faster training (long intervals, pace training) will train fast oxidative glycolytic fibers and raise the anaerobic (lactate) threshold.

Anaerobic Training

You develop anaerobic capabilities at higher intensities, when you exceed the anaerobic threshold. Because high-intensity effort is fatiguing, it is best to alternate short periods of intense exertion with periods of active rest in the technique called **interval training**. Allow a gradual anaerobic buildup, beginning with longer intervals and rest periods. Increase the pace and shorten the distances as training progresses. Always use active rest (walk or slow jog) to hasten the removal of lactic acid (see Table 15.3).

The interval training prescription includes the rate and distance of the work interval, the length of the rest period, and the total number of repetitions (e.g., run 6 × 440 yd at 75 s with 2 min active rest). Rest intervals can be individually tailored by using the recovery heart rate. For example, your heart rate should return to 110 or 120 bpm before you attempt the next interval. Because interval runs are accomplished at a faster pace, they require a period of psychological adjustment. Some never learn to enjoy this form of training; I find it more tolerable when shared with others of similar ability.

The interval training concept allows a great deal of manipulation to suit individual needs and abilities. It can be relatively mild (e.g., 4 × 440 m at 90 s) for the neophyte, and it can be made more interesting with a variety of distances (e.g., 200, 400, 600, 800 m) and paces. It can also be mind numbing, like the program used by Buddy Edelen to prepare for the Tokyo Olympic Marathon. Buddy would run as many as 25 × 400 m to "break the monotony" of long-distance training. Roger Bannister trained until he could run 10 × 440 yd at 60 s to prepare for the first 4-min mile. You, too, can use interval training to prepare for athletic competition. But use it and all intense training in moderation, and never do more than two or three intense workouts a week.

Muscular Fitness Training

As sport becomes more competitive at every level, we must invest more time in muscular fitness training. You should evaluate the muscular demands of your sport as well as your strengths and weak points then proceed to develop a program to improve the strength, muscular endurance, power, or speed you need to reach your goals.

Off Season. This is the time for strength training. Select important muscle groups in the upper body, trunk, and legs and engage in a program following the prescriptions presented in chapter 6. Don't develop more strength than you need; when your strength is adequate for the sport, move on to the next phase of training.

For endurance sports (e.g., swimming or cross-country skiing) strength in a muscle group is adequate when it exceeds 2.5 times the force used in a typical stroke. For example, if you need 20 lb of force in the freestyle arm pull, you should have at least 50 lb (20 lb × 2.5 = 50 lb) of strength in the muscle group. Additional strength isn't likely to improve performance (Sharkey, 1984).

Table 15.3 Interval Training Suggestions

Intervals	Train	Repetitions	Duration	Work/rest ratio*	Max speed (%)	Max heart rate (%)
Long	Anaerobic threshold	4-6	2-5 min	1:1	70-80	85-90
Medium	Glycogen pathway	8-12	60-90 s	1:2	80-90	95
Short	High energy	15-20	30-60 s	1:3	95	100
Sprint	Speed	25+	10-30 s	1:3	100	100

*1:1 means the rest lasts as long as the work interval. 1:3 means the rest is 3 times as long as the work interval.

Preseason. By now you should be moving into power and endurance training. As the season approaches make the exercises more sport specific, more like the movements of the sport. Power is developed in 15 to 25 RM sets done as *fast* as possible. Short-term (anaerobic) endurance is improved in sets of 15 to 25 RM also, so this phase of muscular fitness training can achieve two goals.

Early Season. From now on the emphasis is on speed and the maintenance of gains in strength, endurance, and power. Practice sport skills at high speed to become more comfortable with speed and to improve neuromuscular coordination. Once-a-week maintenance sessions will retain strength and power gains.

When I took up cross-country ski racing I found that my upper body lacked the strength, power, and endurance to maintain vigorous poling throughout a race. So I undertook an off-season strength program to build up the triceps, deltoids, lats, and abdominal muscles used in poling. I did the bench press, dips, and other general exercises for the triceps, along with the more ski-specific exercise (see Figures 15.5 and 15.6). And I increased attention to my usually sagging abdominal muscles, using weighted sit-ups, the basket hang, and the Nautilus abdominal machine (see Figures 15.7 and 15.8).

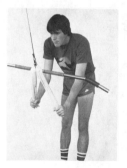

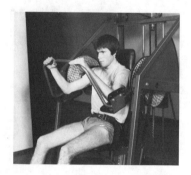

Figure 15.5. Universal; modified for cross-country (towel).

Figure 15.6. Nautilus; pull-over.

In the preseason I switched to even more specific exercises, including the roller-board (see Figure 15.9) and Exergenie for power and short-term endurance, and extended sessions on roller skis for long-term endurance. The early season included power training with short sprints, using only poles for propulsion.

What did all this effort yield? Well, my technique and race times improved significantly, as did my enjoyment of the sport. Evaluate the muscular demands of your sport and get started on a program. As you proceed to develop particular muscle groups, don't ignore flexibility and don't forget to maintain balance by training opposite sides of the joint. Excessive attention to one group, such as the quadricep group on the front of the thigh, could lead to muscle imbalance

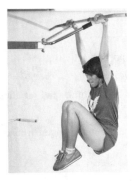

Figure 15.7. Universal; basket hang.

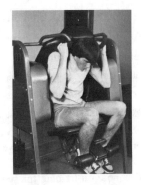

Figure 15.8. Nautilus; weighted sit-ups.

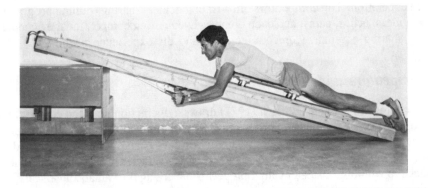

Figure 15.9. Rollerboard.

and a greater risk of injury. For more on training for sports see *Coaches' Guide to Sport Physiology* (Sharkey, 1986).

In Table 15.4 you'll find a format you can use to develop a program for your sport. Table 15.5 provides a work sheet for program development, and Table 15.6 includes a sample program that illustrates the use of the format and the work sheet.

The Psychology of Performance

Sport is a study in cooperation and competition. The quality of the overall experience depends on cooperation. Tennis opponents agree to cooperate by calling lines fairly, keeping track of the score, and observing the written and unwritten

Table 15.4 Developing Your Muscular Fitness Program

1. Determine the muscular fitness requirements of the sport or activity.
2. Identify the major muscle groups and movements involved.
3. Select exercises to develop muscular fitness in upper body, trunk, and leg muscles.
4. Make adjustments for strengths and weaknesses.[a]
5. Establish training goals, set up a schedule, and get started. Remember to keep good records and to test progress every few weeks.

Note. For more on training for sports see Sharkey (1986).

[a]Use fewer sets for strong areas, more for those in need of extra help.

rules of the game. Fair, enjoyable competition is impossible without a high degree of cooperation. Top competitors often train together, sharing training programs, new ideas, aches, pains, and even dreams. Even during competition they cooperate, sharing equipment, encouragement, and the experience itself.

Competitors and Performers

Psychologist Nathaniel Ehrlich (1971) draws a distinction between competitors and performers in athletic competition. **Competitors** evaluate their performances in athletic contests strictly on a relative, win-loss basis, giving little regard to the absolute level of performance. **Performers** attach only secondary importance to winning, instead evaluating performances against an absolute scale, an ideal (Ehrlich, 1971).

The competitor subscribes to the Vince Lombardi school, which says, "Winning isn't everything, it's the *only* thing." The performer, on the other hand, would say, "It isn't whether you win or lose, it's how (and how well) you play the game." Ehrlich draws an analogy between Maslow's self-esteem and self-actualization levels of motivation; the competitor seeks esteem, whereas the performer seeks to realize his or her potential. One would hope to find a more mature, self-actualizing approach to competition among adult athletes, in which each would seek his or her potential, with competition serving as a means to that end. Performers seek good competition because it helps them achieve their potential. Competitors fear good competition because it threatens their win-loss record, their self-esteem.

Statistics tell us that someone loses 50% of the time. If you value your mental health, if you don't want to be frustrated by defeat and lose your self-esteem, become a performer. Competitors realize that someone will soon be able to defeat them, thus their many hours of practice and competition ultimately will end in failure. Performers never fail. If their performance is flawed, they know that time and practice will bring them closer to their goal.

Table 15.5 Muscular Fitness Program Planner

Sport _____ Position _____

Season _____ Goals _____

Individual strengths _____

Weak points _____

Body part	Exercises	Muscle group	Purpose
Arm and shoulder			
Trunk			
Legs			
Other:			

Table 15.6 Sample Muscular Fitness Program

Sport ___ Basketball ___ Position ___ Forward ___

Season ___ Off-season ___ Goals ___ Strength and power ___

Individual strengths ___ Shooting ___

Weak points ___ Rebounding ___

Body part	Exercise	Muscle group	Purpose
Upper body	Lat pull-downs (with basketball)	Hands, arms, chest, and lats	Pull-down rebounds
	Curls	Arm flexors	Rebounding
Trunk	Abdominal curl (Nautilus)	Abdominals	Pull-down rebounds
	Back-ups	Lower back	Back strength
Legs	Leaper or power squats	Leg extension and jumping muscles	Sustained power for jumping
	Plyometrics (down jumping)	Leg extension and jumping muscles	Preload and jumping
	Hill (or stair) running	Leg extension and jumping muscles	Sustained power
	Rebounding and fast break drills		Sustained power and endurance in game situations

Note. When sufficient strength is acquired, shift to an endurance, power, or power-endurance program in the preseason (achieve power-endurance with 15-25 reps as fast as possible).

Try becoming a performer by focusing on the quality of the experience, not the final outcome. Don't get angry when you lose, rather realize that you need good competition. Without it, you would soon lose interest in the sport. Analyze, but don't judge your performance. Approach weaknesses positively ("I need to get my racket back earlier"), not negatively ("my forehand is lousy"). Set goals in terms of performance instead of wins, medals, or trophies. You may find that the wins and trophies come as performance improves. If not, you can still find satisfaction in the game, and you won't feel regret when it's over.

Playing the Game

Have you noticed how you do well on some days and poorly on others? Did you ever wish you could play your best game all of the time? Sport psychologists Tutko and Tosi (1976) offer suggestions to help you do just that, and to improve your ability to deal with the emotional side of your game.

To play your best game more often, try these steps.

- **Relax. Contract then relax muscles, and say "let go" as you learn muscle relaxation (as in Jacobson's *Progressive Relaxation*). Concentrate on breathing, and say "easy" with each exhalation (as in Benson's *The Relaxation Response*). Eventually, you can use these relaxation techniques in competition to help relieve tension.**
- **Concentrate. Focus your attention on an object in the game (e.g., a tennis ball) to free your mind of fears and negative judgments and to allow your best performance.**
- **Mentally rehearse. Rehearse mentally before and during practice and before competition to help focus on key elements of the game. Imagine yourself performing well.**
- **Physically rehearse. Rehearse physically to hone skills in days preceding competition and at skill rehearsal prior to the event.**

You will notice that these sport psychologists neglected to include advice on how to "psych" yourself up for the game. Did they forget it? Of course not. The fact is that most of us fail because we are overly aroused. We are so psyched up and concerned that we are literally tied in knots, unable to execute the skills we worked so hard to perfect. If we think too much and try too hard, we are bound to fail. So Tutko and Tosi provide advice aimed at helping you free your mind, relax, concentrate. Then and only then can you produce your best performance. You'll find yourself saying things like, "I played over my head," "I was out of my mind," or "I couldn't miss; everything I hit went in." Don't get me wrong; I'm not suggesting that you enter an event and then forget why you're there. On the contrary, you're there to play well and have fun, and you should savor every moment.

The theory behind this approach is based on the different roles played by the right and left brains. The left brain is absorbed with details, and is analytical and judgmental, whereas the right brain is concerned with movements, patterns, and the overall picture. Once skills are learned they should be performed without the critical review of the left brain. Relaxation and concentration allow us to play our best game more often.

Successful distance runners tend to "associate" during a race. They periodically tune in to their bodies so they will know how fast they dare run. They are consciously aware of pace, position, key opponents, and features along the course. Less successful runners tend to "disassociate," to lose track of time and place. Form becomes less efficient, and the pace lags.

Learn to handle your emotions, and you'll enjoy the game more. Eliminate your tensions, fears, and frustrations, and you may win more often. Become a performer, and you won't feel you've wasted a day just because you've lost. If you can do all these things and devote sufficient time to practice and training, you will be well on your way to achieving your potential. More importantly, the enjoyment and success you experience will keep you involved in a lifelong pursuit of excellence.

Performance Potential

I will conclude with some surprising insights concerning performance limits, insights gleaned from a careful analysis of the human assault on world records in running. In 1976 researchers at the University of Cincinnati published a fascinating account of the restraints on performance in running (Ryder, Carr, & Herget, 1976). Using running records from the past 50 years, the researchers plotted the rate of improvement and made some surprising conclusions.

On the average, the rate of improvements in distances ranging from 100 m to 30 km has been a steady but slow 0.75 m per minute per year. Because record breakers seldom participate in further assaults on the record, the authors concluded that good runners just don't work as hard after they have set a record. In fact, the authors contend that running records are still far below human physiological limits and that the restraints on performance largely are physiological and pathological. The major obstacle is not the race but the amount of daily training. In recent years, athletes have had to train several hours a day to achieve record-breaking status. Once the runner sets the record, he or she is likely to turn to other goals.

Thus, *time* is the major obstacle—time and the injuries associated with overuse and overtraining. If you feel stymied in your training or if you are stuck on a plateau, invest more time and progress will resume. Barring injury, you should be able to improve with more training. Following this line of reasoning, progress in world records will grind to a halt when athletes have invested all the training time that is humanly possible. For world-class athletes, training is already a full-time job. Of course, you and I cannot continue to invest more and more time in training, so we may define our potential as the level we attain following the maximum possible investment of time and effort.

As athletes spend more time training, new injuries arise. Young women now experience stress fractures from excessive running, and athletes in other sports develop a wide range of overuse injuries, all of which create a demand for athletic trainers, physical therapists, and physicians trained in sports medicine. Progress seldom comes without a cost—or an opportunity.

Given the limitations imposed by job and family as well as heredity, physique, sex, and age, you can still make dramatic progress toward your potential best performances. Consider the case of petite Michiko Suwa from Japan. She came to the United States at the age of 28, met and married Mike Gorman, and changed her first name to Miki. Five years later she began jogging, and in 1973 at the age of 38 she ran her first marathon. Later that same year she astounded the running world by setting a woman's world record; neither physique nor age predicted her potential. Or look at Priscella Welch, a former two-pack-a-day smoker who started running in her 30s and went on to win the women's division of the New York City Marathon. Or consider Sister Marion, a nun who qualified for the 1984 Olympic marathon trials at age 54, only 5 years after her first run!

Overtraining

Training, when overdone, can be a stressor that reduces resistance to infection, yet athletes at all levels seem prone to overtrain. They grew up believing the old adage of no pain, no gain, yet the risk of overtraining are many, including illness, injury, and lost time. So if you undertake serious training, you should become familiar with and use some simple ways to detect overtraining (see Table 15.7).

Table 15.7 Overtraining Indexes

Index	How it's used
Pulse index	Take the pulse rate daily (for 60 s), in the morning before rising. Average the daily rates. When the morning pulse is 5 or more beats above normal you should suspect illness or overtraining.

(Cont.)

Table 15.7 (Continued)

Index	How it's used
Weight index	Take the weight daily, in the morning (after toilet but before breakfast). Average daily weights. A rapid or persistent weight loss could indicate impending problems due to poor eating habits, failure to replace fluids, nervousness, or excessive fatigue.
Temperature index	Take the a.m. temperature daily for a week to establish the "normal." Then use it when the a.m. pulse is elevated. A fever usually indicates infection. Take a day off.
Fatigue index	Rate your tiredness after you arise.

Ready to drop	9
Extremely tired	8
Very tired	7
Slightly tired	6
About average	5
Somewhat fresh	4
Very fresh	3
Extremely fresh	2
Full of life	1

Note. Other useful signs include boredom, weakness, pain in joints, color of urine (dark, concentrated, or cloudy), and skin color (pasty, pale).

Remember, training should be approached as a gentle pastime. Make haste slowly and you will eventually reach your goals; overtrain and you risk illness or injury.

CHAPTER

16

LIFESTYLE

This chapter will help you

become familiar with beneficial health habits,

understand how fitness influences your physiological age, and

learn how you can create a supportive climate for the active lifestyle.

The daily habits of people have a great deal more to do with what makes them sick and when they die than all the influences of medicine.

Lester Breslow, MD, MPH (1980)

Health Habits

Since 1962, researchers at the Human Population Laboratory of the California Department of Health have studied the relationship of health to various health habits. According to their report (Breslow & Enstrom, 1980), health and longevity are associated with the following habits.

RECOMMENDATIONS FOR HEALTH AND LONG LIFE

Get adequate sleep (7 to 8 hr).

Eat a good breakfast.

Eat regular meals and avoid snacks.

Control your weight.

Abstain from smoking.

| **Drink moderately or not at all.**
| **Exercise regularly.**

The study found that men can add 11 years to their lives and women 7 years just by following six of the rules. Let's examine each practice to see if it fits your current lifestyle; then you can decide if changes are in order.

Sleep

Men or women who sleep 6 hr or less are not as healthy as those who sleep 7 or 8 hr nightly; those who sleep 9 hr or more are slightly below average in health. Thus 7 to 8 hr of sleep is most favorable and, as you might expect, too little sleep is more of a problem than too much.

Sleep is characterized by alternating stages. One stage involves rapid eye movements (REM) and changes in heart rate, blood pressure, and muscle tone. This stage may serve as a rest period for the inhibitory nerve cells of the brain; REM usually is accompanied by dreams, and if it is interrupted we become anxious and irritable. This REM sleep constitutes about 20% of the night's total, whereas deeper or quieter periods provide the rest necessary for recovery from fatigue (see Figure 16.1). If you miss some sleep one night, your body will not make any serious attempt to recover the sleep deprivation. However, if a substantial amount of the loss is REM sleep, the REM phase will be longer on subsequent nights. Going without sleep seems to impair creative capabilities, which suggests that another function of sleep is to restore a cerebral cortex fatigued by consciousness.

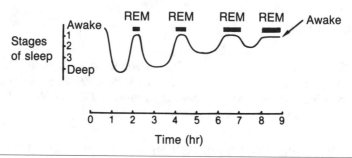

Figure 16.1. The stages of sleep.

Moderate physical activity seems to enhance the ability to fall into deep sleep without altering the time spent in REM sleep. Too little or too much exercise appears to result in sleep disturbance, and significant sleep loss seems to suppress the immune system.

Breakfast

In the California study, those who ate breakfast almost every day experienced better health than those who ate breakfast some of the time. Furthermore, a good breakfast may be a prerequisite to good performance in work and sport. Breakfast often comes 12 hr after the evening meal, so you can see why breakfast is important for energy and cellular metabolism. A few researchers suggest that breakfast should be the largest and most important meal, and everyone agrees that it should include more than a cup of coffee and a doughnut.

Regular Meals

Erratic eaters have poorer health than those who eat regular meals. Those who seldom or never eat between meals have better health than those who eat between meals regularly. Unfortunately, this study did not compare the health status of those who *regularly* eat smaller but more numerous meals, but it does indicate the effects of erratic eating behavior and snacking. We can only guess at the content of the between-meal snacks, but chances are that they were junk foods high in simple sugars and fat and low in nutrients.

Weight Control

When weight is more than 20% above or more than 10% below the desirable weight, health status declines. For example, if your desirable weight is 150 lb, your health status is most favorable when you maintain your weight between 135 lb (-10%) and 180 lb ($+20\%$), a broad margin of error indeed. It would be interesting to compare the effects on health of low body weight (more than 10% below desirable) due to malnutrition, illness, or smoking, and low weight due to habitual vigorous exercise. My personal observations indicate that a low body weight associated with vigorous exercise and good nutrition is at least as healthy as being above the desirable weight.

Smoking

Smoking, especially cigarette smoking, is dangerous to your health. If you don't smoke, don't start. If you do smoke, stop; it may be the best thing you ever do for yourself. And if you can't stop for your own health, think of loved ones, especially children, who are exposed to your habit. Is quitting worth the trouble? Data from numerous studies show that quitting has many benefits, including better oxygen-carrying capacity, lower blood pressure, improved night vision, and increased effectiveness of prescription drugs. And although some diseases, such as emphysema, can't be reversed, others seem to repair with time.

Repair time for smoking-induced illnesses are as follows.

Heart Disease	10 years
Cancer, Lung	10 to 15 years
Larynx	10 years
Mouth	10 to 15 years
Bladder	7 years

Quit today and help make the nation smoke-free by the year 2000.

Alcohol

Breslow and Enstrom (1980) found that poor health is associated with heavy alcohol consumption (five or more drinks at one sitting), and that those who never drink and those who drink moderately enjoy the same level of good health. This should not be construed as an endorsement of moderate alcohol consumption (one to two drinks a day). Even moderate alcoholic consumption, if continued for a sufficient period, can lead to effects on the liver even with adequate nutrition. The best advice is to drink moderately and infrequently, or don't drink at all.

Regular Exercise

The California study compared the health benefits of five types of activity: active sports, swimming or long walks, garden work, physical exercises, and hunting and fishing. Only hunting and fishing (seasonal and infrequent) were *not* associated with improved health. The best health was associated with active sports, followed by swimming or walking, physical exercise, and gardening, and the subjects who participated most often experienced the best physical health. Lowest death rates were recorded for those who were often active in sports, and the highest rates were for those who did *not* engage in exercise.

In summary, daily health habits and lifestyle affect physical health and longevity, even more than do all the influences of medicine. The California study indicated that a 55-year-old who follows all seven health habits has the same health status as a person 25 to 30 years younger who follows less than two of the health practices. Moreover, the researchers found a positive relationship between physical and mental health; so adherence to the seven health habits could contribute to good mental health. You know that an association or relationship between variables does not imply cause and effect, thus good physical health doesn't necessarily cause good mental health. But we are all familiar with psychosomatic illnesses and should realize that a healthy body is an important aid to good mental health. You can help maintain physical (and possibly mental) health by following the recommended health habits.

Physiological Versus Chronological Age

As I have suggested, chronological age is a poor predictor of health or performance. Health is a function of health habits, heredity, environment, and previous illness. Performance in work or sport is a function of the physiological age. The best single measure of physiological age is probably the aerobic fitness score, which tells you about the health and capacity of the respiratory, circulatory, and muscular systems. Moreover, a considerable body of evidence shows inverse relationships between aerobic fitness and a number of risk factors. Thus it is possible at age 60 to have the physiological and performance capabilities of the average 30 year old. This fact has considerable relevance when it comes to age restrictions in hiring; when physical performance is important, the physiological age is a more accurate predictor of performance potential than chronological age (Sharkey, 1987).

Other indicators of physiological age include the health risk age (see Appendix E) and measures of strength, reaction time, vision, hearing, and other variables influenced by age.

Fitness and Age

Cross-sectional and longitudinal studies show that fitness for the general population declines at the rate of 8 to 9% per decade. However, the decline for moderately active individuals is but 4%, and for trained individuals the rate of decline is 2% or less (see Figure 16.2). When weight and body fat gain is avoided, the rate of decline in fitness is minimized. Dr. Paul Davis of the Institute of Human Performance has shown that the major reason for the decline in fitness and performance with age is a rise in percent body fat (Davis & Starck, 1980).

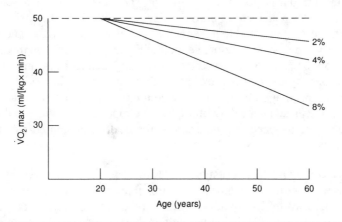

Figure 16.2. Decline in fitness with age. From Sharkey (1987).

Aerobic fitness is usually reported as milliliters of oxygen per kilogram of body weight. If weight goes up, fitness goes down. On the other hand, loss of *fat* weight constitutes the easiest way to improve aerobic fitness; a 10-kg (22-lb) loss from 90 to 80 kg will increase fitness from 40 to 45 ml/[kg × min], an improvement of more than 10% without working up a sweat!

The beneficial effects of a weight and fat control program on fitness, performance, and health are clear. The quality of life depends on the ability to pursue a variety of activities. Negative factors that affect this capacity for activity, such as excess body fat, should receive attention before irreversible physiological deterioration occurs. Excess fat restricts exercise capacity, causing a decline in fitness, which further reduces activity and results in additional fat accumulation—a vicious cycle indeed. A reduction in body fat allows, and may even promote, a more active lifestyle and minimizes the decrease in performance previously blamed on aging.

Caloric Restriction. Animal studies show that eating fewer calories (up to 40% less) can extend survival time dramatically (28% in one study where test animals were put on a low-protein diet after reaching adulthood). Some researchers feel that the most important factors determining life span are those that influence body fatness. Animals fed fewer calories also had a lower tumor incidence and less chronic disease (Comfort, 1979).

When Alexander Leaf studied healthy old people in three remote parts of the world, he found their diets low in calories and fat (1973). Leaf felt that the low-calorie diet, combined with regular physical activity and a productive and respected role in society, contributed to good health and long life. Indeed, although life expectancy has increased dramatically, the maximal attainable human life span remains unchanged at about 114 years, with the life expectancy approaching 85 years. Postponement of chronic illness has extended the period of adult vigor so more people are able to remain physically, emotionally, and intellectually vigorous until shortly before death (see Figure 16.3). We can modify many of the factors believed to be associated with age, such as heart and lung function, bone density, blood pressure, cholesterol, and other factors. Those of us who choose not to age rapidly can reduce morbidity and extend our vigorous years by living an active healthy life (Fries & Crapo, 1984), whereas those who decide to age rapidly become a burden on the health care and community support systems.

Free Radicals. One theory of aging holds that so-called **free radicals** (reactive molecules with one or more unpaired electrons) prove toxic to vulnerable tissues. In the biologic world, life span is inversely related to metabolic rate. Exercise produces oxygen radicals that could help or harm the body. Moderate activity enhances immune response by improving the ability of white blood cells to fight

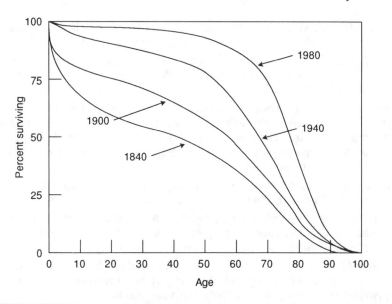

Figure 16.3. Survival curves. With less infant mortality and trauma (accidental death), more survive to the attainable life expectancy, 85 years. With good health habits, more are able to postpone chronic debilitating illness, to remain vigorous until the last years or months of life. *Note.* Adapted from *Vital Statistics of the United States*, 1977 (Vol. 2, Section 5). DHEW Publication PHS 80-1104, National Center for Health Statistics.

infection, but chronic heavy training may produce an excess of free radicals and depress the immune response (Demopolus, Santomier, Seligman, Pietrogro, & Hogan, 1986). The role of free radicals in exercise and aging requires more study. In the meantime, some scientists believe that vitamins A, C, and E provide some protection against the potentially toxic by-products of oxidative metabolism.

Longevity

One key to longevity, to what it takes to live well beyond normal life expectancy, is your lifestyle. Gerontologists, and others who work with healthy older survivors (over 75 years of age) will recognize the following traits and living habits associated with long-term survival.

PERSONAL CHARACTERISTICS ASSOCIATED WITH LONGEVITY

Moderation. **Long-term "survivors" make moderation a common denominator in phases of life, including diet, vices, work, and physical activity. Long-term survival, whether in a foot race or the human race, depends on pacing.**

Flexibility. Survivors have psychological flexibility, which implies the ability to bend but not break, to accept change, and to avoid rigid habits.

Challenge. Survivors accept challenges, create them if necessary, and don't allow life to become too easy. But when the challenge becomes too great, they say so and seek an alternative.

Health Habits. Survivors have a relaxed attitude toward health and are rather unconcerned about their health. They eat a wide variety of foods, do not seek out organic or other fad foods, and are not terribly concerned about avoiding items such as cholesterol. They are moderate in their use of alcohol and some even smoke now and then.

Relationships. Survivors enjoy other people and maintain an interest and continuous contact with friends and family. They enjoy their marriages.

Outlook. Survivors maintain a positive outlook; they recognize the effects of advancing age and *plan* to enjoy each phase of life. They realize that long life means growing old, and they are prepared to enjoy both life and aging.

Active Lifestyle. Survivors engage in daily routines that require activity and find reasons to be socially and physically active. Involvement in daily chores provides the rhythm and activity everyone needs.

The Active Lifestyle

The active lifestyle can benefit you in a number of ways.

- **Health**. Regular activity enhances both physical and mental health.
- **Economy**. Walking, jogging, or cycling to work or to shop saves money.
- **Ecology**. The active lifestyle helps conserve limited energy supplies, and physically active individuals have less impact on the environment than energy-consuming recreational vehicles.
- **Adaptability**. The active individual retains the ability to adapt to changes in the economy or the environment.
- **Survival**. Activity means survival. Senior citizens are survivors who have accumulated wisdom and insights that have value to future generations. The axiom in nature applies to the human race as well: The *fittest* survive.

Active individuals view each moment as one to be lived. They avoid people who depress them; when they feel moody or depressed they *do* something. They take risks, engage in life, and enjoy it; they don't waste the present with moods, worry, or immobilizing thoughts about the future. Depression, worry, guilt, and anger can lead to (or be caused by) subtle changes in brain chemistry and hormone levels. Physical activity can have a direct effect on moods and the chemistry of behavior; activity can also divert the attention and provide enjoyment and a sense of self-satisfaction that minimizes or eliminates self-defeating behavior.

You are free to think, feel, and act as you desire. You are not bound by circumstances, biorhythms, behavior traits, or deep-seated psychological problems. You can create the lifestyle you desire, if you really want to. Don't fall back on excuses like, "I haven't got the time; I'll start a program next week (month, year), I'm too busy right now; when the kids are a little older . . ."

Creating the Climate

With maturation comes the satisfaction of lower-order needs and the opportunity to seek self-actualization. The self-actualized individual is free to determine his or her lifestyle and personal goals and to pursue them without anxiety and without the necessity to conform, except superficially, to society's conventions and restraints. Self-actualized individuals seek to *be*, not to *become*; they enjoy their lives and realize their capacity. They require not the attention and adulation of the crowd, only a personal sense of satisfaction and achievement.

Sometimes making sacrifices is difficult, even for the self-actualized. Pursuing any goal is hard when those around you are nonsupportive. Fitness studies show that the emotional climate created by significant others is highly related to the participant's adherence to the program. When wives, husbands, and loved ones offer encouragement and support, the participant is likely to continue.

Why would anyone deprecate a loved one's efforts in a fitness or sport training program? Spouses often complain about the amount of time involved, the cost, and upset schedules and vacations. Of course, it is possible that some complain because they secretly envy their spouse's dedication and satisfaction, because they fear losing their rejuvenated loved one, or because they lose other shared experiences.

To avoid emotional conflicts, discuss your interests and goals with loved ones. Realize how your participation may affect them and try to minimize the effects. Substitute shared experiences to replace those lost in your personal quest for excellence. A supportive emotional climate is certain to prevail when *both* husband and wife are happily involved in active lifestyles. It isn't necessary for both to be involved in the same sport, although there are many such cases. If both seek excellence in tennis, it isn't absolutely necessary that they play together. What matters is that each understands how important participation is to the other, and that the emotional climate they create can influence both enjoyment and performance.

Climate and geography can enhance or detract from the enjoyment of participation, or in extreme cases they can eliminate it entirely. Tennis buffs able to play only 6 months a year play poorly against opponents from warmer climates or those who enjoy indoor facilities. Distance running can be cruel and inhuman punishment in hot, humid environments, unless you are able to train at night or in the early morning. Skiing is impossible in some parts of the country; if you want to participate, you'll have to move north or take expensive vacations.

The answer, albeit a simple one, is often ignored by many: If possible, move to where the climate and geography are best suited to your interests. Ridiculous, you say! Perhaps, but I've met hundreds who have done just that—left high-paying jobs amid the urban sprawl to seek a better way. I've met them by mountain lakes, on ski lifts, running in the desert, and while ski touring in the wilderness. Do they have regrets? Of course they do. Sometimes they wonder what might have been; some discover they made the wrong move and return.

If you are looking for a change in lifestyle, decide on your goals, your priorities and the kind of life you want to live and then give it your best effort. In time, if you feel the need to change, do it. It's all a part of the process of achieving your potential. With 85 years at your disposal, you will be able to try out several careers and locations. Don't lament time that you must spend away from a favored environment. Enjoy the present as much as possible and realize that future careers and locations await. Active, creative lifestyles are available everywhere, not just at distant holiday resorts. Adapt to the environment you are in and utilize it to learn new skills, not to regret the ones that don't fit the setting. But never give up on the dream that unites vocation, avocation, and location.

Seasonal Activity Planner

Physical activity should be spontaneous and enjoyable. Excessive planning can inhibit spontaneity and induce the kind of drudgery found in many fitness programs. On the other hand, a well-conceived program can add rhythm and substance to the flow of life, and help one season melt into the next. Using Table 16.1,

Table 16.1 Seasonal Activity Planner

	Winter	Spring	Summer	Fall
Major activities				
Minor activities				
Supplements				

sit down and outline your activity plan. Plan to give your chosen activities the same attention you regularly spend on other phases of your life, such as finance, education, or travel. You won't be sorry you did.

Fill in the sports or activities you enjoy each season. When you find a blank spot consider a new activity, supplement, or preparation for an upcoming season. This brief mental exercise will also show you how one activity can blend into the next, thereby removing the need for extensive physical preparation. Hiking or biking in the summer is excellent preparation for skiing. Year-round activity is the ideal way to maintain a desired level of fitness, because it minimizes the pains and soreness associated with the first few days of activity. It also keeps fitness at an optimal level and maximizes the weight control benefits of physical activity.

Life/Styles

Too busy to do all the things you want to do? Some activities, such as football, can only be enjoyed by the young, whereas others are perfectly suited for adults. Still others can be enjoyed at any stage of life (e.g., flyfishing, sailing, or golf). So relax, there is time for everything you want to do. Take a moment to list current and future activities and when you'll be able to enjoy them.

As you advance in years you will find new challenges and new adventures, and although you might temporarily put aside favorite activities, you'll never forget well-learned skills. Competition becomes more difficult as you approach the top of an age group, but when you enter a new age group, it's like being a kid again. Eventually you'll seek less competition and more cooperation; you'll discover the quiet world of sailing, the solitude of wilderness, or companionship with golf or tennis partners. For everything there is a season, so keep active and you'll find time to enjoy them all.

Physical Activity Versus Physical Fitness

Throughout this book I've hinted at an important question: Is it necessary to become fit to achieve health benefits, or is physical activity sufficient? Physicians, physiologists, epidemiologists and other health professionals actively seek an answer to this important question. As researchers do a better job of measuring activity and fitness we come closer to the answer. In the meantime, here is my opinion.

Physical activity and fitness are related to health. However, the major benefits seem to be associated with activity, with less emphasis on fitness. Blair and Kohl (1988) showed that the age-adjusted death rate drops to one third of the rate for inactive individuals when one becomes active, and that little further benefit occurs above a modest level of fitness (35 ml [kg × min] for men, 31.5 for women).

The implications of this finding, if it holds up in subsequent studies, are far-reaching, because less emphasis on fitness minimizes the risk associated with the vigorous training required to raise aerobic fitness. If you want to improve your fitness, you should, but you won't have to in order to gain health benefits. Aerobic fitness is defined and tested by a maximal oxygen consumption test. Most training studies use the $\dot{V}O_2$max as the measure of improvement. Virtually all our information on the prescription of exercise for aerobic fitness is aimed at improving the $\dot{V}O_2$max. If a high $\dot{V}O_2$max isn't necessary, the intense and sometimes more dangerous high-intensity training isn't necessary either.

> **The risks of exercise increase with intensity and duration. At the same time the health benefits of activity and fitness plateau as exercise increases beyond a moderate level. So to maximize health and minimize risk, engage in *regular, moderate activity*.**

Minimizing the $\dot{V}O_2$max

Studies on the relationship of aerobic fitness to performance in sports like running provide additional reasons to minimize the value of the maximal oxygen consumption test. Several studies show that performance in a 10-K (6.2-mi) run is more highly related to the lactate or ventilatory (anaerobic) threshold than to the $\dot{V}O_2$max test. The $\dot{V}O_2$max test indicates the maximal intensity that can only briefly be sustained. The threshold measurements provide information on the oxidative state of the muscles, which is far more related to *sustained performance* or endurance.

Conclusion

If your goal is health, become active and remain active. If you want to improve health *and* fitness, use the exercise prescriptions in this book. But remember, a high level of fitness isn't necessary to achieve the health benefits of exercise. In fact, health and performance may be better served by lower intensity, longer duration activities that burn fat and improve cellular oxidation and endurance.

EPILOGUE

This book began with a physiological analysis of fitness and its benefits, then discussed less measurable but no less meaningful aspects of psychology and their relationship to fitness and health. As I close I want you to know about another dimension of exercise and fitness, a dimension that provides meanings far beyond the measurable. I refer to the transcendent, peak, or even mystical experiences frequently reported by those who regularly engage in exercise and sport.

These moments of perfection are characterized by total involvement, total control, total concentration, ease of movement, and a sense of flow, described as a smooth sequence of movement without conscious effort. These rare moments can occur in training or competition, in individual or team sports, and at all levels of ability. They are more likely to occur when you are relaxed and non-judgmental than when you are critical or dissatisfied, and they impart meaning and satisfaction that transcend the physiological benefits of exercise.

So as you pursue the pleasures and values of exercise and fitness, remain open to peak experiences and flow. Don't become too preoccupied with time, distance, or pulse rates. Set aside a time during each exercise session when you just let things happen. Ignore form so you can enjoy sensations; forget time so you can experience the timeless state called flow. Because once you experience these things you will come back day after day to repeat the experience. And physical activity will be an integral part of your life.

Each of us is engaged in a lifelong search for meaning. The seasons of our lives are marked by an ebb and flow of purpose and confidence; periods of intense satisfaction are followed by periods of doubt. We need an arsenal of coping strategies to help us through the lows, as we regain confidence and establish new goals. Although faith and friends provide the major source of support, fitness provides discipline, challenge, and time for reflection. I hope this book helps you experience and appreciate all the dimensions of fitness.

A

THE PHYSIOLOGY OF EXERCISE: MUSCLES, ENERGY, AND OXYGEN

- **Energy Sources**
- **Oxygen and Energy Metabolism**
- **Muscle Contraction**
- **Respiratory System**
- **Circulatory System**

Fitness is earned during extended periods of movement, and movement re-quires muscles, energy, and oxygen. The brain tells the muscles to contract, then nervous impulses from the motor cortex are routed through neurons that descend the spinal cord and contact the motor nerves that stimulate muscle contractions (see Figure A.1). As they descend the cord, the impulses can

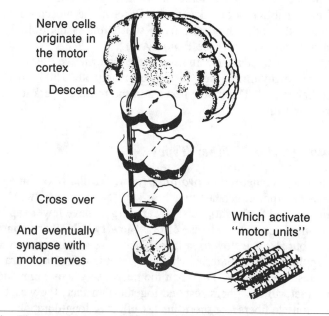

Nerve cells
originate in
the motor
cortex

Descend

Cross over

And eventually
synapse with
motor nerves

Which activate
"motor units"

Figure A.1. The motor cortex and the control of muscles.

be inhibited by other areas of the brain or by reflex mechanisms located in the spinal cord. Thus the body is able to ignore (or inhibit) direct orders from the top. We may tell ourselves to lean out over the hill, to angle our bodies so our skis will better edge on an icy slope, but inhibitions nullify the instructions and cause a fall. Or we may want to let loose on the dance floor, but our inhibitions won't allow this.

But inhibitions are not the only deterrent to regular activity. The use of exercise as a punishment or embarrassing experiences may limit future participation. Exercise is a conscious choice, and intelligent humans select enjoyable activities and avoid the unpleasant. So exercise must be enjoyable if it is to be continued. Keep this point in mind as you examine the physiology of exercise.

Muscle Fibers

Each muscle contains many thousands of spaghetti-like muscle fibers, ranging from 1 to 45 mm long. The fibers contain the contractile proteins actin and myosin. Muscles shorten and produce movement when the actin and myosin filaments creep along each other. The creeping is accomplished by tiny cross bridges extending from the thicker myosin to the thinner actin filaments. The cross bridges reach out, make contact, and pull like oars. The barely perceptible movement produced in one location is added to movement produced along the length of the fiber, and visible motion takes place. Because the muscles attach to bony lever systems, the rather modest muscle shortening is multiplied to produce familiar movement patterns (see Figure A.2).

Muscle fibers contract at the command of the motor nerve. Because each motor nerve branches many times, the typical neuron activates 150 individual muscle fibers simultaneously. The motor nerve and the muscle fibers it commands is called a **motor unit**.

The Motor Unit and Fiber Types

Human muscle is composed of two fiber types. All the fibers in a motor unit are of the same type, either fast twitch or slow twitch. **Fast twitch fibers** are fast contracting and fast to fatigue. They are larger, have fewer capillaries, and seem best suited for short, intense effort. **Slow twitch fibers** contract somewhat slower but also are slow to fatigue. They have a rich capillary supply and are well supplied with the internal chemistry required for long-duration endurance activities (see Table A.1). When the nervous system commands a motor unit to contract, all the fibers respond together. In fact, the way the nervous system uses muscle fibers (for short, intense effort or long-duration effort) seems to dictate their characteristics (see Figure A.3).

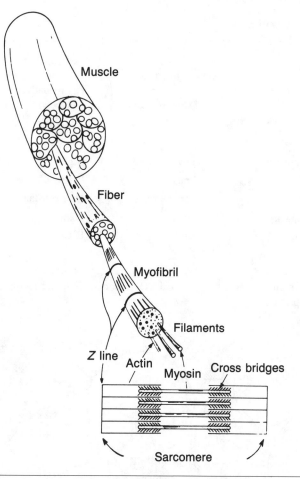

Figure A.2.   The architecture of muscle. *Note*. From Sharkey (1975).

Table A.1   Characteristics of Muscle Fibers

Characteristics	Slow twitch or slow oxidative (SO)	Fast twitch A or fast oxidative glycolytic (FOG)	Fast twitch B or fast glycolytic (FG)
Average fiber percentage	50%	35%	15%
Speed of contraction	Slow	Fast	Fast

(Cont.)

Table A.1 (Continued)

Characteristics	Slow twitch or slow oxidative (SO)	Fast twitch A or fast oxidative glycolytic (FOG)	Fast twitch B or fast glycolytic (FG)
Force of contraction	Low	High	High
Size	Smaller	Large	Large
Fatigability	Fatigue resistant	Less resistant	Easily fatigued
Aerobic capacity	High	Medium	Low
Capillary density	High	High	Low
Anaerobic capacity	Low	Medium	High

Note. We recruit SO fibers to jog, and FOG fibers to run, and recruit remaining FG fibers to sprint.

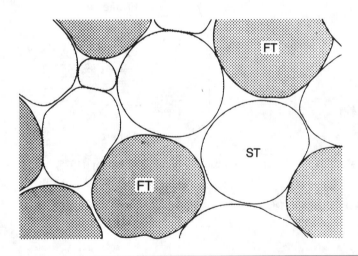

Figure A.3. Fast and slow twitch fibers intermingle in human muscle.

Heredity. A study of world class distance runners showed that these runners had an average of 80% slow twitch muscle fibers. Sprinters, long jumpers, and high jumpers have a high percentage of fast twitch fibers (Saltin, Henriksson, Nygaard, & Andersen, 1977). It may be that you will have to pick your parents carefully if you want to excel in either endurance or high-speed sporting events. Heredity dictates the *ratio* of slow and fast twitch fibers.

Training.   The current research on humans shows that training can improve the performance of either fiber type, but research doesn't prove that you can transform a fast fiber into a slow one, or vice versa. The nervous system recruits slow twitch fibers for endurance activities such as distance running and begins to recruit the fast twitch fibers when the slow fibers have fatigued or when the pace picks up. So any improvement in the fast fibers will be accompanied by change in the slow fibers, usually allowing the slow fibers to retain their original advantage. Training exerts its influence on the percentage area of the fibers. Strength training will make fast twitch fibers larger, but it won't change a slow fiber to a fast one. And although endurance training can increase the oxidative abilities of slow and fast fibers, it won't necessarily change a fast fiber to a slow one.

Recent animal studies show that prolonged activity can transform fast fibers to slow fibers. Metabolic changes occur first, with the fast fibers becoming more oxidative. Then come changes in the myosin subunits that dictate contractile speed (Pette, 1984). Although the contractile changes have not been replicated in human subjects, studies show that the metabolic changes do take place, indicating the adaptability of muscle with training.

Energy for Muscles

Energy—the ability to do work—comes from the sun, is converted into chemical compounds by plants and animals, and eventually finds its way into your body in the form of carbohydrate, fat, or protein molecules. The chemical breakdown of these molecules, oxidation, releases the stored energy and uses it to power the human machine.

Protein

Protein provides the amino acid building blocks we need to build and repair tissue and to synthesize important enzymes and hormones. Protein is usually a minor source of energy, but it becomes an important source during periods of dieting or starvation. For more information about this important nutrient see Part III.

Carbohydrate and Fat

The muscles cannot directly use carbohydrate and fat. They are processed enzymatically to release energy that is used to form the important high-energy compound adenosine triphosphate (ATP), the "energy currency." When the motor nerve tells a muscle fiber to pull, the body expends ATP to provide the immediate energy for contraction. However, because the amount of stored ATP is small, exercise would last only a few seconds if the muscle couldn't begin immediately to produce more ATP by the breakdown of carbohydrate and fat. Following is a brief summary of the pathways that provide the energy for muscular contractions.

1. A nerve impulse triggers splitting of ATP to provide energy for contraction.
2. High-energy creatine phosphate (CP) splits to provide energy for resynthesis of ATP.
3. Glucose or its storage form, glycogen (carbohydrates), is broken down in a pathway called glycolysis to form lactic acid and ATP.
4. Glucose, glycogen, or free fatty acids (fat) are systematically broken down or oxidized by a series of enzymes and finally combine with oxygen to form carbon dioxide and water; the energy released is used to form ATP.

Steps 1, 2, and 3 are nonoxidative, or **anaerobic**; they do not require the presence of oxygen. Step 4 requires oxygen, so it is called **aerobic**.

Anaerobic metabolism of glucose leads to the formation of 2 molecules of ATP, whereas the aerobic metabolism of glucose yields 38 molecules of ATP. This is why you are able to exercise indefinitely at a moderate rate (aerobic) but are limited to a minute or less of all-out anaerobic effort.

Production of Energy

Energy can be neither created nor destroyed, so it is more appropriate to speak of **energy transfer**. We can view muscle as a controlled combustion chamber where the energy stored in carbohydrate and fat is slowly transferred to ATP. The key to this process is **enzyme action**. Enzymes are organic catalysts that release and transfer energy. The 6-carbon glucose molecule is systematically cleaved to form 3-carbon pyruvic acid molecules in the pathway called glycolysis (see Figure A.4).

When sufficient oxygen is available, the 3-carbon skeleton continues into the cell's energy factory, the **mitochondria**, where all oxidative metabolism takes place. There it passes along metabolic pathways (citric acid cycle and the electron transport pathway) to eventually join with oxygen ($C_6H_{12}O_6 + 6O_2 \rightarrow 6CO_2 + H_2O$). Fragments of fat molecules (called free fatty acids, or FFA) enter the mitochondria, and the long carbon chains (e.g., C_{16}) are enzymatically reduced to 2-carbon fragments. These segments then enter the citric acid and electron transport pathways and end up as carbon dioxide and water.

The enzymes that catalyze these reactions are most interesting. Each contains a larger protein portion and a smaller coenzyme. Although the shape of the protein portion dictates the substrate to be acted upon, the coenzyme is the important active portion of the complex. It may surprise you that many vitamins are

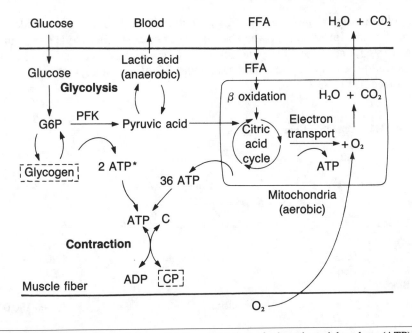

Figure A.4. Metabolic pathways and the production of adenosine triphosphate (ATP). Limited glycogen and creatine phosphate (CP) supplies are depleted at the start of exercise, during high-intensity effort and during the transition to exhaustion. Blood glucose is spared for use by the central nervous system. Free fatty acids (FFA) provide the major fuel for prolonged exercise. *Anaerobic: Glucose → pyruvate = gain of 2 ATP; Aerobic: Glucose → CO_2 + H_2O = 38 ATP. *Note.* From Sharkey (1975).

coenzymes. Each enzyme has a simple job such as adding or taking away water or hydrogen. Enzyme activity can be influenced by several factors.

- *Temperature*: Enzyme activity increases when the muscles are warmed, so energy production is enhanced following warm-up.
- *Acidity*: Each enzyme works best at a particular acid-base level. Vigorous exercise produces lactic acid and hydrogen ions, and the increased acidity (lower pH) reduces enzyme activity and energy production, leading to fatigue.
- *Availability of fuel*: Enzymes seem to work faster when more fuel (substrate) is available. In the text I tell you how to eat to make more fuel available and, as a special bonus, how to train to increase the concentration of enzymes.

Availability of Energy

ATP and CP are good only for 3 to 4 cal of energy and can be exhausted in a few seconds of maximal effort, such as running up stairs. A limited supply of glucose is available in the blood, but it is needed for brain and nerve metabolism, for which it is the sole source of energy. Glucose is stored in the liver (80 g) and muscle (15 g per kilogram of muscle) as glycogen. If you could use it all for exercise, you would have about 1,200 cal, enough to fuel a 10-mile run (see Table A.2).

Table A.2 Available Energy Sources

Source	Supply	Energy (cal)
ATP and CP	Small quantities stored in muscle	5
Carbohydrate		
Muscle glycogen	15 g (per kg of muscle)	1,200
Liver glycogen	80 g	320
Blood glucose	4 g	16
Fat	Adipose tissue	50,000-100,000[a]

Note. Adapted from Sharkey (1984).

[a]Depends on % body fat and body weight: for example, 15% fat × 150 lb = 22.5 lb fat; 22.5 lb × 3,500 cal/lb = 78,750 cal of energy stored as fat.

Fat is the most abundant source of energy. Young men average 12.5% body fat; young women average 25%. If you weigh 121 lb (55 kg) and have 25% fat, you'll have about 30 lb of fat. Because each pound of fat yields 3,500 cal of energy, 30 lb of fat would yield 105,000 cal of energy. When you consider that you burn up about 100 cal per mile, you realize that you have enough energy in the form of fat to run more than 1,000 miles! Most of us have more fat than we need, so all we need to do is learn how to burn fat during exercise. In so doing, we extend our endurance dramatically, eliminate the problem of excess weight, and improve overall health.

Use of Energy

To delay fatigue we must use aerobic pathways. They are more efficient than anaerobic pathways, and the fuels are abundant. As exercise intensifies from a walk to a jog, we switch from fat as the predominant source of energy to a fat-carbohydrate (glycogen) mixture. Switch from a jog to a run, and glycogen becomes the main source of energy. Sprint, and glycogen is the sole source of energy.

The intensity of exercise dictates the fuel used for exercise. Carbohydrate ($C_6H_{12}O_6$) has more oxygen per atom of carbon than a typical fatty acid ($C_{16}H_{32}O_2$), which is oxygen poor. Because oxygen supply is critical during intense effort, it is not surprising to find we switch to the fuel less likely to strain the oxygen delivery system (see Figure A.5).

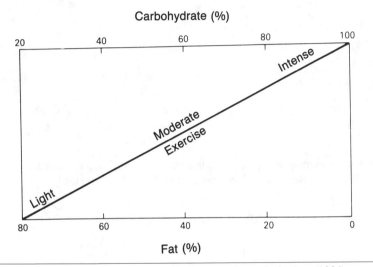

Carbohydrate (%)

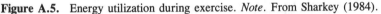

Fat (%)

Figure A.5. Energy utilization during exercise. *Note.* From Sharkey (1984).

The sources of energy include the following:

For rest, FFA and glucose

When exercise begins, CP and glycogen

At steady state, FFA/glycogen/glucose

At exhaustion, CP and/or glycogen
  (short intense depletes CP; prolonged depletes glycogen).

Glycogen in the muscles is preferred over blood glucose as a fuel during exercise. One molecule of ATP is used when glucose enters the muscle, so previously stored glycogen yields more energy just when it is needed (see Figure A.6).

In long-duration exercise (over 80 min) the use of blood glucose increases as muscle glycogen is depleted. Eventually, liver glycogen stores decline, the blood glucose concentration falls (the condition is known as hypoglycemia or low blood sugar), and you become severely fatigued. Glucose feeding will restore energy and allow continued activity (see Figure A.7).

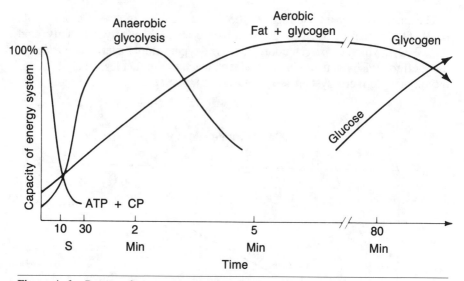

Figure A.6. Pattern of energy use. As muscle glycogen is used up, blood glucose temporarily fills the demand for carbohydrates. *Note.* From Sharkey (1984).

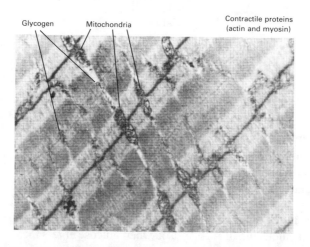

Figure A.7. Skeletal muscle. Note the actin and myosin filaments. Observe the oblong mitochondria where all oxidative energy production takes place. The small dark particles are granules of glycogen × 11,000. *Note.* From "Effect of Exercise and Training on Mitochondria of Skeletal Muscle" by P.D. Gollnick and D.W. King, 1969, *American Journal of Physiology*, **216**, p. 1505.

During long-duration exercise, fat utilization increases with time. Fat mobilization from adipose tissue is delayed in the first half-hour of exercise. But as the activity continues, fat use increases. Training increases fat utilization, with early supplies coming from triglyceride stored in muscle (Holloszy et al., 1986). As I have said, fat is so abundant it cannot be depleted during exercise.

Oxygen and Exercise

Oxygen is the key to aerobic exercise. When you can't supply sufficient oxygen, you are forced to use inefficient anaerobic pathways and limited sources of energy, such as ATP, CP, and glycogen. When you begin to exercise, oxygen intake does not immediately meet demands. An oxygen deficit results as you rely on ATP, CP, and anaerobic glycolysis (leading to formation of lactic acid). When oxygen intake meets the demands, a steady state is achieved, and exercise can continue as long as you are able to meet the fuel and oxygen requirements. After exercise, oxygen returns slowly to resting levels. Recovery oxygen intake in excess of resting needs is called the **oxygen debt**. The debt or excess postexercise oxygen consumption is used to repay the oxygen deficit, to replace ATP and CP, to remove lactic acid, and to replace some of the energy used during exercise (see Figure A.8).

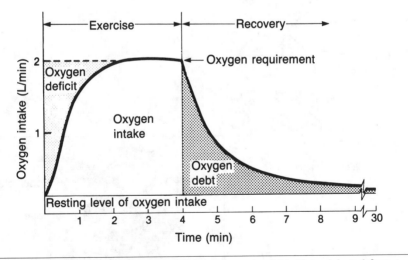

Figure A.8. Oxygen intake, oxygen deficit, and oxygen debt. *Note.* Adapted from Sharkey (1975).

Oxygen, then, is the key to prolonged activity. Now let's see how air gets into the lungs and how blood and circulation carry oxygen and energy to working muscles.

Respiration

Most people have said, "I ran out of wind" or "I couldn't catch my breath." There is no doubting the sensation of fatigue associated with breathing during exercise, but that sensation doesn't necessarily mean that you lack sufficient oxygen. Respiration has two major functions: getting oxygen into the body and getting rid of carbon dioxide. We tend to ignore the latter, but we shouldn't. Insufficient removal of carbon dioxide may impose limits on our ability to sustain vigorous activity.

Atmospheric air contains 20.93% oxygen. Air enters the lungs when the diaphragm contracts and creates an area of lower pressure, allowing air to rush in. When the diaphragm relaxes, air is exhaled. During exercise exhalation is assisted by abdominal and intercostal (between rib) muscles. Breathing takes more energy and oxygen during exercise (see Figure A.9).

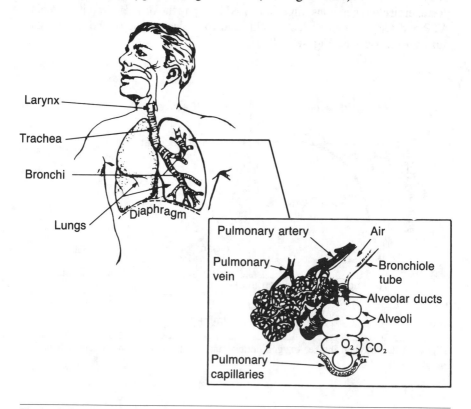

Figure A.9. Respiratory system.

Ventilation

Ventilation describes the volume (V) of air you inhale or exhale per minute. It is the product of respiratory rate or frequency (f) and the volume of air per breath (tidal volume, or TV): $V = f \times TV$. A resting ventilation of 6 L results from a rate of 12 breaths per minute and tidal volume of 0.5 L. During moderate effort, ventilation increases to 40 or 50 L/min and reaches 120 L at maximal exertion (e.g., 120 L = 40 breaths $\times$ 3 L air).

Although we can control the rate and depth of respiration consciously, we usually leave control to the autonomic nervous system, which seems quite able to fine tune air intake to the demands of exercise. Sensory receptors in the joints first signal the need for increased ventilation. Then chemical receptors sense rising levels of carbon dioxide in the blood and use that information to regulate the rate and depth of respiration. Proof of the importance of carbon dioxide is easily demonstrated. Inhale and exhale deeply (hyperventilate) about 10 times or until dizzy, then take one more deep breath and hold it as long as you can. You'll find you can hold your breath much longer after "blowing off" carbon dioxide, the respiratory stimulus.

Some of the air we inhale never gets to the tiny air sacs (alveoli) where diffusion takes place. Air that remains in the passageways (nose, mouth, pharynx, larynx, trachea, bronchi, and bronchioles) cannot transfer its oxygen into the blood. This volume of air in the so-called **dead space** amounts to about 0.15 L, or almost one third of the resting tidal volume. Because of the dead space, taking deeper breaths so more air reaches the lungs is more efficient. Although rate and depth of respiration are self-adjusting, they can be influenced. Trained respiratory muscles are able to take in more air per breath.

Diffusion

To reach the blood, oxygen must cross the thin alveolar and capillary membranes. The physical process of diffusion, by which molecules move from an area of higher concentration to a lower one, explains the movement of oxygen into the blood and carbon dioxide from the blood.

The concentration or molecular activity of a gas is referred to as its partial pressure. Partial pressure of a gas depends on the percentage of that gas in the atmosphere. Thus the partial pressure of oxygen (PO_2) is equal to its percentage (20.93%) times the atmospheric pressure (760 mmHg at sea level) or: $PO_2 = .2093 \times 760 = 159$ mmHg.

Oxygen passes from the atmosphere ($PO_2 = 159$ mmHg) into the alveoli ($PO_2 = 100$ mmHg). The decline in partial pressure is due to a mixing effect with old air in the dead space and lungs. Oxygen then goes into the blood and finds its way to the muscles where the PO_2 may be 40 mmHg or less. The carbon dioxide goes in the other direction, from muscles, to blood, to lungs, and to the atmosphere.

Gas Transport

How are oxygen and carbon dioxide transported by the blood to or from the working muscles?

Oxygen Transport.   A small amount of oxygen that diffuses into the blood is carried in simple solution. If that were all we could transport, we would be in serious trouble. Fortunately, hemoglobin is available to increase the oxygen-carrying capacity of the blood about 70 times. This large protein molecule contains four subunits containing iron. Each iron atom can temporarily bind a molecule of oxygen (O_2) in loose association.

Men average 15 to 16 g of hemoglobin per 100 ml of blood; women average 13 to 14 g. Each gram of hemoglobin holds 1.34 ml of oxygen, so under normal conditions the hemoglobin has about 19.5 ml of oxygen. With the 0.29 ml that is carried in solution, the blood has about 19.8 ml of oxygen per 100 ml of blood.

Arteriovenous Oxygen Difference.   After the blood passes by the tissues, the oxygen content of venous blood drops to 15.2 ml. This resting arteriovenous oxygen difference of 4.6 ml (19.8 − 15.2 = 4.6 ml of oxygen) describes how much oxygen is dropped off at the tissues. Thus the tissues have taken 4.6 ml of oxygen from each 100 ml of blood. During vigorous exercise the arteriovenous oxygen difference can increase over 3 times, providing more than 16 ml of oxygen per 100 ml of blood. When you realize that blood flow to muscles also increases dramatically, you can begin to understand how oxygen utilization can be increased as much as 20 times above resting levels.

Hemoglobin Saturation.   Each red blood cell flows through the tiny lung capillary in less than a second. During vigorous effort the cell has less than half a second to pick up oxygen. Even then oxygen saturation returns to 97% of capacity. Will breathing pure oxygen further increase the saturation? Not enough to improve performance and hardly enough to justify the cost.

Carbon Dioxide Transport.   Physical activity increases production of carbon dioxide. As it diffuses from muscle fibers into the blood, carbon dioxide unites with water to form carbonic acid.

$$CO_2 + H_2O = H_2CO_3$$

Carbonic acid then splits (dissociates) to form hydrogen and bicarbonate ions.

$$H_2CO_3 = H^+ + HCO_3^-$$

This presents a problem, because the free hydrogen ions (H^+) are very reactive (acidic). They must be soaked up (or buffered) by other compounds, or they cause problems. Remember that enzymes are less effective when the acid-base balance goes down. Because vigorous exercise also increases muscle and blood lactic acid levels, you can see how important acid-base balance is during physical activity.

Acid-Base Balance (pH)

We have three lines of defense against marked changes in the acid-base balance (pH): buffers, respiration, and the kidneys. The kidneys receive a diminished blood supply during vigorous effort so they must do their job of hydrogen ion removal after exercise stops.

Hemoglobin, buffer systems, and protein molecules in the blood are able to buffer free hydrogen ions without a noticeable effect on the pH. One important buffer works closely with respiration to keep the pH of the blood close to 7.4. This buffer soaks up hydrogen ions and carbon dioxide and, when the blood reaches the lungs, blows them off as carbon dioxide and water. By working together, buffers and respiration minimize the undesirable by-products of vigorous effort. However, intense exercise eventually produces enough acidic by-products to interfere with the contractile process, slow enzyme activity, and cause fatigue.

Attempts to improve buffering capacity with the ingestion of bicarbonate solutions have shown some promise, especially in short events such as an 800-m run.

Circulation

We have followed oxygen from the atmosphere to the blood. Now let us consider the blood, heart, and blood vessels that transport oxygen to the working muscles.

Blood

Could you perform better with more red blood cells and hemoglobin? Swedish researchers took 800 or 1,200 cm³ of blood from two groups of subjects who then engaged in endurance training (Ekblom, Goldbarg, & Gullbring, 1973). After several weeks the subjects received a reinfusion of their own red cells. The following day they were able to double endurance running time and increase maximal oxygen intake 9%! Although I would never advocate the use of "blood doping" to achieve an edge in athletics, I mention the study to emphasize the importance of blood volume, red cells, and hemoglobin.

The blood serves to transport oxygen and carbon dioxide as well as foods, waste products, hormones, antibodies, and even heat. Blood also helps to regulate the pH. Studying the cells and plasma of this complex fluid will aid your understanding of its role in exercise and training.

Blood Cells. The cellular components of blood, including red cells, white cells, and platelets, compose about 45% of the total blood volume. Blood volume averages 5 L, about 7 to 8% of body weight for a 70-kg (154-lb) person.

Red Cells. Red cells number about 5 million per cubic millimeter; they are formed in bone marrow and survive approximately 120 days. Red cell production can be stimulated by the diminished oxygen supply encountered at high altitude. The red cells, or **erythrocytes**, contain all the hemoglobin found in the blood. The hemoglobin is degraded when the red cell completes its life cycle, but the iron portion can be reused for red cell synthesis. Growing young people are sometimes iron deficient, as are adult females, so a good diet or regular iron supplement is recommended for women and young men engaged in vigorous endurance activity.

White Cells. White cells are involved in phagocytosis and antibody reactions and number 4,000 to 11,000 per cubic millimeter. Platelets (300,000 per cubic millimeter) are important for clot formation; substances contained within their walls cause local vasoconstriction when a vessel is injured. The platelets themselves also serve to clog the forming clot.

Blood Plasma. Plasma is remarkable, both for what it carries and for what it does. Plasma makes heat transfer and temperature regulation possible, because the fluid that forms the basis of blood plasma is water. Although water is known as the universal solvent, not all the constituents of the blood are in true solution. Some very large protein molecules are suspended in solution. These proteins are important because they help provide buffering capacity and because they exert an osmotic force that tends to keep water from leaving the bloodstream.

Albumin is the protein most responsible for the osmotic pressure of the blood. The **globulin** protein fraction is involved in antibody formation. **Fibrinogen**, the largest of the plasma proteins, is an essential element in the clotting mechanism.

Blood Clotting. The development of a clot involves a series of steps that eventually leads to the formation of insoluble fibrin threads from once-soluble fibrinogen. Once formed, the fibrin branches catch sticky platelets like leaves in a stream. To counteract the tendency for premature clotting, the blood has a clot-busting system called the fibrinolytic system. Premature clots could clog vessels in the heart or brain and cause a heart attack or stroke. Thus, enhancing the fibrinolytic system seems most desirable.

Exercise of moderate intensity seems to enhance fibrinolysis. The effect lasts a day or two, but no longer, thus it is necessary to engage in moderate exercise on a regular basis. If the exercise is too intense or stressful, the effect is lost and clotting time is reduced. Stress increases the production of the adreno-corticotrophic hormone (ACTH), which inhibits the fibrinolytic system. Also, stress leads to an increased secretion of epinephrine, which has long been known to hasten blood clotting.

I cannot leave this brief discussion of clotting without a warning to women. Some years ago evidence implicated the birth control pill in clotting disorders, and some labels warned of a twofold increase in the incidence of clotting disorders among women using the pill. The improved pill used today is much safer. However, those who elect to use the pill should be aware of the added effects of emotional and physical stress and smoking on blood clotting. Moderate physical activity does not seem to significantly influence clotting time for regularly active *nonsmoking* women who use the pill.

The Heart

The heart is the ultimate endurance muscle, amply supplied with mitochondria for oxygen utilization. It has a well-developed system of blood vessels (coronary arteries) for delivery of oxygen and fuel to the cardiac muscle. In simple terms, the heart consists of two pumps: the right side (pulmonary pump), which sends blood to the lungs, and the left side (systemic pump), which pumps blood through the rest of the body (see Figure A.10).

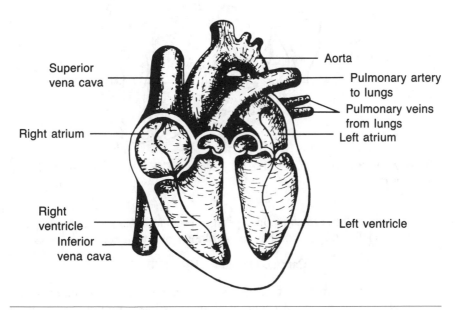

Figure A.10. The heart.

As a red blood cell returns to the heart after delivering oxygen to working muscles in the leg, the red blood cell ascends the inferior vena cava to the right side of the heart, mixes with blood coming from above by way of the superior vena cava, and enters the right atrium. As the atria contract, the blood moves to the right ventricle. Contraction of the ventricles sends the red blood cell to the lungs by way of the pulmonary circulation. The cell passes through ever smaller channels until it reaches a capillary no wider than itself (8 microns). During the cell's brief residence in the capillary (about 0.75 s), it picks up a supply of oxygen. Then the cell returns to the left atrium and is pushed down into the thickly muscled left ventricle and sent swiftly on its way with a vigorous contraction. Coursing upward in the aorta, the cell may pass into one of the branches serving the upper body, or it could continue in the down-curving aorta to serve the trunk or lower extremities. One other possibility exists: The cell could pass quickly into the coronary circulation to provide the oxygen necessary for the heart itself (see Figure A.11).

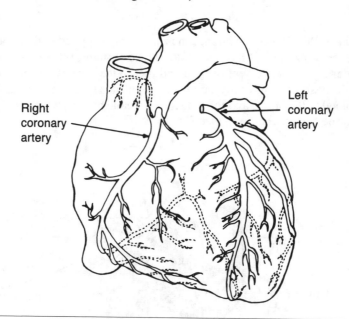

Figure A.11. Coronary arteries. The left coronary artery branches to serve the muscular left ventricle.

The output of the cardiac pump depends on two factors: the rate of the pump (heart rate, HR) and the volume per stroke (stroke volume, SV). Thus:

$$\text{Cardiac Output} = \text{HR} \times \text{SV}$$

With a resting heart rate of 72 bpm and a stroke volume of 70 ml of blood, the cardiac output is about 5 L/min of blood. It is interesting to observe what happens to these factors with exercise, when the need for blood flow increases.

__Heart Rate and Exercise__. As the intensity of work increases, the HR rises in a linear fashion (see Figure A.12). HR is controlled by impulses arriving at the sinoatrial node. When exercise begins, blood vessels in the skeletal muscles dilate to allow more blood to flow. This dilation leads to a drop in blood pressure, which pressure receptors sense and the information is relayed to the cardiac control center in the brain. The center then sends a call for a faster, stronger heart beat. When pressure becomes too high in the arteries, the cardiac control centers tells the heart to slow down. In this way the HR is fine tuned to the demands of exercise. The HR is an excellent barometer of the intensity of exercise.

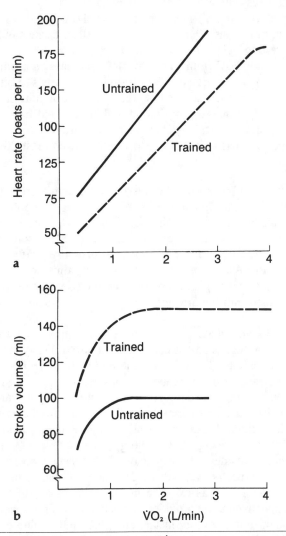

Figure A.12. Relationship of oxygen intake ($\dot{V}O_2$) to heart rate (a) and stroke volume (b). At work loads above 1.4 L/min any increase in the cardiac output results from an increase in the heart rate. *Note*. From Sharkey (1975).

Stroke Volume and Exercise. SV also rises during exercise. However, the increase plateaus at relatively low work loads (see Figure A.12). Beyond that point no further increase in SV takes place. Because cardiac output is the product of HR and SV, it seems clear that further increases in cardiac output are due to changes in HR alone. This point is of considerable importance, because it supports the use of exercise heart rate as an indicator of cardiac output, as well as the energy expenditure of exercise. This one simple measure provides accurate information regarding the intensity of exercise, an important factor in the prescription of exercise. It can serve as a guide to caloric expenditure during exercise and to assess the effects of aerobic training.

Cardiac output (HR × SV) increases to meet the demands of exercise. At a moderate level of exercise (HR = 150; SV = 100), cardiac output is 15 L, or 3 times the resting value. At maximal effort (HR = 200; SV = 100), the pump is pushing out 20 L/min. This fourfold increase in cardiac output is accompanied by a *redistribution* of blood from inactive areas to active muscles. The intensity of exercise dictates the degree of redistribution. Some digestion may go on during light activity, but blood will be diverted from the digestive organs during maximal effort. Together, increased cardiac output and the redistribution of blood increase blood flow to the muscles almost 20 times above resting values!

Oxygen and Fuel. Oxygen for the heart muscle comes from the coronary circulation (see Figure A.11). Maintenance of the oxygen supply is crucial because the heart cannot utilize anaerobic energy sources. During exercise the heart gets the additional oxygen it needs by increasing coronary blood flow. The best indicator of myocardial oxygen needs is the **rate-pressure product**: HR × Systolic Blood Pressure. As HR increases, the working time per minute goes up, hence a greater need for oxygen. As blood pressure rises, the heart has to pump harder to send blood into the arteries, and more work means more oxygen is needed.

Because both HR and blood pressure increase dramatically during maximal lifting efforts, physiologists advise caution in the use of heavy resistance exercises for untrained adults. The strong static contractions increase the oxygen needs of the heart and also can reduce venous return to the right side of the heart. Thus when blood flow and oxygen needs increase, supply can be reduced. These events can be alarming for those with already narrowed coronary arteries. However, healthy individuals can actually use resistance training to lower coronary risk factors (Hurley, Hagberg, & Goldberg, 1988).

Fuel for the heart includes free fatty acids (FFA), lactate, and glucose (about 40, 30, and 30%, respectively, at rest). This doesn't change much with light effort such as walking, but as exercise intensity increases, FFA and glucose metabolism decline, and lactate provides as much as 60% of the energy required. During exercise of long duration, lactate and glucose contributions eventually decline and FFA utilization rises to almost 70% of the total energy production (Keul, 1971). It appears that the heart is adaptable as far as energy is concerned.

Blood Vessels

Blood leaves the heart and travels through strong, elastic arteries. As the blood approaches the muscles, the vessels branch and arterial diameter diminishes. Traveling through ever-smaller arterioles, the blood finally reaches the capillary bed, where oxygen and fuels are exchanged for carbon dioxide and metabolic waste products. On the return journey the blood passes through tiny veins and on through larger veins to the vena cava. Veins are not well muscled and tend to allow blood to pool. Valves within veins keep blood from backing up. With the help of skeletal muscle contractions squeezing on the vessels, the blood is moved back toward the heart. This "muscular pump" is a vital component of venous return. Remember what happens to a soldier forced to stand at attention for a long period? Blood pools in the large veins of the legs, venous return is diminished, and cardiac output declines. As a result, the brain lacks blood and oxygen, and the soldier falls to the ground in a faint.

Blood flow depends on the pressure (P) driving blood through the vascular system and the resistance (R) acting to oppose that flow. This relationship may be viewed as a simple equation:

$$\text{Blood Flow} = \frac{P}{R}$$

As pressure increases, blood flow increases. As resistance declines, flow increases. Conversely, as pressure falls or resistance increases, the flow declines.

Blood Pressure.   Forceful contraction of the left ventricle sends a surge of blood into the aorta; the peak pressure is called **systolic pressure**. Arterial blood pressure falls when the ventricle is refilling, to a low point called the **diastolic pressure**. Blood pressure typically averages about 120/80 mmHg at rest. During exercise involving rhythmic contractions (e.g., jogging, cycling, and swimming), systolic pressure increases and diastolic pressure remains relatively unchanged (see Figure A.13). During forceful, sustained (static) contractions, both the systolic and diastolic pressures increase. The rise in diastolic pressure is due to the increased resistance caused by the contracting muscles.

Resistance.   Vessel constriction (vasoconstriction) or relaxation (vasodilation) can increase or decrease resistance. Vasoconstriction and vasodilation take place in the arterioles. These adjustments are local reflexes, but they are also subject to control by the central nervous system. During exercise, vasodilation occurs in working muscles, first because of local changes (e.g., less oxygen, more carbon dioxide, more lactic acid, and increased temperature) and later at the command of the central nervous system. Vasoconstriction occurs in less active regions to help *redistribute* blood to the muscles. Veins also constrict (venoconstriction) to avoid pooling and to assist in the return of the blood to the heart.

Static muscular contractions stop blood flow in a muscle when they exceed 60% of maximal force. Thus, near-maximal contractions have a marked influence

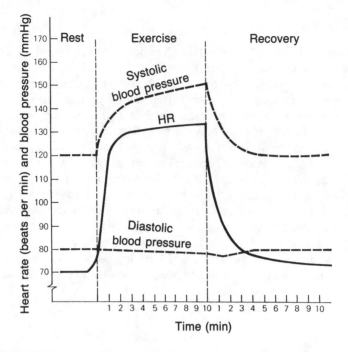

Figure A.13. Typical heart rate and blood pressure response to a submaximal work load (such as jogging). Notice the slight rise in HR just prior to exercise, the so-called anticipatory increase. The HR and systolic blood pressure begin to level off after about 2 min of exercise. The continued rise in HR illustrates the need to increase the circulation of blood to the skin in order to dissipate the heat generated during exercise. During a rhythmic exercise (jogging, cycling), the diastolic blood pressure declines a bit or remains unchanged. During strong static contractions, the diastolic pressure increases markedly (to 100 mmHg and beyond). Immediately after exercise, the systolic blood pressure declines quickly toward resting levels, whereas the HR remains elevated for some time to help remove waste products and to supply the postexercise demands for oxygen and fuel. The diastolic pressure sometimes exhibits a postexercise depression lasting up to a few minutes. Fit individuals demonstrate less dramatic changes in HR and blood pressure (for the same work load) and a more rapid return to resting values. *Note.* From Sharkey (1975).

on resistance and blood pressure—both go up. The cold air of a winter day can cause vasoconstriction and increase peripheral resistance. Add the task of lifting heavy shovelfuls of snow (static contractions), and you increase the resistance. Thus blood pressure must climb to dangerous heights to maintain flow to the muscles. When these events occur in a heart already limited by narrowed coronary arteries, you may expect to find angina pectoris (chest pain) or worse. The answer is to use a smaller shovel, take your time, and make the effort aerobic. Better yet, read Part I on aerobic fitness and get started on your personal fitness and health program.

APPENDIX

B

AEROBIC FITNESS

- **Aerobic Fitness Tests**
  - *Step Test*
  - *1.5-Mi Run*
  - *Montana Bicycle Test*
  - *V̇O₂max Test Protocol*
  - *Lactate Threshold Test*
- **Aerobic Fitness Programs**
  - *Starter Programs*
  - *Intermediate Program*
  - *Advanced Program*
  - *Aerobic Fitness Log*
  - *Training Tips*
  - *Aerobic Alternatives*

Aerobic Fitness Tests

You can estimate your fitness score with the step test or 1-1/2-mi run. The step test is submaximal so you can take it before you start training. The 1-1/2-mi-run test requires maximal effort, so it should wait until you have had 6 to 8 weeks of serious training. I've added a 5-mi bicycle test for those who prefer cycling, a maximal treadmill protocol for the serious fitness enthusiast, and a way to predict the lactate (anaerobic) threshold.

Step Test

If you've been inactive this is the test for you. The 5-min test was designed to be submaximal, so it will not place undue stress on an older or less fit individual. After a rest, step up and down on a bench (15-3/4 in. high for men; 13 in. for women) at the rate of 22-1/2 steps per minute. After 5 min sit down and take a postexercise count (from 15 to 30 s after the test). The body weight and postexercise pulse are used to determine aerobic fitness (see Tables B.1 and B.2 on pages 296-297).

The step test, originally developed by researchers at the Harvard Fatigue Laboratory in the 1930s, was later adapted by Swedish medical physiologists Irma and Per Olaf Åstrand in 1954. Further adaptations were made and a scoring calculator was added for use by the U.S. Forest Service. In laboratories throughout the world researchers have compared the procedure to the actual laboratory test and found the test to be a valid and reliable predictor of aerobic fitness. Thousands of individuals have taken the test without incident. Even so, should you experience excessive fatigue or nausea during the test you should stop and rest. See your physician if you are concerned about your health. Remember, the test can wait for 6 to 8 weeks of progressive conditioning (use the Prefit questionnaire in chapter 3).

Equipment Required for Test.   Plywood box—15-3/4 in. (40 cm) high for men; 13 in. (33 cm) for women.

Metronome or other device programmed for 90 beats per minute (tape record a metronome).

Watch with sweep second hand (or digital watch).

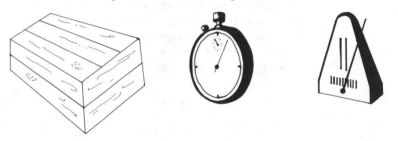

Testing Procedure.   Enter a quiet room (temperature 65° to 75°) and rest for about 5 min. Remove heavy clothing. It is permissible to take the test in street shoes. Start the signaling device programmed for 90 beats per minute, and begin.

Follow the beat of the timer, stepping up onto the bench and back onto the floor. If you cannot stay in step with the timer because of poor coordination

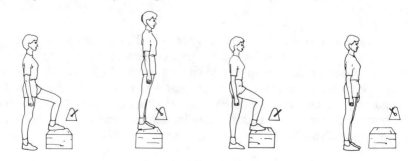

or physical exhaustion, stop and take the test again after several weeks. This test does not place undue stress on respiratory and circulatory systems and should be safe even for those in relatively poor physical condition.

You may change the leading foot by marking time for one beat of the timing device. When you complete 5 min of exercise, sit down. Take your pulse for *exactly* 15 s, starting *exactly* at 15 s and ending *exactly* at 30 s after exercise. Weigh yourself in the outfit worn during the test. With practice you will be able to take the test by yourself.

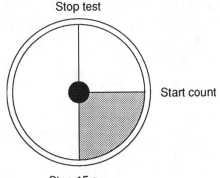

Checking the Pulse Rate.
Place the four fingertips in the groove directly above the base of the thumb on the underside of the wrist. Count the pulse rate for 15 s. Once you know the postexercise rate, you can find your fitness level in the tables. Practice counting pulse rates to gain skill.

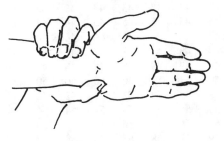

Remember to count the pulse for exactly 15 s, beginning 15 s after exercise and stopping at 30 s after the exercise test.

Note: Some find it easier to count the postexercise pulse by placing the fingers along the forward side of the throat. Because excessive pressure on the carotid artery can slow the pulse momentarily, be sure to use gentle contact.

Scoring the Test

1. Locate your body weight (Table B.1 or B.2).
2. Locate your postexercise pulse count in the appropriate column.
3. Opposite the pulse count, find your fitness score.
4. Turn to Table B.3 and enter your fitness score.
5. Find the age-adjusted score opposite the nearest age. (Because the step test relies on the pulse rate to predict aerobic capacity, and because the maximal pulse declines with age, you must adjust the score for age.)
6. With the adjusted fitness score, find your physical fitness rating.
7. Consult the fitness rating to see how you compare with others your age (Table B.4).

Table B.1 Men's Fitness Scores

Postexercise pulse [2] count	[3] Fitness score												
45	33	33	33	33	33	32	32	32	32	32	32	32	32
44	34	34	34	34	33	33	33	33	33	33	33	33	33
43	35	35	35	34	34	34	34	34	34	34	34	34	34
42	36	35	35	35	35	35	35	35	35	35	35	34	34
41	36	36	36	36	36	36	36	36	36	36	36	35	35
40	37	37	37	37	37	37	37	37	36	36	36	36	36
39	38	38	38	38	38	38	38	38	38	38	38	37	37
38	39	39	39	39	39	39	39	39	39	39	39	38	38
37	41	40	40	40	40	40	40	40	40	40	40	39	39
36	42	42	41	41	41	41	41	41	41	41	41	40	40
35	43	43	42	42	42	42	42	42	42	42	42	42	41
34	44	44	43	43	43	43	43	43	43	43	43	43	43
33	46	45	45	45	45	45	44	44	44	44	44	44	44
32	47	47	46	46	46	46	46	46	46	46	46	46	46
31	48	48	48	47	47	47	47	47	47	47	47	47	47
30	50	49	49	49	48	48	48	48	48	48	48	48	48
29	52	51	51	51	50	50	50	50	50	50	50	50	50
28	53	53	53	53	52	52	52	52	52	52	51	51	51
27	55	55	55	54	54	54	54	54	54	53	53	53	52
26	57	57	56	56	56	56	56	56	56	55	55	54	54
25	59	59	58	58	58	58	58	58	58	56	56	55	55
24	60	60	60	60	60	60	60	59	59	58	58	57	
23	62	62	61	61	61	61	61	60	60	60	59		
22	64	64	63	63	63	63	62	62	61	61			
21	66	66	65	65	65	64	64	64	62				
20	68	68	67	67	67	66	66	65					
[1] Body weight	120	130	140	150	160	170	180	190	200	210	220	230	240

Table B.2   Women's Fitness Scores

Postexercise pulse [2] count	[3] Fitness score											
45										29	29	29
44								30	30	30	30	30
43							31	31	31	31	31	31
42			32	32	32	32	32	32	32	32	32	32
41			33	33	33	33	33	33	33	33	33	33
40			34	34	34	34	34	34	34	34	34	34
39			35	35	35	35	35	35	35	35	35	35
38			36	36	36	36	36	36	36	36	36	36
37			37	37	37	37	37	37	37	37	37	37
36		37	38	38	38	38	38	38	38	38	38	38
35	38	38	39	39	39	39	39	39	39	39	39	39
34	39	39	40	40	40	40	40	40	40	40	40	40
33	40	40	41	41	41	41	41	41	41	41	41	41
32	41	41	42	42	42	42	42	42	42	42	42	42
31	42	42	43	43	43	43	43	43	43	43	43	43
30	43	43	44	44	44	44	44	44	44	44	44	44
29	44	44	45	45	45	45	45	45	45	45	45	45
28	45	45	46	46	46	47	47	47	47	47	47	47
27	46	46	47	48	48	49	49	49	49	49		
26	47	48	49	50	50	51	51	51	51			
25	49	50	51	52	52	53	53					
24	51	52	53	54	54	55						
23	53	54	55	56	56	57						
[1] Body weight	80	90	100	110	120	130	140	150	160	170	180	190

Although the fitness test is *no substitute* for a comprehensive medical examination, it is an excellent means for predicting fitness and physical working capacity. Its simplicity and ease of scoring make it adaptable to a wide variety of situations and needs.

Test Accuracy.   When properly administered, the test will give an accurate estimate of the *maximal oxygen intake*, or aerobic fitness. Scores do not fluctuate even with extreme differences in resting heart rate. The bench height does not seem to discriminate against persons who are very short. The test closely follows common laboratory tests of fitness and work capacity. Physicians approve the test because it does not place undue stress on respiratory and circulatory systems.

Table B.3 Age-Adjusted Scores*

④ Enter fitness score

⑤ Age-adjusted score

Nearest age	30	31	32	33	34	35	36	37	38	39	40	41	42	43	44	45	46	47	48	49	50
15	32	33	34	35	36	37	38	39	40	41	42	43	44	45	46	47	48	49	50	51	53
20	31	32	33	34	35	36	37	38	39	40	41	42	43	44	45	46	47	48	49	50	51
25	30	31	32	33	34	35	36	37	38	39	40	41	42	43	44	45	46	47	48	49	50
30	29	30	31	32	33	34	35	36	37	38	39	40	41	42	43	44	45	46	47	48	49
35	27	28	29	31	32	33	34	35	36	37	38	39	40	41	42	43	44	45	46	47	48
40	26	27	28	30	31	32	33	34	35	36	37	38	39	40	41	42	43	44	45	46	47
45	25	26	27	29	30	31	32	33	34	35	36	37	38	39	40	41	42	43	44	45	46
50	24	25	26	28	29	30	31	32	33	34	35	36	37	38	39	40	41	42	43	44	45
55	23	24	25	27	28	29	30	31	32	33	34	35	36	37	38	39	40	41	41	42	43
60	22	23	24	25	26	27	28	30	31	32	33	34	35	36	37	37	38	39	40	41	42
65	21	22	23	24	25	26	27	28	29	30	31	32	33	34	35	36	37	38	38	39	40

4 Enter fitness score

5 Age-adjusted score

Nearest age	51	52	53	54	55	56	57	58	59	60	61	62	63	64	65	66	67	68	69	70	71	72
15	54	55	56	57	58	59	60	61	62	63	64	65	66	67	68	69	70	71	72	74	75	76
20	52	53	54	55	56	57	58	59	60	61	62	63	64	65	66	67	68	69	70	71	72	73
25	51	52	53	54	55	56	57	58	59	60	61	62	63	64	65	66	67	68	69	70	71	72
30	50	51	52	53	54	55	56	57	58	59	60	61	62	63	64	65	66	67	68	69	70	71
35	49	50	51	52	53	54	55	56	57	58	59	60	60	61	62	63	64	65	66	67	68	69
40	48	49	50	51	52	53	54	55	55	56	57	58	59	60	61	62	63	64	65	66	67	68
45	47	48	49	50	51	52	52	53	54	55	56	57	58	59	60	61	62	63	64	65	65	66
50	45	46	47	48	49	50	51	52	53	53	54	55	56	57	58	58	59	61	61	62	63	64
55	44	45	46	46	47	48	49	50	51	52	53	53	54	55	56	57	58	59	59	60	61	62
60	42	43	44	45	46	46	47	48	49	50	51	51	52	53	54	55	56	57	57	58	59	60
65	41	42	42	43	44	45	46	46	47	48	49	50	50	51	52	53	54	54	55	56	57	58

*Example: If your age is 40 years and you score 50 on the step test, your age-adjusted score is 47.

Improper test administration is the most common reason for inaccurate scores. Pulse counting errors are common among inexperienced test takers. The post-exercise pulse is extremely regular. The individual counting the pulse should establish the rhythm of the beat and be sure to count each beat, even those that seem to be missing. The heart is working to supply the recovering muscles with oxygen and will not be interrupted during recovery. If you suspect a scoring error, retake the test another day.

Table B.4 Physical Fitness Rating—Men

(Use age-adjusted score) 6 7

Nearest age	Superior	Excellent	Very good	Good	Fair	Poor	Very poor
15	57+	56-52	51-47	46-42	41-37	36-32	31−
20	56+	55-51	50-46	45-41	40-36	35-31	30−
25	55+	54-50	49-45	44-40	39-35	34-30	29−
30	54+	53-49	48-44	43-39	38-34	33-29	28−
35	53+	52-48	47-43	42-38	37-33	32-28	27−
40	52+	51-47	46-42	41-37	36-32	31-27	26−
45	51+	50-46	45-41	40-36	35-31	30-26	25−
50	50+	49-45	44-40	39-35	34-30	29-25	24−
55	49+	48-44	43-39	38-34	33-29	28-24	23−
60	48+	47-43	42-38	37-33	32-28	27-23	22−
65	47+	48-42	41-37	36-32	31-27	26-22	21−

Table B.5 Physical Fitness Rating—Women

(Use age-adjusted score) 6 7

Nearest age	Superior	Excellent	Very good	Good	Fair	Poor	Very poor
15	54+	53-49	48-44	43-39	38-34	33-29	28−
20	53+	52-48	47-43	42-38	37-33	32-28	27−
25	52+	51-47	46-42	41-37	36-32	31-27	26−
30	51+	50-46	45-41	40-36	35-31	30-26	25−
35	50+	49-45	44-40	39-35	34-30	29-25	24−
40	49+	48-44	43-39	38-34	33-29	28-24	23−
45	48+	47-43	42-38	37-33	32-28	27-23	22−
50	47+	46-42	41-37	36-32	31-27	26-22	21−
55	46+	45-41	40-36	35-31	30-26	25-21	20−
60	45+	44-40	39-35	34-30	29-25	24-20	19−
65	44+	43-49	38-34	33-29	28-24	23-20	19−

Tests *should not* be taken

- after strenuous physical activity,
- immediately after you drink coffee or smoke,
- in an extremely warm room (above 78 °F), or
- when you are anxious or excited.

Running Test

The 1-1/2-mi-run test requires a maximal effort. Before the run, go through a light warm-up, then rest. Run the 1-1/2 mi over a level course. Pacing and high motivation are essential for best performance. Use your time for the run to predict aerobic fitness and work capacity. If you've been inactive, precede the test with at least 8 weeks of training (walk-jog-run program). Those over 35 years of age should consider a medical examination, including an exercise electrocardiogram. The time for the run is used to predict aerobic fitness (see Figure B.1).

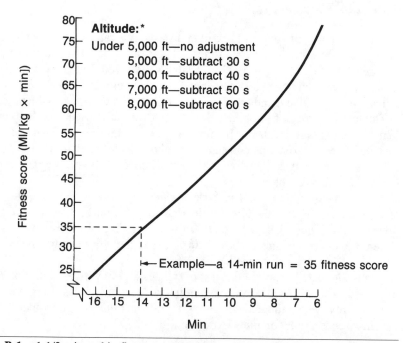

Figure B.1. 1-1/2-mi aerobic fitness test. *Subtract altitude adjustment from 1.5-mi run time. Then use the graph to find your score. *Note.* Adapted from *A Simple Field Test for the Assessment of Physical Fitness* (p. 65) by B. Balke, 1963, Oklahoma City: Civic Aeronautic Research Institute, Federal Aviation Agency; *The New Aerobics* (p. 85) by K.H. Cooper, 1970, New York: Bantam; Daniels, personal communication, 1972; and Sharkey (1977).

This prediction is based on the oxygen cost of running at certain speeds. The data for the test were first published by Dr. Bruno Balke in 1963; an adaptation of the test appeared in Dr. Cooper's book *Aerobics* (1968). Additional data for top flight endurance runners have been provided by Dr. Jack Daniels. I arranged a simplified scoring method and established test validity in the laboratory (see Figure B.1). When highly motivated subjects take the test it proves to be an excellent predictor of aerobic fitness.

Studies show that running tests lasting 12 min or more are best for the prediction of aerobic fitness. When highly fit individuals are able to run the 1-1/2-mi distance in 10 min or less the results may reflect basic speed or anaerobic power *as well as* aerobic fitness. For this reason, the step test and 1-1/2-mi-run scores may not always agree. However, the running test is an excellent predictor of aerobic fitness. It is most suitable for active individuals and lends itself well to group testing situations. Unlike other running tests, this method yields an aerobic fitness score instead of just a category such as good or bad. Your score can be compared with others, regardless of age, sex, or body size, and you can use your score to document the effects of training.

Montana Bicycle Test

Because a number of you don't like running tests, several people set out to develop a bicycle test to predict aerobic fitness. The result, the Montana Bicycle Test, was developed jointly by Jim Tobin, Kathy Miller, Ted Coladarci, and me. This is an early version of the test developed on male subjects. I decided to include it to see how you like it and so others can evaluate and improve on the procedure.

The test involves a 5-mi bike ride over a level out-and-back or loop course. Wind speed should be under 10 mph. The test is taken on a 27-in., 10-speed bicycle. The gear remains constant throughout with the chain on the 50-tooth chainwheel in front and 18-tooth rear sprocket. Use the drop position on the handlebars throughout the test.

After a warm-up, rest and prepare for the 5-mi ride. Then ride the course as fast as possible. Use the time for the ride and your percent body fat to predict your aerobic fitness. Use Figure D.2 in Appendix D to estimate your body fat. When the test is conducted above 5,000 ft, use the altitude adjustments found on the 1-1/2-mi run test (see Table B.6).

When conducted properly this test correlates highly with treadmill or bicycle ergometer tests of the maximal oxygen intake (aerobic fitness). Remember, the test has only been validated for young men. But I encourage women to use it as a reference point for bicycle training.

Bicycle Ergometer Test

This is a submaximal test that predicts fitness ($\dot{V}O_2max$). It uses several work loads to determine the relationship between HR and work load, then extrapolates

Table B.6   The Montana Bicycle Test

% Fat	\multicolumn{11}{c}{Time for the 5-mi bicycle test (min*)}
	12.0	12.4	12.8	13.2	13.6	14.0	14.4	14.8	15.2	15.6	16.0
4	65.2	64.1	63.2	61.0	60.7	59.6	58.5	57.3	56.2	55.1	54.0
6	63.9	62.8	61.7	60.6	59.4	58.3	57.2	56.0	54.9	53.8	52.7
8	62.6	61.5	60.4	59.3	58.1	57.0	55.9	54.7	53.6	52.5	54.4
10	61.4	60.2	59.1	58.0	56.8	55.7	54.6	53.4	52.3	51.2	50.1
12	60.1	58.9	57.2	56.7	55.5	54.4	53.3	52.1	51.0	49.9	48.8
14	58.8	57.6	56.5	55.4	54.2	53.1	52.0	50.8	49.7	48.6	47.5
16	57.5	56.3	55.2	54.1	52.9	51.8	50.7	49.5	48.4	47.3	46.2
18	56.2	55.0	53.9	52.8	51.6	50.5	49.4	48.2	47.1	46.0	44.9
20	54.9	53.7	52.6	51.5	50.3	49.2	48.1	47.0	45.8	44.7	43.6
22	53.6	52.4	51.3	50.2	49.0	47.9	46.8	45.7	44.5	43.4	42.3

*Minutes and decimal fractions: 12.4 = 12 min 24 s; 12.8 = 12:48, etc.

to the maximum HR to predict the maximal working capacity and $\dot{V}O_2$max. The test requires a bicycle ergometer, a stationary bicycle that allows precise measurement of the work load. The Monark or Tuntari ergometers are found at most health clubs.

The work load per minute (power in kilogram meters per minute—kgm/min) is calculated using the following.

Pedal rpm—this test uses 60 rpm
Force—the resistance to pedaling (from 1 to 7 kg)
Distance—a combination of mechanical advantage and wheel circumference (totals 6 on the Monark bicycle)

Thus the work load is 60 rpm $\times$ 1 kg $\times$ 6 = 360 kgm/min
60 rpm $\times$ 2 kg $\times$ 6 = 720 kgm/min
60 rpm $\times$ 3 kg $\times$ 6 = 1,080 kgm/min

The Test

1. Adjust the seat height so your leg is *almost* extended when the pedal is in its lowest position (ball of foot on pedal).
2. Warm up for 2 min with easy pedaling at a low resistance.
3. Become familiar with cadence—use a metronome set at 60 to pace your cadence or watch a clock and push down with your right foot every second.
4. After a brief rest begin the test.

   Stage 1: Begin the first of three 2-min stages with a setting of 1 kg. Maintain the cadence; in the last 30 s of the first stage carefully take a 15-s HR reading at the throat (use gentle contact on carotid). Multiply by 4 and record HR and setting (1 kg).

Stage 2: Increase the resistance (see the following guide to selection) and take HR as in Stage 1. Record HR and setting.

Stage 3: Increase the resistance and take HR as in Stage 1. Record HR and setting.

Cool down with easy cycling.

Guide to selection of work loads

Men: **Stage 1—Begin at 1 kg (360 kgm/min).**

Stage 2—HR below 95, set at 3 kg.
HR 95 to 110, set at 2.5 kg.
HR over 110, set at 2 kg.

Stage 3—Increase 1 kg for Stage 3.

Women: **Stage 1—Begin at 0.5 kg (180 kgm/min)*.**

Stage 2—HR below 110, set at 1.5 kg.
HR above 110, set at 1 kg.

Stage 3—Increase 1 kg for Stage 3.

*Note: Active women can follow the men's protocol.

Scoring.   Plot the HR and corresponding work loads on graph paper (see Figure B.2). Then draw a line that comes closest to all three points and extrapolate the line to the estimated maximal heart rate (220 − age). Now draw a vertical line down to the baseline to read the maximal working capacity (in kgm/m).

Example: for 30-year-old individual
        120 HR = 360 kgm/m
        138 HR = 720 kgm/m
        162 HR = 1,080 kgm/m

Then enter the correct value from Table B.7 to predict aerobic fitness ($\dot{V}O_2$max) in milliliters per kilogram of body weight per minute, or ml/[kg × min].

Use the table located with the step test instructions to evaluate your aerobic fitness score.

$\dot{V}O_2$max Test Protocol

The protocol described in Figure B.3 is the result of many years of experimentation in my lab. The protocol is suitable for a wide range of subjects, from the sedentary to elite athletes. The actual test, which takes from 8 to 12 min, can utilize actual metabolic measurements or serve as a prediction of the $\dot{V}O_2$max. The protocol allows the test to be tailored to the subject in terms of level of fitness, walking versus running, and work load increases in the final minutes

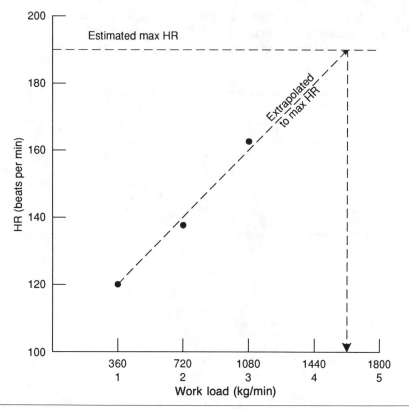

Figure B.2.   Heart-rate–work-load relationship. For a 30-year-old the estimated max HR is 220 − 30 = 190. Max work load is 1,620 kgm/min. Now consult Table B.7 to determine aerobic fitness.

Table B.7   Predicting Aerobic Fitness from Max Work Load on Bicycle Test

Weight (kg)	Work load (kg/min)								
	600	750	900	1,050	1,200	1,350	1,500	1,650	1,800*
50	30**	36	42	48	54	60	66	72	
60	25	30	35	40	45	50	55	60	65
70		26	30	34	39	43	48	52	57
80		22	26	30	34	38	42	46	50
90			23	27	31	35	39	43	46
100				24	27	31	34	38	42

*Extrapolate for values above 1.800 kg/m.

**Tabled values are aerobic fitness scores in ml/[kg × min].

of the test. Figure B.3 describes the protocol and provides data to estimate the $\dot{V}O_2$max if metabolic equipment isn't available. The subject should not be allowed to hold onto the railing of the treadmill if you plan to predict the $\dot{V}O_2$max.

Predicting Aerobic Fitness From Final Rate and Grade on Treadmill Test

	MPH	8%*	10%	12%	14%	15%
W	3.0		26**	30	34	
A	3.5		29	34	39	
L	4.0		32	38	44	(48)
K	—	—	—	—	—	—
R	6.0	(47)	50	53	56	
U	7.0		58	61	65	
N	8.0		66	70	74	

(RATE) · Grade (header over grade columns)

*Extrapolate for intermediate rates and grades.
**Tabled values are aerobic fitness scores in ml/[kg × min].

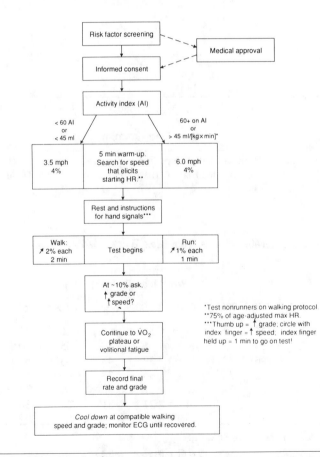

Figure B.3. Flowchart for $\dot{V}O_2$max test protocol.

Predicting the Lactate Threshold

The lactate threshold is a better indicator of endurance performance than aerobic fitness ($\dot{V}O_2$max) in events like a 10-k road race. The lactate threshold indicates the oxygen utilization capabilities of the muscles. You can predict your threshold using equations developed by Dr. Art Weltman (1989) at the University of Virginia.

The prediction equation uses the time for a 3,200-m run to predict the lactate threshold—expressed as the $\dot{V}O_2$ at the threshold (4 mM lactate). You can use this value and the results of your aerobic capacity test to determine the percentage of the maximum that you can sustain.

> **For men:** $\dot{V}O_2$ **(ml/[kg × min]) = 122.0 − (5.310 × [3,200-m time in min*])**
> ***in minutes and decimal fractions; e.g., 30 s = .5 min**
>
> **For women:** $\dot{V}O_2$ **= − 1.12 × [3,200-m time]) + 61.57 (note negative in equation)**
>
> **Example: 40-year-old male with 3,200-m time of 14 min:**
>
> $\dot{V}O_2$ **= 122 − 5.31 × 14**
> **= 122 − 74.34**
> **= 47.66**
>
> **Divide the result (47.66) by the max (56) to get the lactate threshold as a percentage of the max = 85% of the $\dot{V}O_2$max. Use the aerobic fitness and threshold tests to gauge the progress of your training.**

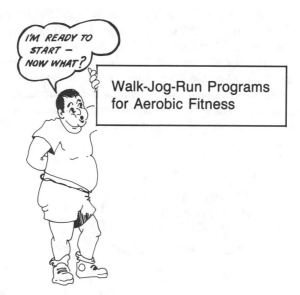

Your fitness prescription gives you the freedom to tailor a fitness program to meet your specific needs. You have a wide choice of exercises and many options as far as the length of time you want to exercise and the intensity of that activity. Some of you may prefer a more detailed, step-by-step approach. For this reason, I've included some walk-jog-run programs.

I'll describe programs for three levels of ability: a starter program for those in low-fitness categories (under 35 fitness score), an intermediate program (35 to 45), and one for those in the high-fitness categories (46 or better). The starter program was prepared by the President's Council on Physical Fitness and Sports and appears in the booklet *An Introduction to Physical Fitness*.

Starter Programs (Walk-Jog-Run)

Take the walk test to determine your exercise level.

Walk Test. The object of this test is to determine how many minutes (up to 10) you can walk at a brisk pace, on a level surface, without undue difficulty or discomfort.

If you can't walk for 5 min, begin with the *red* walking program.

If you can walk more than 5 min, but less than 10, begin with the third week of the *red* walking program.

If you can walk for the full 10 min, but are somewhat tired and sore as a result, start with the *white* walk-jog program. If you can breeze through the full 10 min, you're ready for bigger things. Wait until the next day and take the 10-min walk-jog test.

Walk-Jog Test. In this test you alternately walk 50 steps (left foot strikes ground 25 times) and jog 50 steps for a total of 10 min. Walk at the rate of 120 steps per minute (left foot strikes the ground at 1-s intervals). Jog at the rate of 144 steps per minute (left foot strikes ground 18 times every 15 s).

If you can't complete the 10-min test, begin at the third week of the *white* program. If you can complete the 10-min test but are tired and winded as a result, start with the last week of the *white* program before moving to the *blue* program. If you can perform the 10-min walk-jog test without difficulty, start with the *blue* program.

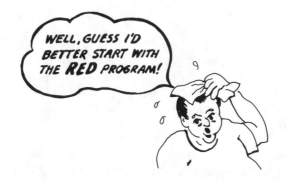

Red Walking Program

Do each activity every other day at first.

Week 1.   Walk at a brisk pace for 5 min or for a shorter time if you become uncomfortably tired. Walk slowly or rest for 3 min. Again walk briskly for 5 min or until you become uncomfortably tired.

MON	TUE	WED	THU	FRI	SAT	SUN

Week 2.   Same as Week 1, but increase pace as soon as you can walk 5 min without soreness or fatigue.

MON	TUE	WED	THU	FRI	SAT	SUN

Week 3.   Walk at a brisk pace for 8 min or for a shorter time if you become uncomfortably tired. Walk slowly or rest for 3 min. Again walk briskly for 8 min or until you become uncomfortably tired.

MON	TUE	WED	THU	FRI	SAT	SUN

Week 4.   Same as Week 3, but increase pace as soon as you can walk 8 min without soreness or fatigue.

When you've completed Week 4 for the *red* program, begin at Week 1 of the *white* program.

MON	TUE	WED	THU	FRI	SAT	SUN

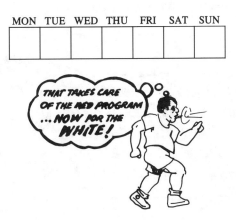

White Walk-Jog Program

Do each activity 4 times a week.

Week 1. Walk at a brisk pace for 10 min or for a shorter time if you become uncomfortably tired. Walk slowly or rest for 3 min. Again, walk briskly for 10 min or until you become uncomfortably tired.

MON	TUE	WED	THU	FRI	SAT	SUN

Week 2. Walk at a brisk pace for 15 min or for a shorter time if you become uncomfortably tired. Walk slowly or rest for 3 min.

MON	TUE	WED	THU	FRI	SAT	SUN

Week 3. Jog 10 s (25 yd). Walk 1 min (100 yd). Do 12 times.

MON	TUE	WED	THU	FRI	SAT	SUN

Week 4. Jog 20 s (50 yd). Walk 1 min (100 yd). Do 12 times.

MON	TUE	WED	THU	FRI	SAT	SUN

When you've completed Week 4 of the *white* program, begin at Week 1 of the *blue* program.

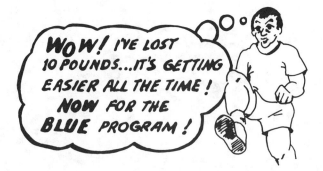

Blue Jogging Program

Do each activity 5 times a week.

Week 1. Jog 40 s (100 yd). Walk 1 min (100 yd). Do 9 times.

MON	TUE	WED	THU	FRI	SAT	SUN

Week 2. Jog 1 min (150 yd). Walk 1 min (100 yd). Do 8 times.

MON	TUE	WED	THU	FRI	SAT	SUN

Week 3. Jog 2 min (300 yd). Walk 1 min (100 yd). Do 6 times.

MON	TUE	WED	THU	FRI	SAT	SUN

Week 4. Jog 4 min (600 yd). Walk 1 min (100 yd). Do 4 times.

MON	TUE	WED	THU	FRI	SAT	SUN

Week 5. Jog 6 min (900 yd). Walk 1 min (100 yd). Do 3 times.

MON	TUE	WED	THU	FRI	SAT	SUN

Week 6. Jog 8 min (1,200 yd). Walk 2 min (200 yd). Do 2 times.

MON	TUE	WED	THU	FRI	SAT	SUN

Week 7. Jog 10 min (1,500 yd). Walk 2 min (200 yd). Do 2 times.

MON	TUE	WED	THU	FRI	SAT	SUN

**Week 8**. Jog 12 min (1,760 yd). Walk 2 min (200 yd). Do 2 times.

MON	TUE	WED	THU	FRI	SAT	SUN

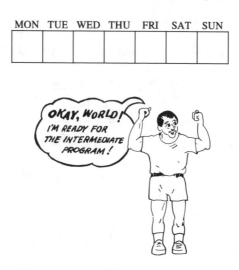

Intermediate Program (Jog-Run)

If you've followed the starter program or are already reasonably active, you're ready for the intermediate program. You're able to jog 1 mi slowly without undue fatigue, rest 2 min, and do it again. Your sessions consume about 250 cal.

You're ready to increase both the intensity and the duration of your runs. You'll be using the heart rate training zone for those of medium fitness (35 to 45 ml/[kg × min]). You'll begin jogging 1 mi in 12 min, and when you finish this program you may be able to complete 3 mi or more at a pace approaching 8 min per mile. Each week's program includes three phases—the basic workout, longer runs (overdistance), and shorter runs (underdistance). If a week's program seems too easy, move ahead; if it seems too hard, move back a week or two. Remember to warm up and cool down as a part of every exercise session (see Table B.8).

Table B.8 Pace Guide for Gauging Speed Over Various Distances

	Pace	1 mi	1/2 mi	1/4 mi	220 yd	100 yd	50 yd
				(min:s)			
Slow jog	10 cal/min (120 cal/mi)[a]	12:00	6:00	3:00	1:30	0:40	0:20
Jog	12 cal/min (120 cal/mi)	10:00	5:00	2:30	1:15	0:34	0:17

	Pace	1 mi	1/2 mi	1/4 mi	220 yd	100 yd	50 yd
					(min:s)		
Run	15 cal/min (120 cal/mi)	8:00	4:00	2:00	1:00	0:27	0:13
Fast run	20 cal/min (120 cal/mi)	6:00	3:00	1:30	0:45	0:20	0:10

ªDepends on efficiency and body size; add 10% for each 15 lb over 150; subtract 10% for each 15 lb under 150.

Note. Adapted from Sharkey (1974, 1975).

Week 1

Basic Workout.   Monday, Thursday

1 mi in 11 min; active recovery (walk). Run twice.

MON	THUR

Underdistance.   Tuesday, Friday.

1/4 to 1/2 mi slowly.
1/2 mi in 5 min 30 s. Run twice (recover between repeats).
1/4 mi in 2 min 45 s. Run 4 times (recover between repeats).
Jog 1/4 to 1/2 mi slowly.

TUE	FRI

Overdistance.   Wednesday, Saturday (or Sunday)

2 mi slowly. (Use the talk test: Jog at a pace that allows you to converse.)

	SAT
WED	SUN

Week 2

Basic Workout.   Monday, Thursday

1 mi in 10 min 30 s; active recovery. Run twice.

MON	THUR

Underdistance.   Tuesday, Friday.

1/4 to 1/2 mi slowly.
1/2 mi in 5 min.

TUE	FRI

1/4 mi in 2 min 30 s. Run 2 times (recover between repeats).
1/4 mi in 2 min 45 s. Run 2 times (recover between repeats).
220 yd in 1 min 20 s. Run 4 times (recover between repeats).
1/4 to 1/2 mi slowly.

Overdistance. Wednesday, Saturday (or Sunday).

2-1/4 mi slowly.

| SAT |
| WED SUN |
| | |

Week 3

Basic Workout. Monday, Thursday.

| MON THUR |
| | |

1 mi in 10 min 30 s; active recovery. Run twice.

Underdistance. Tuesday, Friday.

| TUE FRI |
| | |

1/4 to 1/2 mi slowly.
1/2 mi in 4 min 45 s.
1/4 mi in 2 min 30 s. Run 4 times (recover between repeats).
220 yd in 1 min 10 s. Run 4 times (recover between repeats).
100 yd in 30 s. Run 4 times (recover between repeats).
1/4 to 1/2 mi slowly.

Overdistance. Wednesday, Saturday (or Sunday).

2-1/2 mi slowly.

| SAT |
| WED SUN |
| | |

Week 4

Basic Workout. Monday, Thursday.

| MON THUR |
| | |

1 mi in 10 min; active recovery. Run twice.

Underdistance. Tuesday, Friday.

| TUE FRI |
| | |

1/4 to 1/2 mi slowly.
1/2 mi in 4 min 45 s. Run twice (recover between repeats).
1/4 mi in 2 min 20 s. Run 4 times (recover between repeats).
220 yd in 1 min. Run 4 times (recover between repeats).
1/4 to 1/2 mi slowly.

Overdistance. Wednesday, Saturday (or Sunday).

2-3/4 mi slowly.

| SAT |
| WED SUN |
| | |

Week 5

Basic Workout.   Monday, Thursday.

MON THUR

1 mi in 9 min 30 s; active recovery. Run twice.

Underdistance.   Tuesday, Friday.

TUE   FRI

1/4 to 1/2 mi slowly.
1/2 mi in 4 min 30 s.
1/4 mi in 2 min 20 s. Run 4 times (recover between repeats).
220 yd in 60 s. Run 4 times (recover between repeats).
100 yd in 27 s. Run 4 times (recover between repeats).
1/4 to 1/2 mi slowly.

Overdistance.   Wednesday, Saturday (or Sunday).

SAT
WED   SUN

3 mi slowly.

Week 6

Basic Workout.   Monday, Thursday.

MON THUR

1-1/2 mi in 13 min 30 s; active recovery. Run twice.

Underdistance.   Tuesday, Friday.

TUE   FRI

1/4 to 1/2 mi slowly.
1/2 mi in 4 min 30 s. Run twice (recover between repeats).
1/4 mi in 2 min 10 s. Run 4 times (recover between repeats).
220 yd in 60 s. Run 4 times (recover between repeats).
100 yd in 25 s. Run 4 times (recover between repeats).
1/4 to 1/2 mi slowly.

Overdistance.   Wednesday, Saturday (or Sunday).

SAT
WED   SUN

3 mi slowly; _increase pace_ last 1/4 mi.

Week 7

Basic Workout.   Monday, Thursday.

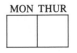

1-1/2 mi in 13 min; active recovery. Run twice.

Underdistance. Tuesday, Friday.

TUE   FRI

1/4 to 1/2 mi slowly.
1/2 mi in 4 min 15 s. Run twice (recover between repeats).
1/4 mi in 2 min. Run 4 times (recover between repeats).
220 yd in 55 s. Run 4 times (recover between repeats).
1/4 to 1/2 mi slowly.

Overdistance. Wednesday, Saturday (or Sunday).

SAT
WED   SUN

3-1/2 mi slowly; always increase pace near finish.

Week 8

Basic Workout. Monday, Thursday.

MON THUR

1 mi in 8 min; active recovery. Run 1 mi in 8 min 30 s; active
recovery; repeat (total of 3 mi).

Underdistance. Tuesday, Friday.

TUE   FRI

1/4 to 1/2 mi slowly.
1/2 mi in 4 min. Run twice (recover between repeats).
1/4 mi in 1 min 50 s. Run 4 times (recover between repeats).
220 yd in 55 s. Run 4 times (recover between repeats).
100 yd in 23 s. Run 4 times (recover between repeats).
1/4 to 1/2 mi slowly.

Overdistance. Wednesday, Saturday (or Sunday)

SAT
WED   SUN

3-1/2 mi slowly.

Week 9

Basic Workout. Monday, Thursday.

MON THUR

1 mi in 8 min. Run 3 times (recover between repeats).

Underdistance. Tuesday, Friday.

TUE   FRI

1/4 to 1/2 mi slowly.
1/2 mi in 4 min.
1/4 mi in 1 min 50 s. Run 4 times (recover between repeats).
220 yd in 50 s. Run 4 times (recover between repeats).

100 yd in 20 s. Run 4 times (recover between repeats).
50 yd in 10 s. Run 4 times (recover between repeats).
1/4 to 1/2 mi slowly.

Overdistance.   Wednesday, Saturday (or Sunday).

4 mi slowly.

Week 10

Basic Workout.   Monday, Thursday.

1-1/2 mi in 12 min. Run twice (recover between repeats).

Underdistance.   Tuesday, Friday.

1/4 to 1/2 mi slowly.
1/2 mi in 3 min 45 s. Run 2 times (recover between repeats).
1/4 mi in 1 min 50 s. Run 6 times (recover between repeats).
220 yd in 45 s. Run twice (recover between repeats).
1/4 to 1/2 mi slowly.

Overdistance.   Wednesday, Saturday (or Sunday).

4 mi; increase pace last 1/2 mi.

Week 11

Basic Workout.   Monday, Thursday.

1 mi in 7 min 30 s. Run 3 times (recover between repeats).

Underdistance.   Tuesday, Friday.

1/4 to 1/2 mi slowly.
1/2 mi in 3 min 30 s. Run 4 times (recover between repeats).
1/4 mi in 1 min 45 s. Run 4 times (recover between repeats).
220 yd in 45 s. Run 2 times (recover between repeats).
1/4 to 1/2 mi slowly.

Overdistance.   Wednesday, Saturday (or Sunday).

4 mi slowly (more than 400 cal per workout).

Week 12

Basic Workout.

1-1/2 mi in 11 min 40 s (fitness score = 45).

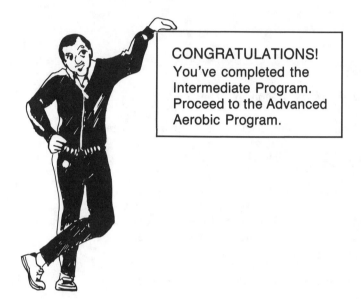

CONGRATULATIONS!
You've completed the
Intermediate Program.
Proceed to the Advanced
Aerobic Program.

Aerobic Training Programs

This section provides training programs for walkers, cyclists, and swimmers. The programs combine the training concepts outlined in chapter 15 and the principles of training described in Appendix F to provide safe, effective, and interesting approaches to fitness. Use the programs to improve fitness, but when you are satisfied with your level of fitness, switch to a maintenance program. It isn't necessary to improve fitness to a high level; the health benefits are available to those who remain active.

Walking Program

Begin with the walk test on p. 308 of this appendix. If you can walk for the full 10 min you are ready for this program. If not, complete the 4-week red walking program (p. 309).

The weekly training menu includes the following.

Monday:	Easy distance—walk at a comfortable pace (PE = 12).*
Tuesday:	Pace—stride briskly (PE = 15).

YOUR WEEKLY WALKING PROGRAM

	Week							
	1	2	3	4	5	6	7	8
Monday	15 min	20	25	20	25	30	35	30
Tuesday	2 × 8 min*	2 × 9	2 × 10	3 × 7	3 × 8	3 × 9	3 × 10	4 × 10
Wednesday	10 min	11	12	13	2 × 10	2 × 12	2 × 14	3 × 10
Thursday	3 × 2 min	3 × 3	3 × 4	4 × 2	4 × 3	4 × 4	5 × 2	5 × 3
Friday	30 min	35	40	35	40	45	50	60

*2 sets at 8 min each.

Always warm up and stretch before each workout.

Pace: Do one set, walk slowly to recover, and do the next.

Hills: Optional; try not to exceed PE = 13.

Intervals: Do one set, walk slowly to recover, and do another.

Wednesday: Hills (or Stairs)—walk briskly uphill to build stamina (PE = 13).
Thursday: Intervals—walk intervals at PE = 16.**
Friday: Overdistance—walk slowly for a long distance (PE = 11).
Saturday: Variety—try a different activity or hike a trail at a leisurely pace.
Sunday: Rest—or try light activity (e.g., gardening).

---

*PE = perceived exertion, from Table 13.3, p. 211.
**Increase to PE = 17 after 4 weeks.

After you have completed the 8-week program, design your own using this or another format or switch to a walk-jog program. If you prefer one type of training, such as easy distance, use that and forget the other items I've mentioned. Remember, you should enjoy your regular activity.

Plan a hiking trip with friends and train together to prepare for the outing. You may even want to take up race walking, that curious gait that requires the heel of one foot to touch the ground before the toe of the other foot leaves the ground.

Cycling Program

This program utilizes a training menu to guide your progress. The weekly training menu includes the following.

Monday: Easy distance—ride at a comfortable pace (PE = 13).
Tuesday: Pace—cycle at a brisk pace (PE = 15).
Wednesday: Hills—include hills to build stamina (PE = 14).
Thursday: Intervals—push harder for brief intervals PE = 16.*
Friday: Overdistance—go easy to develop endurance (PE = 11).
Saturday: Variety—try a different activity (e.g., tennis or hiking) or ride a trail.
Sunday: Rest—or try light activity (e.g., gardening or walking).

---

*Increase to PE = 17 after 4 weeks.

After 8 weeks design your own program using elements from this plan or others you enjoy. Plan a long trip with friends and do training rides together.

Swimming Program

This program assumes a certain amount of skill in swimming (see p. 323). If the program seems too difficult for your level of ability, scale down the program and take lessons to improve your skill and efficiency.

YOUR WEEKLY CYCLING PROGRAM

	Week							
	1	2	3	4	5	6	7	8
Monday	30 min	40	50	40	50	60	70	60
Tuesday	2 × 10 min	2 × 15	2 × 20	3 × 10	3 × 15	3 × 20	4 × 10	4 × 15
Wednesday	15 min	20	25	20	15	20	25	20
Thursday	3 × 3 min	3 × 4	3 × 5	3 × 6	4 × 3	4 × 4	4 × 5	5 × 5
Friday	60 min	70	80	75	90	100	110	120

Always wear a helmet; ride easy to warm up.

Pace: Ride 10 min, relax and recover, ride another set.

Hills: Include some standing but try to keep PE = 14.

Intervals: Ride one, cycle easy to recover, and ride the next.

Overdistance: Ride easy; stop for rest and fluids every 30 min.

The weekly training menu includes the following.

Monday: Easy distance—go easy at a comfortable pace (PE = 12).
Tuesday: Pace—swim at a firm pace (PE = 15).
Wednesday: Arms/Legs—swim with arms and legs only (PE = 13).
Thursday: Intervals—swim harder for brief intervals PE = 16.*
Friday: Overdistance—relax on a longer swim (PE = 11).
Saturday: Variety—try a different activity or water games (e.g., water polo).
Sunday: Rest—or try light activity (e.g., gardening or walking).

---

*Increase to PE = 17 after 4 weeks.

When you have completed 8 weeks, design your own program using the types of training you most enjoy. You could even decide to take up triathlon training.

Triathlon Training Tips

This combination of swimming, cycling, and running has become very popular in recent years. The variety in training makes it a safer sport than the marathon. For those who crave a challenge, the triathlon is just the ticket.

The triathlon requires a high level of performance in each event. Although some enthusiasts are able to train each event 4 or more times per week, most participants are happy to train each event 3 times each week (nine training sessions per week is about all the time most can afford). Because it takes more than 3 sessions per week to improve in each event, I recommend that you raise your best event to a high level with five training sessions per week (leaving only two sessions each for the other events). Then switch to maintenance (2 to 3 times per week) and raise the next best event. When this event is satisfactory, place it on a maintenance schedule and focus on your weakest event.

When you feel ready to experience the entire triathlon, enter a small, local event, preferably one where the swimming is conducted in a pool. Then hone your sports, transitional skills, and conditioning in more competitive events. Along the way you'll probably also want to upgrade your equipment to be more competitive in your age group. Someday you may be ready for the grueling Ironman Triathlon in Hawaii (over 2 mi of swimming, 116 mi of cycling, and a full marathon—26.2 mi—of running). Even if not, you will certainly be a more fit, versatile, and adaptable athlete.

Advanced Aerobic Training

This section is for the well-trained individual. I'll provide some suggestions for advanced training, but keep in mind there is no single way to train. If you enjoy

YOUR WEEKLY SWIMMING PROGRAM

Week

	1	2	3	4	5	6	7	8
Monday	15 min	20	25	20	25	30	35	30
Tuesday	2 × 5 min	2 × 6	2 × 7	2 × 8	3 × 6	3 × 7	3 × 8	4 × 5
Wednesday	5 min/each	6/e	7/e	8/e	9/e	10/e	11/e	12/e
Thursday	3 × 3 min	3 × 4	3 × 5	3 × 4	4 × 3	4 × 4	4 × 5	5 × 4
Friday	25	30	35	40	35	40	45	50

Use good goggles; warm up well on Tuesday, Wednesday, and Thursday, and swim easy laps after those workouts.
Pace: Swim slowly or walk in the water to recover between repeats.
Arms/Legs: Use a kickboard or flotation device for support.
Intervals: Swim slowly or walk to recover between repeats.

underdistance training, by all means use it. If you find that you prefer over-distance, use that approach.

Simply pick up the pace as you approach the end of a long run, and you'll receive an optimal training stimulus. Moreover, because the speed work is limited to a short span near the end of the run, discomfort is brief.

Consider the following suggestions.

- Always warm up before your run.
- Use the high-fitness heart rate training zone.
- Vary the location and distance of the run (long-short, fast-slow, or hilly-flat).
- Set distance goals:

  Phase 1: 20 mi per week
  Phase 2: 25 mi per week (ready for 3- to 5-mi road races)
  Phase 3: 30 mi per week
  Phase 4: 35 mi per week (ready for 5- to 7-mi road races)
  Phase 5: 40 mi per week
  Phase 6:[1] 45 mi per week (ready for 7- to 10-mi road races)
  Phase 7: More than 50 mi per week (consider longer races such as the marathon—26.2 mi)

- Don't be a slave to your goals, and don't increase weekly mileage unless you enjoy it.
- Run 6 days per week if you like; otherwise, try an alternate day schedule with longer runs.
- Try one long run (not over one third of weekly distance) on Saturday or Sunday.
- Try two shorter runs if the long ones seem difficult: 5 + 5 instead of 10.
- Keep records if you like—you'll be surprised (see Table B.9)! Record date, distance, and comments. Note morning pulse and body weight. At least once per year, check your performance over a measured distance to observe progress (use a local road race or the 1-1/2-mi-run test). Check your fitness score on the step test several times per year.
- Don't train with a stopwatch. Wear a wristwatch so you'll know how long you've run.
- Increase speed as you approach the finish of a run.
- Always cool down after a run.

Training Tips

You may wonder why I emphasize walking and running as modes of exercise. For the time invested, they provide a great training stimulus. The intensity and duration are easy to control or to change. These activities can be done at any

---

[1]Beyond health and fitness, for personal and performance goals.

Table B.9   Advanced Aerobic Training Log

Week	Mon	Tue	Wed	Thu	Fri	Sat	Sun	Comments
____								_____
____								_____
____								_____
____								_____
____								_____
____								_____
____								_____
____								_____
____								_____
____								_____
____								_____

time, in almost any weather, with little investment in equipment. The equipment is light and easily transported on vacation or a business trip. You can exercise alone or in a group. Both activities are possible at any stage of life. For these reasons and more, walking and running are fine ways to achieve and maintain aerobic fitness.

Shoes, Socks, and Clothing

Nothing is more essential to your enjoyment than proper shoes, so don't economize when selecting them. Go to your sporting goods dealer or shoe store for advice. Buy a training shoe, not a shoe built for competition. A firm, thick sole, good arch support, and a thick, padded heal are essential. (To test sole firmness, grip shoes on sides and squeeze. If the sole bends, it's probably too soft.) A good shoe will be well padded under the sole but not terribly difficult to flex. A firm heel counter is also important. Never attempt distance runs in an ordinary sneaker; you may get away with it, but it isn't worth the risk. Tube socks help prevent blisters, and some runners prefer to wear a thin sock under a heavier outer one.

Walking and jogging don't require fancy clothing. Nylon or cotton gym shorts and a T-shirt are adequate in summer. For winter, a sweat shirt or jogging suit serves until temperatures fall below 20 °F. Some runners prefer tights or long underwear under their shorts. Several layers of lighter apparel are preferable to a single heavy garment. Add gloves and a knit cap in colder temperatures. When the wind blows, a thin nylon windbreaker helps to reduce heat loss. A cap is particularly important in cold weather, because you lose a great deal of body heat from your head. When temperatures fall below 20 °F, you may choose to wear both the underwear and a sweat suit. Many runners continue to run in subzero temperatures, which is safe provided you are properly clothed, warmed up, and sensitive to signs of wind chill and frostbite. (Many runners and skiers appreciate polypropylene underwear that wicks perspiration away from skin, thereby avoiding rapid cooling.)

Never wear a rubberized sweat suit in *any weather*. The water lost through perspiration doesn't contribute to long-term weight loss, and your body's most effective mode of heat loss is blocked.

Running Technique

An upright posture conserves energy. Run with your back comfortably straight, your head up, and your shoulders relaxed. Bend your arms and hold your hands in a comfortable position. Keep arm swing to a minimum during jogging and slow running; pumping action should increase with speed. Your legs should swing freely from the hip with no attempt to overstride. Many successful runners employ a relatively short stride. Lab studies show that the stride that feels best is usually the most efficient as well.

No aspect of running technique is violated more often by neophytes than the footstrike. Many beginners say they don't like to jog. Observation of their footstrike often reveals the reason: They run on the balls of their feet. Although appropriate for sprints and short distances, this footstrike is inappropriate for distance runs and will probably result in soreness. I recommend the **heel-to-toe** footstrike for most new runners. Upon landing lightly on the heel, the foot rocks forward to push off on the ball of the foot. For faster running, employ a slight forward lean, more knee lift, a quick forceful push off the ball of the foot (toe-off), and more vigorous arm action. The heel-to-toe technique is the least tiring of all, and a large percentage of successful distance runners use it. The flat footstrike is a compromise: The runner lands on the entire foot and rocks onto the ball for push-off. Check your shoes after several weeks of running; if you're using the correct footstrike, the outer border of the heel will show some wear.

Time of Day

Exercise whenever it suits your fancy. Some like to do several miles before break-fast. Others elect to train during lunch hour, then eat a sandwich at their desks. Many prefer to exercise after work to help cleanse the mind of the day's prob-lems. A few night owls brave the dark in their quest for fitness; they are quick to point out that the run and shower help them sleep. I caution you to avoid vigorous activity 1 or 2 hr after a meal, when the digestive organs require an adequate blood supply and when fat in the circulation hastens the risk of clotting.

Unless you enjoy spending time by yourself, consider training with a com-panion. When you find one with similar abilities, interest, and goals, you aren't likely to miss your workout.

Where to Walk or Run

Where should you go? Almost anywhere you please. Avoid hard surfaces for the first few weeks of training. Walk or run in the park, on playing fields, on golf courses, or on running tracks. After a few weeks, you'll be ready to try the back roads and trails in your area. Varying your routes will help you main-tain interest. When the weather prohibits outdoor exercise, try a mall, YMCA, or school gym, or choose an exercise supplement you can do at home, such as running in place or skipping rope.

If your community doesn't already have one, you should encourage your parks and recreation department to consider developing a fitness trail (see Appendix F). This easy-to-build outdoor fitness facility consists of a running trail and exer-cise stations made from inexpensive materials. The trail can be filled with wood chips to provide a soft, springy surface. Exercise stations along the trail en-courage the development of muscular fitness (Sharkey, Jukkala, & Herzberg, 1978).

Other Activities

If running isn't your cup of tea, consider these tips on training program develop-ment for other activities such as rowing or cross-country skiing.

- Review aerobic prescriptions in chapter 3.
- Review fitness for sport in chapter 15.
- Review the walk-jog-run programs in this appendix.

- Review the principles of training in Appendix F.
- If appropriate, plan a SERIOUS training program (see Sleamaker, 1989) that includes the following.

S = speed
E = endurance
R = race or pace
I = intervals
O = overdistance
U = up or vertical (e.g., hills) if applicable
S = strength

If you are not that serious, forget speed and pace, but don't ignore variety in your training. Alternate hard with easy, short with long, and speed with distance, and don't forget to include rest days for recovery. Outline a program and get started. Keep simple records and change the program when your goals change. As your interest grows, seek out books or magazines that focus on your activity. In time you will become an expert on training.

Aerobic Alternatives

When you are unable to engage in your regular aerobic activity (e.g., walking, jogging, or cycling) because of time, weather, or injury, consider an alternative. These activities also are good aerobic supplements if you are on a weight control program.

Skipping rope is a full-time aerobic activity for some. The equipment is inexpensive and easy to transport. You can skip rope anywhere, even in a hotel room. The exercise allows a wide range of intensities. Rope length is important; the ends of the rope should reach your armpits when you hold the rope beneath your feet. Commercial ropes with ball bearings in the handles are easier and smoother to use, but a length of No. 10 sash cord from your local hardware store serves quite well. Rope skipping requires a degree of coordination and if done inappropriately can quickly raise the heart rate above your training zone. If this happens, walk or jog in place slowly, then resume skipping. Besides the aerobic benefits, rope skipping could improve your tennis or racquetball game, where rapid footwork is important.

Race walking has not yet taken the country by storm, but if you are a jogger with an injury or a fitness walker in search of a greater challenge, race walking may be for you. The difference between regular walking and race walking is form. The rules require that the toe of one foot remain on the ground until the heel of the other foot touches, producing the distinctive rolling style of competitive walking. This excellent form of aerobic exercise provides all the benefits of jogging. But because there is less pounding on the feet and knees, it is easier to tolerate. If you like to jog but can't, or if you are in an area where race walking is becoming popular, give it a try.

Joggers and runners can try **running in place** when bad weather or travel prohibits the usual run. Because it's necessary to double the running time to achieve a comparable benefit, running in place can only be viewed as an occasional supplement. You may prefer walking; many shopping malls open early to allow indoor walking.

Several **stationary bicycles** are available for indoor cycling. They range from the less expensive (including my choice, a stand for your bicycle) to the moderate price range for a stationary bicycle, to the expensive (approaching $1,000) for fancy cycles that include the electronics necessary to provide resistance as well as a readout of heart rate responses to work load. You can use your aerobic fitness prescription to achieve training benefits on the bicycle. The indoor cycle must include a mechanism for the control of resistance, because without resistance you won't be able to achieve your heart rate training zone.

Several relatively inexpensive **treadmills** are sold. These nonmotorized devices must have an adjustable grade if they are to serve for aerobic training. Expensive motorized devices are excellent indoor training machines, but price prohibits their general use. The stationary bicycle and the treadmill often are used in post-coronary home rehabilitation programs.

Rowing devices have become popular in recent years. Less expensive models use adjustable shock absorbers to control resistance. More expensive models use a fly wheel or an electronic brake. These devices provide both lower and upper body exercise as do the many versions of cross-country ski simulators.

A sturdy bench or box can become an exercise device by using it for **bench stepping**. By increasing the rate or duration of effort, you can achieve specific training effects. By wearing a loaded pack, you can emphasize the muscular fitness benefits of the exercise. Bench stepping is like push-ups for the legs, but it is dull.

Stair walking or running is another aerobic alternative. Coaches often have their athletes run stadium steps in a combination aerobic-anaerobic muscular-fitness training program. For duration, aerobic training predominates; for speed, strength and anaerobic capabilities are developed. The steps in gym, office, or apartment building provide the opportunity for extended effort.

Other aerobic alternatives include aerobic dance, swimming, rebound exercise devices, and other types of exercise simulators. The rebound devices are easy on the legs and provide a low to moderate training stimulus. They sell for $50 to $100.

Remember, before you buy any piece of equipment, try it out to be sure it is right for you.

APPENDIX

C

MUSCULAR FITNESS

- **Muscular Fitness Tests**
- **Muscular Fitness Programs**
  - *Warm-Up Exercises*
  - *Weight Lifting*
  - *Calisthenics*
  - *Counterforce Exercises*
- **Muscular Fitness Log**

Muscular Fitness Tests

See Table C.1 on p. 332 for tests that measure the fitness of muscle groups, level of contractile capacities, or proportion of muscle fiber types.

A. Warm-Up Exercises

Here are some suggested warm-up exercises for a muscular fitness program. You may wish to use some or substitute your own.

1. Seated Toe Touch for Back and Hamstrings.   With toes pointed, slowly slide hands down legs until you feel stretch; hold position. Grasp ankles and slowly pull until head approaches legs. Relax. Draw toes back and slowly attempt to touch toes. Repeat several times.
   Variation: Try toe touch with legs apart.

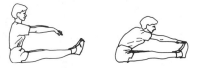

2. Knee Pull for Thigh and Trunk.   Pull leg to chest with arms and hold for count of 5. Repeat with opposite leg (8 to 10 times each leg).
   Variation: Use double knee pull.

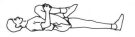

Table C.1 Muscular Fitness Tests

		Men			Women		
		Low	Medium	High	Low	Medium	High
Upper body	Strength	Chin-up[a]	<6	7-9	>10	<20	20-30	>30
	Endurance	Push-up	<20	20-40	>40	<10	10-20	>20
Trunk	Endurance	Sit-up	<30	30-50	>50	<25	25-40	>40
Leg	Strength	Leg press	<400	400-550	>550	<300	300-450	>450
Flexibility (toe touch)	Reach toes		No	Yes	Beyond	No	Yes	Beyond
Power	Vertical jump		<17	17-23	>23	<10	10-15	>15
Speed (50 yd)	Seconds		>7.5	7.5-6.0	<6.0	>9.0	9.0-7.5	<7.5
Muscle fiber type estimation								
	Fast twitch	Vertical jump	<17	17-23	>23	<10	10-15	>15
	Slow twitch	Aerobic fitness (step test or 1.5-mi run)	<40	40-60	>60	<35	35-50	>50

[a]Women do modified chin-up.

3. Ankle Pull for Groin and Inner Thighs.   Pull on ankles while pressing legs down with elbows.

Variation: Lean forward and try to touch head to feet or floor.

4. Stride Stretch for Calf and Thigh Muscles.   Slowly slide into stride position with front foot *flat* on floor, knee aligned over ankle, and rear foot on toes. Put hands on chair or floor for balance. Hold for 10 counts. Switch legs.

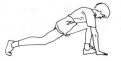

5. Wall Stretch for Legs.   Stand 3 ft from wall, feet slightly apart. Put both hands on wall. With heels on ground, lean forward slowly and feel stretch in calves. Hold position for 15 to 20 s. Repeat several times.

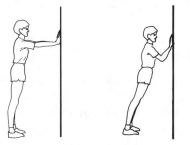

6. Flexed Leg–Back Stretch for Legs and Back.   Stand erect, feet shoulder-width apart. With knees slightly flexed, slowly bend over, touching the ground between the feet. Hold for 10 s. Repeat several times.

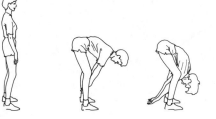

7. Side Bender for Trunk.   Extend one arm overhead, other on hip and keep your knees slightly bent. Slowly bend to side; bob gently. Repeat 5 times each side.

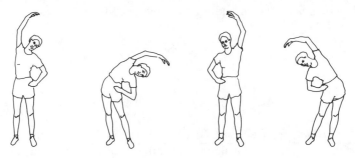

8. Side Twister for Trunk.   With feet comfortably apart, extend arms palms down. Twist to one side as far as possible. Repeat to other side; do 5 repetitions on each side.

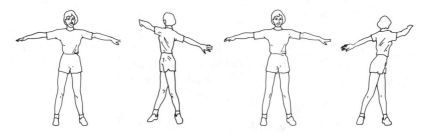

9. Elbow Thrust for Shoulder and Back.   Keep your feet apart, arms bent, hands in front of chest, and elbows out to side. Without arching back, rhythmically thrust elbows backward, then return to starting position. Repeat 15 times.

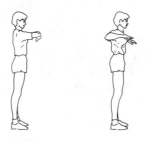

10. Neck Circles for Neck.   With feet apart, gently roll head in half circle, first to one side, then to the other. Repeat 3 times to each side. Do not drop head to back.

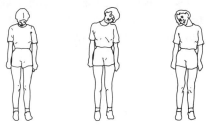

11. Jumping Jacks for Legs and Trunk.   Hold arms at sides. On Count 1, jump and spread feet apart and simultaneously swing arms over head. On Count 2, return to starting position. Use a rhythmic, moderate cadence. Repeat 15 to 25 times. Attempt variations.

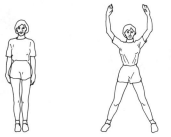

12. Run in Place.   Start slowly, then increase rate, height of leg lift, or both. As training progresses, run in place between subsequent conditioning exercises.

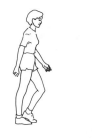

B. Weight Lifting

You can lift weights with conventional barbells or with modern weight machines. Machines are expensive, but have several advantages over barbells; they are safer, and more versatile, they save time, and they eliminate equipment theft.

The Universal Gym

This popular isotonic equipment typically provides stations for (a) bench press and (b) leg press, as well as

- abdomen and trunk exercises,
- military press and curls,
- lat exercises, and
- leg extension and flexion.

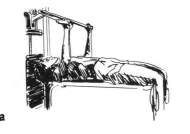
a

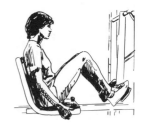
b

Nautilus

Nautilus equipment utilizes a cam to adjust resistance throughout the lift. Most clubs have stations for (a) triceps, (b) chest, (c) leg press, as well as

- biceps curl,
- bench press,
- lat pull over and pull down,
- leg flexion and extension, and
- abdominals and trunk.

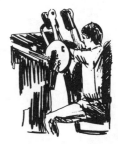
a

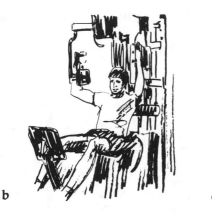

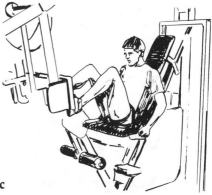

b   c

Mini Gym

This company makes a variety of variable resistance devices, such as the ''leaper'' shown here. The company has devices specifically designed for certain sports such as basketball and volleyball (e.g., leaper) and for swimming.

Excellent equipment is also manufactured by Paramount, Hydra Gym, Kiefer, Polaris, and others. And sturdy home devices are now available at a cost ranging from under $100 for free weights to $500 and more for home training centers.

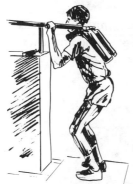

The following exercises are offered as suggestions for a weight training program. Use free weights or machines to accomplish your muscular fitness goals. For each exercise do 3 sets of up to 6 to 8 repetitions each for strength; do more repetitions with lighter weights for endurance. Exhale while raising weight; inhale while lowering it.

Bench Press for Chest, Arm Extensor Muscles. Lie flat on back with feet on floor astride bench. Grasp bar wider than shoulder-width apart with arms extended. Lower bar to chest. Press bar back up to starting position. Inhale while lowering weight, exhale while pressing it. Partner should assist with weight before and after exercise.

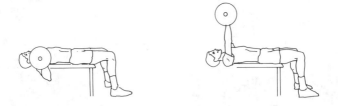

Tricep Extension for Triceps. Sit astride bench with back straight. Grasp bar with hands about 2 in. apart, using overhand grip. Bring bar to full arm extension above head. Lower bar behind head, keeping elbows stationary.

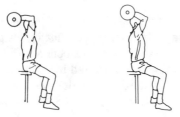

Military Press for Arm and Shoulder Muscles. Stand erect with feet comfortably apart. Grasp barbell overhand grip and raise to upper chest. Then press bar overhead, until elbows are fully extended. Lower bar to chest position; repeat.

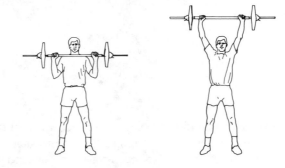

Curls for Biceps.   Stand erect, feet comfortably apart, knees slightly flexed. Hold bar in front of thighs with underhand grip shoulder-width apart, arms straight. Flex elbows fully, lifting bar toward chest. Keep elbows close to sides and avoid raising shoulders. Don't lean backward or "bounce" bar with leg motion. Return to starting position.

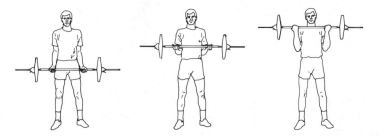

Bent Rowing for Back Muscles.   Stand in bent-over position, back flat and slightly above parallel with floor. Spread feet shoulder width, with knees comfortably bent. Grasp barbell with an overhand grip; hands should be slightly wider than shoulder width. Keep buttocks lower than shoulders. Pull bar to chest. Lower bar to starting position. Keep upper body stationary.

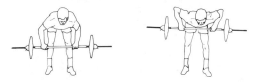

Pull Down for Lats.   Kneel on one or both knees, grasp handles. Pull bar down and return to starting position.

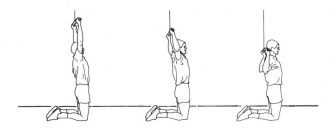

Leg Press for Quadriceps. Place feet on pedals, grasp handles on seat. Press feet forward to elevate weight, return. Inhale while lowering weight and exhale while lifting it.

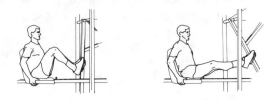

Leg Flexion for Hamstrings. Lie face down on table with heels positioned behind padded bar. Flex legs to elevate weight. Return to starting position. Watch for leg cramps.

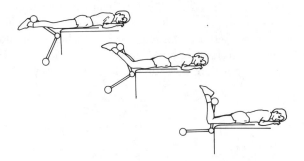

Leg Extension for Quadriceps. Sit on table with instep under padded bar. Extend leg to elevate weight. Return to starting position.

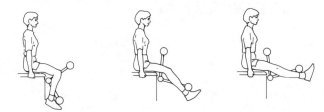

C. Calisthenics

Chest and Triceps: Strength and Endurance

Knee Push-Up (beginner).   With hands outside shoulders and knees bent, push up keeping back straight. Do as many as possible.

Push-Up (intermediate).   With hands outside shoulders, push up keeping back straight; return until chest almost touches floor. Do as many as possible.

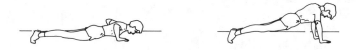

Chair Dips (advanced).   Be sure chair is stationary. Grasp sides of chair, slide feet forward while supporting weight on arms. Lower body and return. Do as many as possible.
    Variation: Use parallel bars if available.

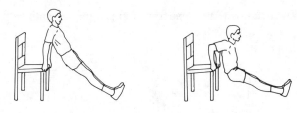

Biceps and Back: Strength and Endurance

Modified Chin-Up (beginner). Stand with bar about chest height. With underhand grasp, hang from bar with body straight and feet on ground. Pull up and return. Do as many as possible.

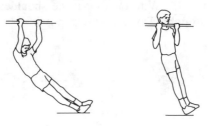

Flexed Arm Hang (beginner).   With underhand grasp and the assistance of a companion, raise body until chin is above bar and arms flexed. Hold position as long as possible. Let down as slowly as possible.

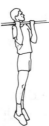

Chin-Up (intermediate).   With underhand grasp, pull up until chin is over bar; return. Do as many as possible.
Variation: Rope climb.

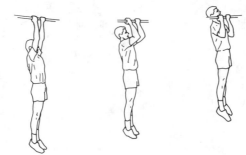

Pike Chin-Up (advanced).   Chin up with legs in pike position.

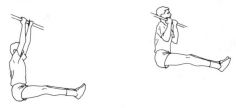

Abdominal: Strength and Endurance

Sit-Up With Arms Crossed.   On back with arms crossed on chest and knees bent, curl up to semisitting position and return. Do 10 to 15 times.

Variation: Do repetitions very fast; do on an inclined board; hold weight on chest.

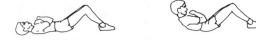

Basket Hang (advanced).   Hang from bar with underhand grasp. Raise legs into "basket" and return. Do as many as possible.

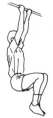

Back: Strength and Endurance

Leg Lifts.   Lying face down on floor with partner holding trunk down, raise legs 5 to 10 times.

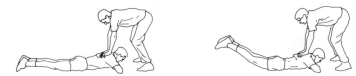

Trunk Lifts. Lying face down on floor with fingers laced behind head and ankles anchored to the ground, raise trunk 5 to 10 times.

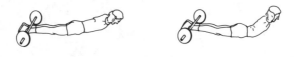

Leg: Strength and Endurance

Half Knee Bends. With feet apart and hands on hips, squat until thighs are parallel to ground; return. Do as many as possible. Try 2-in. block under heels to aid balance.

Variation: Do with weight on back (e.g., a backpack or a friend).

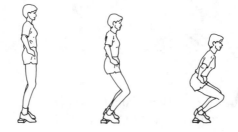

Bench Stepping. Step up and down on bench as fast as possible for 30 s. Switch lead leg and repeat.

Variation: Do with loaded pack.

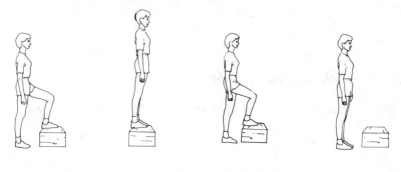

Heel Raises.   Stand erect, hands at sides or on hips, feet close together. Raise up on toes 20 to 40 times.

   Variation: Do with toes on 2-in. platform; do with loaded pack.

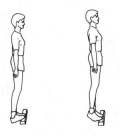

Hill Running.   Run up and down a steep hill.

   Variation: Use the stairs of a gym, stadium, or office building. Wear a weighted pack.

Leg Strength and Power

Build power with calistheniclike jumping exercises known as plyometrics. Do on a mat or on grass.

Squat Jumps.   Stand with hands on hips, one foot a step ahead of the other. Squat until front leg is at a 90° angle, jump as high as possible, extending the knees. Switch position of feet on way down and jump again; 10 to 20 repetitions.

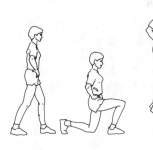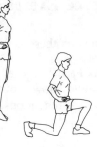

**Hops**.   Do one-leg hops, alternate legs with a balance step between hops. Do 10 with each leg; work up to 2 sets of 20.

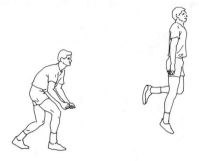

**Two-Leg Jumps**.   Do 10 to 20 explosive two-leg jumps. Jump as high as possible on each attempt.

D. Counterforce Exercises

Work with a partner on these isokinetic exercises.

**Arm Flexion**.   As Partner 1 tries to move arms up, Partner 2 resists movement; Partner 2 should allow movement to progress slowly (range of motion in 3 s). Do 3 sets of 8 repetitions.

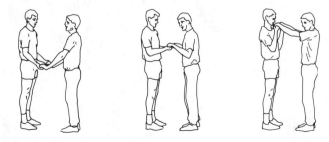

Arm Extension.   As Partner 1 tries to extend arms down, Partner 2 resists movement; Partner 2 should allow movement to progress slowly (range of motion in 3 s). Do 3 sets of 8 repetitions.

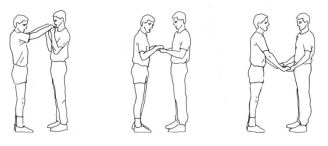

Push-Up.   As Partner 1 does conventional push-up, Partner 2 provides resistance. Do 3 sets of 8 repetitions. Switch places between sets to allow time to rest.

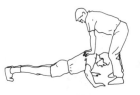

Leg Flexion.   As Partner 1 tries to flex leg, Partner 2 resists movement; Partner 2 should allow movement to progress slowly through range of motion in 3 s. Switch legs and repeat. Do 3 sets of 8 repetitions each. Switch positions between sets; watch out for leg cramps.

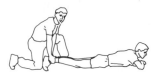 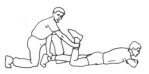

Leg Extension. As Partner 1 tries to extend leg, Partner 2 resists movement; Partner 2 should allow movement to progress slowly through range of motion in 3 s. Switch legs and repeat. Do 3 sets of 8 repetitions each. Switch positions between sets.

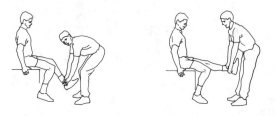

Use your imagination to devise additional isokinetic exercises. Isokinetic exercise devices are commercially available.

Note: See Appendix F for more exercises on the "Fitness Trail."

Record your muscular fitness training in a log, like the one in Table C.2.

Table C.2   Muscular Fitness Log

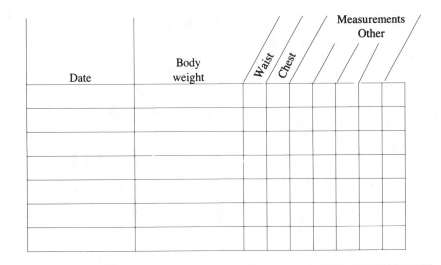

APPENDIX

D

FITNESS AND WEIGHT CONTROL

- **Determining Caloric Intake**
- **Determining Energy Expenditure**
- **Predicting Caloric Expenditure**
- **Determining Body Composition**

Determining Caloric Intake

The determination of daily caloric intake is the first step toward the calculation of the energy balance. Table D.1 includes comprehensive calorie charts organized according to general categories (e.g., vegetables, meats). Calories contained in each portion are given. Remember:

- 3 teaspoons = 1 tablespoon
- 2 tablespoons = 1 fluid ounce
- 16 tablespoons = 1 cup
- 1 cup = 8 fluid ounces or 1/2 pint
- 4 cups = 1 quart
- 1 lb = 16 ounces

Carry a small notepad so you can jot down any food, drink, or snack. At the end of the day sit down with the calorie charts and figure your daily intake. Many computer programs are available to simplify the calculations and provide information on the nutritional value of your diet. You should attempt to assess your caloric intake for at least several days; it is a most educational experience.

In Table D.1, I've included the grams of fat contained in each portion of food or beverage. This should help you avoid unwanted fat if you decide to pursue a low-fat diet. The low-fat diet helps reduce body weight as well as cholesterol. Each gram of fat contains 9.3 cal. If your goal is to reduce fat intake from the typical 40% of calories, try to stay within the following targets:

For a daily calorie intake of 2,000 cal, 40% fat = 86 g of fat (40% × 2,000 = 800 cal ÷ 9.3 = 86 g).

30% fat = 65 g
20% fat = 43 g
10% fat = 22 g

Table D.1   Caloric Content of Foods

Food	Portion	Fat[a] (grams)	Calories
Beverages, alcoholic			
Beer	12 ounces	0	150
Beer, light	12 ounces	0	100
Brandy	1 ounce	0	70
Eggnog	1 cup	19	335
Highball	1 cup	0	165
Port, vermouth, muscatel	1/2 cup	0	155
Rum	1 jigger (1-1/2 ounces)	0	140
Whiskey	1 jigger (1-1/2 ounces)	0	130
Wine, white, rose	1/2 cup	0	85-105
Beverages, nonalcoholic			
Carbonated soft drinks	1 cup	0	80
Chocolate milk	1 cup	10.5	200
Cocoa	1 cup	11	175
Coffee, black	1 cup	0	1
with cream and sugar			
(1 teaspoon each)	1 cup	3	45
Tea	1 cup	0	1
Cereals, cereal products			
Bread			
Boston, enriched, brown	2 large slices	1.2	200
corn or muffins, enriched	2	6	220
raisin, enriched	2 slices	1.5	130
rye, American	2 slices	0.6	110
white, enriched	2 slices	1.5	120
whole wheat	2 slices	1.5	110
Bread, rolls, sweet, unenriched	1	3	320
Cornflakes	1 cup	0.1	100
Crackers, graham	2	1.0	60
saltines	2	1.5	50
soda	10 oyster	1.3	40
Macaroni, cooked	1/2 cup	0.3	70
Noodles, cooked	1 cup	2.0	150
Oatflakes, cooked	1 cup	1.0	75
Pancakes, wheat	2 cakes	6.0	150
Popcorn, popped	1 cup	0.8	60
Pretzels	Handful	1.0	110
Rice, cooked	1/2 cup	0.1	100
Spaghetti with tomato sauce	1 cup	7.0	220

Food	Portion	Fat[a] (grams)	Calories
Tapioca, cooked	1/2 cup	4.0	130
Waffles, baked (frozen or mix)	1 waffle	4-8	225
Wheat germ	1 oz	3.5	120
Confectionery, sugar			
Chocolate	1 ounce	16	150
Fudge	1 piece	5	120
Honey	1 tablespoon	0	65
Jams	1 tablespoon	0	55
Jellies	1 tablespoon	0	50
Molasses	1 tablespoon	0	50
Syrup (chiefly corn syrup)	1 tablespoon	0	60
Sugar, maple	1 tablespoon	0	55
cane or beet	1 tablespoon	0	50
Dairy products, eggs			
Cheese, cheddar	1 ounce	9.5	115
cottage	1/2 cup	5	100
cream	2 tablespoons	10	100
Limburger	1 ounce	8	100
Parmesan	1 ounce	8.5	110
Roquefort	1 ounce	8	105
Swiss	1 ounce	8	105
Cream, light	1 tablespoon	3	30
heavy or whipping	1 tablespoon	5.5	50
Eggs, whole	1 medium	5	75
Egg white, raw	1 medium	0	15
Egg yolk, raw	1 medium	5	60
Milk, pasteurized, whole	1 cup	8.5	165
buttermilk, cultured	1 cup	0.4	80
canned, evaporated, unsweetened	1/2 cup	10.0	140
condensed, sweetened	1/2 cup	14	480
nonfat	1 cup	0.4	80
Ice cream	1/2 cup	9-13	155-225
Sherbet	1/2 cup	2-3	135
Yogurt, low fat	1 cup	2.0	61
regular	1 cup	8.5	152
Fats, Oils			
Butter	1 tablespoon	4.0	35

(Cont.)

Table D.1 (Continued)

Food	Portion	Fat[a] (grams)	Calories
Mayonnaise	1 tablespoon	11.0	100
Olive oil	1 tablespoon	12.0	125
Peanut butter	1 tablespoon	8.0	85
Fruit, fruit juices			
Apples	1	0.8	60-90
Apple juice, fresh	1 cup	0	120
Apple sauce, sweetened	1/2 cup	0	80
Apricots	1 medium	0	18
Avocados, fresh	1/2	18	190
Bananas	1 (about 6 in.)	0	94
Blackberries, fresh	1/2 cup	0.6	40
Blueberries, fresh	1/2 cup	0.4	45
Cantaloupe, fresh	1/2	0.2	40
Cherries, canned, sweetened	1/2 cup	0.2	100
Cranberry sauce	2 tablespoons	0	60
Dates, dried, pitted	5	0.2	100
Fruit cocktail, canned	1/2 cup	0.2	90
Grapes, fresh	20	0.8	45
Grape juice	1/2 cup	0	80
Grapefruit	1/2 (4-1/4 in. dia.)	0.1	75
Grapefruit juice, fresh	1/2 cup	0.2	45
Lemons, fresh	1 (2 in.)	0	30
Olives, green or ripe	5 large	2.5/4.0	20/35
Oranges, fresh	1 (3 in.)	0.1	70
Orange juice, fresh	1/2 cup	0.3	55
Peaches, fresh	1 (2-1/2 in.)	0.1	45
canned, sweetened	2 halves	0.2	85
Pears	1 (2-1/2 in.)	0.7	95
Pineapple, canned, sweetened	1/2 cup	0.2	100
Pineapple juice, canned	1/2 cup	0.1	60
Plums	1 (2 in.)	0.1	30
Prunes, dried, uncooked	4 large	0.3	110
Raisins, dried	1/4 cup	0.1	100
Raspberries, fresh	1/2 cup	0.5	50
Strawberries, fresh	10 large	0.5	35
frozen, sweetened	1/2 cup	0.2	125
Sorbet	1/2 cup	0.2	110

Food	Portion	Fat[a] (grams)	Calories
Meat, poultry (raw unless otherwise stated)			
Bacon, medium fat, cooked	2 strips	9.0	100
Beef (medium fat), hamburger, cooked	1/4 lb	15	225
rib roast, cooked	3 ounces	33	335
sirloin, cooked	3 ounces	27	330
canned, corned	4 ounces	11	240
liver, fried	3 ounces	9.0	200
Chicken, fried	1/4 lb	9.0	275
roasted	1/4 lb	3.0	170
liver	3 ounces	15.0	235
Ham, baked	3 ounces	19	250
canned, spiced	3 ounces	21	245
Lamb (medium fat), leg roast	3 ounces	6.0	160
rib chop	1	15.0	230
Pork (see also bacon and ham), medium fat	3 ounces	24	310
loin or chops	1	24.5	300
Turkey, light and dark	3 ounces	3.5-7.0	150/170
Veal	3 ounces	9.5	180
Venison	3 ounces	2.5	120
Nuts			
Almonds	15 nuts	8.0	100
Brazil nuts	5 nuts	12.0	100
Cashew nuts, roasted or cooked	10 nuts	14.0	200
Peanuts, roasted	30	14.0	165
Pecans	1 tablespoon	5	52
Walnuts	2 tablespoons	10	95
Sea food (raw unless otherwise stated)			
Clams	1/4 lb	0.8	80
Cod	4 ounces	6.0	180
Crab, canned or cooked	1/2 cup	2.0	100
Flounder	1/4 lb	7.0	180
Frog legs, fried	4 legs	28.0	418
Haddock	1/4 lb	7.0	180
Halibut	1/4 lb	8.0	200

(Cont.)

Table D.1 (Continued)

Food	Portion	Fat[a] (grams)	Calories
Lobster	1 (3/4 lb)	5.0	300
Oysters	5-8 medium	2.0	80
Salmon, Pacific, cooked	1/4 lb	7.0	180
canned	1/2 cup	7.0	190
Sardines, canned in oil	5 medium	9.0	180
Scallops, fried	4 ounces	10.0	200
Shrimps, canned	3 ounces	0.9	100
Shrimps, fried	3 ounces	9.5	190
Trout	1/4 lb (brook-lake)	10-13	210-290
Soup			
Broth	1 cup	0	25
Bean	1 cup	6.0	170
Beef	1 cup	4.0	115
with vegetables	1 cup	2.0	90
Chicken noodle	1 cup	2.0	68
Pea	1 cup	3.0	140
Tomato	1 cup	2.5	100
Vegetable	1 cup	2.0	90
Vegetables			
Asparagus, canned	1/2 cup	0.4	25
Beans, kidney	1/2 cup	0.5	120
lima, fresh	1/2 cup	0.4	90
snap, fresh	1/2 cup	0.4	35
wax, canned	1/2 cup	0.2	20
Beets (beetroots), peeled, fresh	1/2 cup	0.1	35
Broccoli, fresh	1/2 cup	0.2	30
Brussels sprouts, fresh	1/2 cup	0.3	30
Cabbage, fresh	wedge	0.2	25
Carrots, canned	1/2 cup	0.2	30
fresh	1 carrot (6 in.)	0.1	20
Cauliflower, fresh	1 cup	0.2	25
Celery	2 stalks	0.1	17
Corn, fresh, with butter	1 ear	2.0	90
canned	1/2 cup	0.6	70
Cucumbers	1 (7-1/2 in.)	0.2	20
Eggplant, fresh	1/2 cup	0.2	25
Kale, fresh	1/2 cup	0.4	20
Lentils	1/2 cup	—	110
Lettuce, headed, fresh	1/4 head	0.1	15
Mushrooms	1/2 cup	0.1	10
Onions	1 (2-1/2 in.)	0.1	40

Food	Portion	Fat[a] (grams)	Calories
Peas, green, fresh	1/2 cup	0.2	55
canned	1/2 cup	0.4	70
Peppers, green, fresh	1 large	0.1	24
Potatoes, raw	1 medium	0.2	90
french fried	20 pieces	12	220
Radishes, fresh	4 small	—	10
Rhubarb, fresh	1/2 cup	—	10
Spinach, canned	1/2 cup	0.2	25
Sweet potatoes, fresh	1 small	0.6	150
candied	1 medium	3.5	180
Tomatoes, fresh	1 medium	0.2	25
canned	1/2 cup	0.2	25
Tomato juice, canned	1/2 cup	0.2	35
Miscellaneous			
Gelatin dessert	1/2 cup	0	60
Pie	1 slice	16-18	300-400
Pecan pie	1 slice	31.5	580
Potato chips	7-10	8.0	110
Salad dressing (French, Thousand Island)	1 tablespoon	6-8	60-100
Tomato catsup	2 tablespoons	0.1	40
Yeast, compressed, baker's	1 cake	0.1	20

[a]1 g of fat contains 9.3 calories.

See how quickly calories add up in popular eating establishments (see Table D.2 on page 358).

Consider the amount of running (at about 120 cal per mile) needed to burn off the calories consumed in the following snacks.

Snack	Running
Highball	1-1/3 mi
Beer (12 ounces)	1-1/2 mi
Light beer	1 mi
Potato chips (15)	1-1/2 mi
Peanuts (handful)	2 mi
Peanut butter and jelly (1 tablespoon of each) on crackers	2-1/3 mi

Table D.2 Caloric Values for Fast Food

	Energy (cal)	Protein (g)	Fat (g)	Carbohydrate (g)
McDonald's				
2 hamburgers, fries, shake	1030	40	37	135
Big Mac, fries, shake	1100	40	41	143
Big Mac	550	21	32	45
Quarter pounder	420	25	19	37
Hamburger	260	14	9	30
French fries	180	3	10	20
Chocolate shake	315	9	8	51
Burger King				
Whopper, fries, shake	1200	40	47	147
Whopper	630	29	35	50
Whopper, Jr.	285	16	15	21
Double hamburger	325	24	15	24
Hamburger	230	14	10	21
French fries	220	2	12	10
Chocolate shake	365	8	8	65
Pizza Hut				
10-in. Supreme (cheese, tomato sauce, sausage, pepperoni, mushrooms, etc.)	1200	72	35	152
10-in. pizza (cheese)	1025	65	23	140
Kentucky Fried Chicken				
3-piece dinner (chicken, potatoes, roll, slaw)	1000	55	55	71
Dairy Queen				
4 ounce serving soft ice cream	180	5	6	27
Arby's				
Sliced beef sandwich, 2 potato patties, slaw, shake	1200	27	40	166

Determining Energy and Caloric Expenditure

Short Method—Follow Steps 1 Through 4

1. Calculate Basal Energy Expenditure (Table D.3)

Table D.3   Basal Energy Expenditure for Men and Women

	Men		Women
Weight	Energy expenditure[a] (cal)	Weight	Energy expenditure[b] (cal)
140	1,550	100	1,225
160	1,640	120	1,320
180	1,730	140	1,400
200	1,815	160	1,485
220	1,900	180	1,575

[a]5 ft 10 in. tall (add 20 cal for each inch taller; if shorter subtract 20 cal).

[b]5 ft 6 in. tall (add 20 cal for each inch taller; if shorter subtract 20 cal).

Note. Basal energy = calories expended in 24 hr of complete bed rest.

2. Add Increases in Caloric Expenditure (Table D.4)

Table D.4   Approximate Increases in Caloric Expenditure for Selected Activities

Activity	Percent above basal
Bed rest (eating and reading)	10
Quiet sitting (reading, knitting)	30
Light activity (office work)	40-60
Moderate activity (housekeeping)	60-80
Heavy occupational activity (construction)	100

3. Adjust Total for Age

Subtract 4% of caloric expenditure for each decade (10 years) over 25 years of age.

4. Add Calories Expended in Nonwork (Recreational) Activities

Use caloric expenditure charts (skip ahead to Table D.6, used in the long method). Figure minutes of activity and cost in calories per minute.

Example:

    5 ft 10 in., 200-lb, 45-year-old construction worker
    Basal = 1,815 + 100% = 3,630 − 8% (age) = 3,340
    Table tennis (30 min × 5 kcal/min) = 150   =   150

                                      Total = 3,490 kcal/day

Long Method

You calculated your daily caloric expenditure using a short method. This section provides the information for a minute-by-minute estimation of caloric expenditure that allows the computation of a 24-hr total. You may be interested in comparing the two methods. If so, begin by making a list of your daily activities. Then proceed to determine the cost of each activity in calories per minute. Finally, get the total for each activity and the total for the day. Table D.5 shows how this can be done.

Table D.6, which shows caloric expenditure, also serves as a useful guide to *exercise intensity*, because intensity is directly related to calories expended per minute. Also, the charts can guide you to appropriate weight-control activities. You can readily see that walking burns more calories than recreational volleyball, that jogging requires more energy than calisthenics. Finally, a glance at the charts will tell you how long you must exercise to accomplish a 100-, 200-, or 300-cal workout.

Table D.5 Form for Assessment of Energy Expenditure and Energy Balance

Activity	Kcal/min		Min		Totals
Sleeping	_____	×	_____	=	_____
Working	_____	×	_____	=	_____
Eating	_____	×	_____	=	_____
Personal	_____	×	_____	=	_____
Play or sport	_____	×	_____	=	_____
Relaxation (e.g., TV)	_____	×	_____	=	_____
_____	_____	×	_____	=	_____
_____	_____	×	_____	=	_____
_____	_____	×	_____	=	_____
_____	_____	×	_____	=	_____
			24 hr		cal/day

Adjust total for body size: add 10% for each 15 lb above 150 lb. Subtract 10% for each 15 lb under 150 lb.

Energy balance can now be calculated.

$$\text{Intake} = \underline{\hspace{1.5cm}} \text{ cal} - \text{Expenditure} = \underline{\hspace{1.5cm}} \text{ cal}$$

If intake exceeds expenditure (regularly) you have a positive energy balance. The excess will be stored as fat.

Example

Activity	Kcal/min		Min		Totals
Sleeping	1.2	×	480	=	576
Working	2.6	×	480	=	1,248
Reading	1.3	×	120	=	156
Writing	2.6	×	60	=	156
Eating	1.5	×	60	=	90
Personal	2.5	×	60	=	150
Walking	5.0	×	60	=	300
Talking	1.3	×	60	=	78
Tennis	7.1	×	60	=	426
			24 hr		3,180 cal/day

Table D.6 Caloric Expenditure During Various Activities

Activity	Cal/min[a]
Sleeping	1.2
Resting in bed	1.3
Sitting, normally	1.3
Sitting, reading	1.3
Lying, quietly	1.3
Sitting, eating	1.5

(Cont.)

Table D.6 (Continued)

Activity	Cal/min[a]
Sitting, playing cards	1.5
Standing, normally	1.5
Classwork, lecture (listening)	1.7
Conversing	1.8
Personal toilet	2.0
Sitting, writing	2.6
Standing, light activity	2.6
Washing and dressing	2.6
Washing and shaving	2.6
Driving a car	2.8
Washing clothes	3.1
Walking indoors	3.1
Shining shoes	3.2
Making bed	3.4
Dressing	3.4
Showering	3.4
Driving motorcycle	3.4
Metal working	3.5
House painting	3.5
Cleaning windows	3.7
Carpentry	3.8
Farming chores	3.8
Sweeping floors	3.9
Plastering walls	4.1
Repairing trucks and automobiles	4.2
Ironing clothes	4.2
Farming, planting, hoeing, raking	4.7
Mixing cement	4.7
Mopping floors	4.9
Repaving roads	5.0
Gardening, weeding	5.6
Stacking lumber	5.8
Sawing with chain saw	6.2
Working with stone, masonry	6.3
Working with pick and shovel	6.7
Farming, haying, plowing with horse	6.7
Shoveling (miners)	6.8
Walking down stairs	7.1
Chopping wood	7.5
Sawing with crosscut saw	7.5-10.5
Tree felling (ax)	8.4-12.7
Gardening, digging	8.6
Walking up stairs	10.0-18.0

Activity	Cal/min[a]
Playing pool or billiards	1.8
Canoeing, 2.5 mph-4.0 mph	3.0-7.0
Playing volleyball, recreational to competitive	3.5-8.0
Golfing, foursome to twosome	3.7-5.0
Horseshoes	3.8
Playing baseball (except pitcher)	4.7
Playing ping-pong or table tennis	4.9-7.0
Practicing calisthenics	5.0
Rowing, pleasure to vigorous	5.0-15.0
Cycling, 5-15 mph (10-speed)	5.0-12.0
Skating, recreational to vigorous	5.0-15.0
Practicing archery	5.2
Playing badminton, recreational to competitive	5.2-10.0
Playing basketball, half-full court (more for fast break)	6.0-9.0
Bowling (while active)	7.0
Playing tennis, recreational to competitive	7.0-11.0
Water skiing	8.0
Playing soccer	9.0
Snowshoeing (2.5 mph)	9.0
Playing handball and squash	10.0
Mountain climbing	10.0
Skipping rope	10.0-15.0
Practicing judo and karate	13.0
Playing football (while active)	13.3
Wrestling	14.4
Skiing	
Moderate to steep	8.0-20.0
Downhill racing	16.5
Cross-country; 3-10 mph	9.0-20.0
Swimming	
Leisurely	6.0
Crawl, 25-50 yd/min	6.0-12.5
Butterfly, 50 yd/min	14.0
Backstroke, 25-50 yd/min	6.0-12.5
Breaststroke, 25-50 yd/min	6.0-12.5
Sidestroke, 40 yd/min	11.0
Dancing	
Modern, moderate to vigorous	4.2-5.7
Ballroom, waltz to rumba	5.7-7.0
Square	7.7
Walking	
Road or field (3.5 mph)	5.6-7.0
Snow, hard to soft (3.5-2.5 mph)	10.0-20.0

(Cont.)

Table D.6 (Continued)

Activity	Cal/min[a]
Uphill, 15% grade (3.5 mph)	8.0-11.0-15.0
Downhill, 5-10% grade (2.5 mph)	3.5-3.7
15-20% grade (2.5 mph)	3.7-4.3
Hiking, 40-lb pack (3.0 mph)	6.8
Running	
12-min mile (5 mph)	10.0
8-min mile (7.5 mph)	15.0
6-min mile (10 mph)	20.0
5-min mile (12 mph)	25.0

[a]Depends on efficiency and body size. Add 10% for each 15 lb over 150, subtract 10% for each 15 lb under 150. Use activity pulse rate to confirm the caloric expenditure.

Note. Adapted from *Physiological Measurements of Metabolic Functions in Man* by C.F. Consolazio, R.E. Johnson, and L.J. Pecora, 1963, New York: McGraw-Hill; "Human Energy Expenditure" by R. Passmore and J. Durnin, 1955, *American Journal of Epidemiology,* **108**; and *Compendium of Human Responses to the Aerospace Environment III* by E.M. Roth (Ed.), 1968, Washington, DC: N.A.S.A. Data generated at The Human Performance Laboratory, University of Montana, 1964-1986, is included in this table.

Predicting Caloric Expenditure

Predicting Caloric Expenditure From the Exercise Pulse Rate

Caloric expenditure is directly related to pulse rate. This relationship varies with the level of fitness. For those in the low-fitness categories a high pulse rate does not indicate an extremely high caloric expenditure. For those in the high-fitness categories, a high pulse rate indicates a much higher rate of energy expenditure (see Figure D.1). If you know your fitness category, as you should after taking one of the tests presented in Appendix B, you can check your caloric expenditure in any type of activity.

To use this relationship, you need only engage in an activity for 3 min or more and then stop for a 15-s pulse count. Be ready to start counting the pulse immediately after you cease activity. Count a 15-s period and multiply the count by 4 (or count 10 s and multiply by 6).

$$30 \times 4 = 120 \text{ beats/min}$$

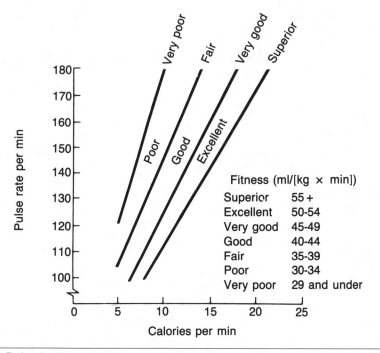

Figure D.1. Predicting calories burned during physical activity from pulse rate. (10-s pulse count taken immediately after exercise—10-s rate × 6 = rate/min.) *Note.* Adapted from Sharkey (1974, 1975).

Then find the prediction line that represents your fitness category and determine your caloric expenditure in calories per minute. This method affords an excellent check on the values listed in the previous section. It also shows you how a gain in fitness corresponds with a gain in caloric expenditure. Use the graph often to become familiar with the energy demands of your favorite activities and to learn more about new activities. Use Table D.7 to record your exercise caloric expenditure.

Table D.7 Exercise Caloric Expenditure

Activity	Typical values (cal/min)	Your HR (bpm)	Your expenditure[a] (cal/min)

(Cont.)

Table D.7   (Continued)

Activity	Typical values (cal/min)	Your HR (bpm)	Your expenditure[a] (cal/min)
_____	_____	_____	_____
_____	_____	_____	_____
_____	_____	_____	_____
_____	_____	_____	_____
_____	_____	_____	_____
_____	_____	_____	_____
_____	_____	_____	_____
_____	_____	_____	_____
_____	_____	_____	_____
_____	_____	_____	_____

[a]From Figure D.1.

Use Table D.6 to see how many calories you burn during your favorite activities. You may find that your active style of play burns more calories than the averages depicted in the tables.

Determining Body Composition

Body weight consists of fat and fat free weight (lean body weight). The percent of body weight composed of fat (percent body fat) is best determined in the laboratory. Body fat can also be predicted from surface measurements made with relatively inexpensive calipers (see Figure D.2 for a skinfold nomogram). However, no one method is valid for all members of the population. Each technique is best suited for the group on which it was developed.

Table D.8 shows average (not desirable or ideal) values for percent body fat according to age and sex.

Skinfold Calipers

Using skinfold calipers or a homemade substitute, measure skinfold thickness and substitute in the appropriate formula. Technique is very important in these measures. Expensive skinfold calipers are not necessary to get accurate results.

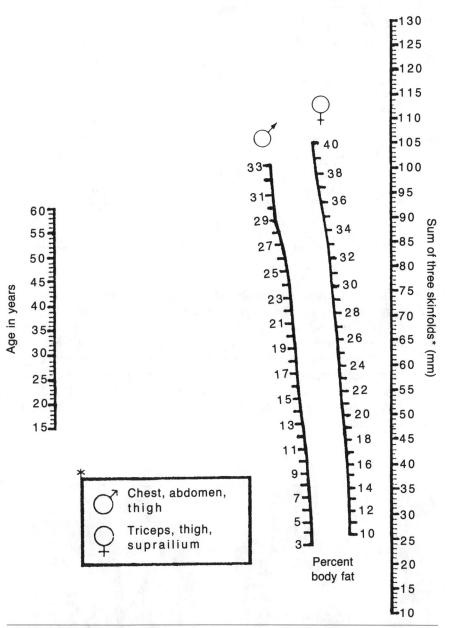

Figure D.2. A nomogram for the estimate of percent body fat for both male and female populations, using age and the sum of three skinfolds. Use a straight edge and draw a line from your age to the sum of three skinfolds and read your percent fat from the appropriate scale. From ''A Nomogram for the Estimate of Percent Body Fat from Generalized Equations'' by W.B. Baun, M.R. Baun, and P.B. Raven, 1981, *Research Quarterly*, **52**, p. 382. Copyright 1981 by the American Alliance for Health, Physical Education, Recreation and Dance, 1900 Association Drive, Reston, VA 22091.

Table D.8 Percentages of Body Fat

Age	Men (%)	Women (%)
15	12.0	21.2
17	12.0	28.9
18-22	12.5	25.7
23-29	14.0	29.0
30-40	16.5	30.0
40-50	21.0	32.0
Minimum	2-5	7-11
Obese	20	30

Grasp skinfolds between the thumb and forefinger, then apply calipers about 1/2 in. from the fingers. The calipers go in about as deep as the fold is wide (if fold is 1/2″ go in 1/2″ with calipers). Take the measurement, release, repeat the measurement, and continue until your measure is consistent.

Figure D.2 provides a simple method for the estimation of percent body fat from the sum of three skinfolds. Use chest, abdomen, and thigh skinfolds for males, and triceps, suprailium, and thigh for females (see Figures D.3 through D.7). *Note*: Inexpensive skinfold calipers are available from Ross Laboratories, Columbus, Ohio.

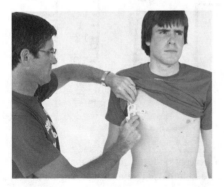

Figure D.3. Chest.

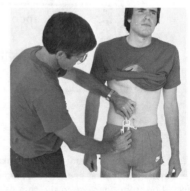

Figure D.4. Abdomen.

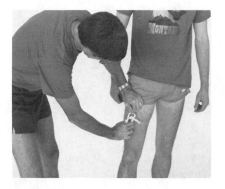

Figure D.5.   Thigh.

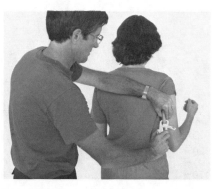

Figure D.6.   Tricep.

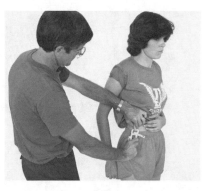

Figure D.7.   Suprailium.

Girth Measurements

Various body dimensions have been used to predict the lean body weight and percent fat. For men, the girth at the waist (or the abdominal skinfold) always seems to be a good predictor of body fat. For this method simply measure the girth of the waist at the level of the navel. Then use a straight edge and go from waist girth to body weight on Figure D.8 to estimate percent fat. For other tape measure methods to estimate percent body fat consult Katch and McArdle (1983) or Hoeger (1989).

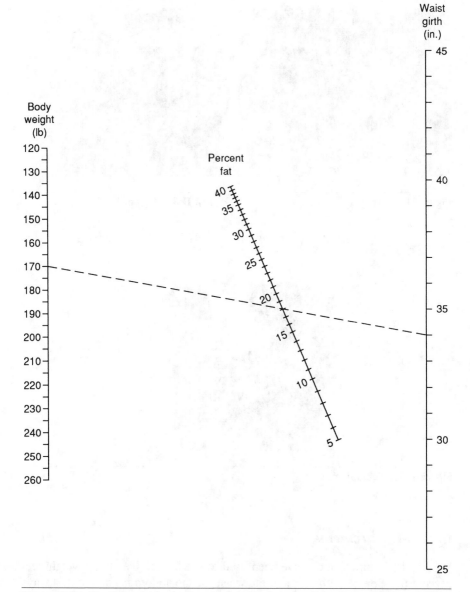

Figure D.8. Predicting body fat from waist girth in men. *Note*. From Sharkey (1977).

APPENDIX
E

FITNESS AND HEALTH

- **Health Risk Analysis and Longevity Estimate**
- **Warning Signs**
- **Exercise Problems**
- **Special Considerations**
- **Low Back Fitness**

Health Risk Analysis and Longevity Estimate

Although it is possible to assign a statistical risk to certain conditions and forms of behavior, no one can predict how long you will live or how you will die. Take this exercise in health risk analysis, but don't take it too seriously. The longevity estimate is just a way to get you to weigh the consequences of your behavior. I make no claims for its accuracy. Although many of the effects are based on real findings from large epidemiological investigations, they are generalized in this example. A more accurate estimate can be achieved by estimating risk according to age, sex, and race. Several organizations use computer scoring to provide more statistically valid estimates.

Complete the following pages (pp. 372-381) and then fill in the boxes in Table E.1 (p. 382).

I Coronary Heart Disease (CHD) Risk Factors

Cholesterol and HDL Cholesterol

Cholesterol under 160	160-200	200-220	220-240	over 240
Cholesterol/HDL ratio under 3	3-4	4-5	5-6	over 6
+2	+1	0	-2	-4

Blood pressure: $\left(\dfrac{systolic}{diastolic}\right)$

110	110-130	130-150	150-170	170
60-80	60-80	80-90	90-100	more than 100
+1	0	-1	-2	-4

Smoking

never	quit	smoke cigar or pipe or close family member smokes	1 pack cigarettes daily	2 or more packs daily
+1	0	-1	-3	-5

Heredity

no family history of CHD	1 close relative over 60 with CHD	2 close relatives over 60 with CHD	1 close relative under 60 with CHD	2 or more close relatives under 60 with CHD
+2	0	-1	-2	-4

Body weight (or fat)

5 lb below desirable weight (less than 10% fat—men; less than 16% fat—women)	5 lb below to 4 lb above desirable weight (10-15% fat—men; 16-22% fat—women)	5-20 lb overweight (15-20% fat—men; 22-30% fat—women)	20-35 lb overweight (20-25% fat—men; 30-35% fat—women)	35 lb overweight (over 25% fat—men; 35% fat—women)
+2	+1	0	-2	-3

Sex

female under 45 years	female over 45 years	male	stocky male	bald, stocky male
0	-1	-1	-2	-4

Stress

phlegmatic, unhurried, generally happy	ambitious but generally relaxed	sometimes hard driving, time conscious, competitive	hard driving, time conscious, competitive (Type "A")	Type "A" with repressed hostility
+1	0	0	-1	-3

Physical activity

high-intensity, over 30 min daily	intermittent, 20-30 minutes 3-5 times/week	moderate, 10-20 minutes 3-5 times/week	light, 10-20 minutes 1-2 times/week	little or none
+2	+2	+1	0	-2

TOTAL: I (CHD) RISK FACTORS.............. ☐

Enter on Table E.1

II Health Habits (associated with good health and longevity)

Breakfast	daily +1	sometimes 0	none −1	coffee −2	coffee and doughnut −3
Regular meals	3 or more +1	2 daily 0	not regular −1	fad diets −2	starve and stuff −3
Body weight					
Smoking		*previously considered in Part I, CHD*			
Physical activity					
Sleep	7-8 hr +1	8-9 hr 0	6-7 hr 0	9 hr −1	6 hr −2
Alcohol	none +1	occasional +1	1-2 drinks daily 0	2-6 drinks daily −2	6 drinks daily −4

TOTAL: II HEALTH HABITS ....

Enter on Table E.1

III Medical Factors

Medical exam and screening tests (blood pressure, diabetes, glaucoma)

regular tests, see doctor when necessary	periodic medical exam and selected tests	periodic medical exam	sometimes get tests	no tests or medical exams
+1	+1	0	0	−1

Heart

no history of problems self or family	some history	rheumatic fever as child, no murmur now	rheumatic fever as child, have murmur	have ECG abnormality and/or angina pectoris
+1	0	−1	−2	−3

Lung (including pneumonia and TB)

no problem	some past problem	mild asthma or bronchitis	emphysema, severe asthma, or bronchitis	severe lung problems
+1	0	−1	−2	−3

Digestive tract

no problem	occasional diarrhea, loss of appetite	frequent diarrhea or stomach upset	ulcers, colitis, gall bladder, or liver problems	severe gastrointestinal disorders
+1	0	−1	−2	−3

(Cont.)

III Medical Factors (Continued)

Diabetes

no problem or family history	controlled hypoglycemia (low blood sugar)	hypoglycemia and family history	mild diabetes (diet and exercise)	diabetes (insulin)
+1	0	−1	−2	−3

Drugs

seldom take	minimal but regular use of aspirin or other drugs	heavy use of aspirin or other drugs	regular use of amphetamines, barbiturates, or psychogenic drugs	heavy use of amphetamines, barbiturates, or psychogenic drugs
+1	0	−1	−2	−3

TOTAL: III MEDICAL . . . . Enter on Table E.1

IV Safety Factors

Driving in car

4,000 mi/year, mostly local	4,000-6,000 mi/year, local and some highway	6,000-8,000 mi/year, local and highway	8,000-10,000 mi/year, highway and some local	10,000 mi/year, mostly highway	
+1	0	0	-1	-2	

Using seat belts

always	most of time (75%)	on highway only	seldom (25%)	never	
+1	0	-1	-2	-3	

Risk-taking behavior
(motorcycle, skydive, mountain climb, fly small plane, etc.)

some with careful preparation	never	occasional	often	try anything for thrills	
+1	0	-1	-1	-2	

TOTAL: IV SAFETY............

Enter on Table E.1

V Personal Factors

Diet

low-fat, high-complex carbohydrates	balanced, moderate fat	balanced, typical fat	fad diets	starve and stuff
+2	+1	0	−1	−2

Longevity

grandparents lived past 90 parents past 80	grandparents lived past 80 parents past 70	grandparents lived past 70 parents past 60	few relatives lived past 60	few relatives lived past 50
+2	+1	0	−1	−3

Love and marriage

happily married	married	unmarried	divorced	extramarital relationship
+2	1	0	−1	−3

Education

postgraduate or master craftsman	college graduate or skilled craftsman	some college or trade school	high school graduate	grade school graduate
+1	+1	0	−1	−2

Job satisfaction

enjoy job, see results, room for advancement	enjoy job, see some results, able to advance	job OK, no results, no where to go	dislike job	hate job
+1	+1	0	−1	−2

Social

have some close friends	have some friends	have no good friends	stuck with people I don't enjoy	have no friends at all
+1	0	−1	−2	−3

Race

white or oriental	black or Hispanic	American Indian
0	−1	−2

TOTAL: V PERSONAL..........

Enter on Table E.1

VI Psychological Factors

Outlook

feel good about present and future	satisfied	unsure about present or future	unhappy in present, don't look forward to future	miserable, rather not get out of bed
+1	0	-1	-2	-3

Depression

no family history of depression	some family history—I feel OK	family history and I am mildly depressed	sometimes feel life isn't worth living	thoughts of suicide
+1	0	-1	-2	-3

Anxiety

seldom anxious	occasionally anxious	often anxious	always anxious	everybody hates me
+1	0	-1	-2	-3

Relaxation

relax or meditate daily	relax often	seldom relax	usually tense	always tense
+1	0	-1	-2	-3

TOTAL: VI PSYCHOLOGICAL ....

Enter on Table E.1

VII For Women Only

Health care

regular breast and pap exam	occasional breast and pap exam	never have exam	treated disorder	untreated cancer
+1	0	−1	−2	−4

Birth control pill

never used	quit 5 years ago	still use, under 30 years of age	use pill and smoke	use pill, smoke, over 35
+1	0	−1	−3	−5

TOTAL: VII FOR WOMEN ONLY ....

Enter on Table E.1

Table E.1 Longevity Estimate Based on Current Lifestyle

Category	Score	Life expectancy	
		Nearest age	Expectancy
I. CHD risk factors		30	74
II. Health habits		35	74
III. Medical factors		40	75
IV. Safety factors		45	76
V. Personal factors		50	76
VI. Psychological factors		55	77
VII. For women only		60	78
		65	80
		70	82

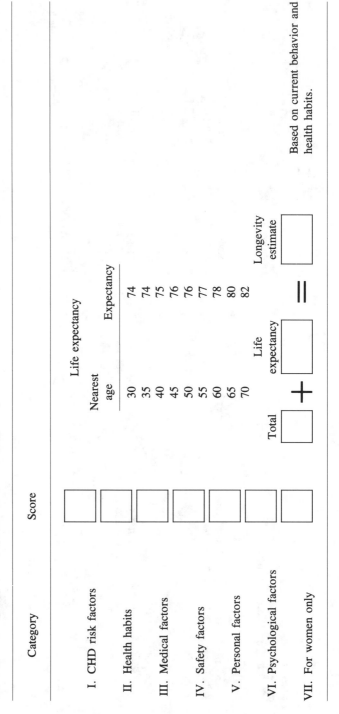

Total $\boxed{}$ $+$ Life expectancy $\boxed{}$ $=$ Longevity estimate $\boxed{}$

Based on current behavior and health habits.

Now, go back and see how you can add years to your life by improving behaviors and lifestyle. Check each category for possible changes you would like
to make in your current lifestyle.

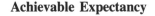

Achievable Expectancy

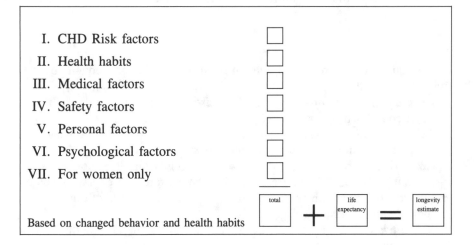

I.   CHD Risk factors ☐

II. Health habits ☐

III. Medical factors ☐

IV. Safety factors ☐

V.   Personal factors ☐

VI. Psychological factors ☐

VII. For women only ☐

Based on changed behavior and health habits   [total] **+** [life expectancy] **=** [longevity estimate]

Warning Signs

As you train or test, be aware of these warning signs.

Group 1

If any of these occur, *even once*, stop exercising and consult your physician
before resuming exercise.

Abnormal heart action. This includes irregular pulse; fluttering, pumping or
palpitations in chest or throat; sudden burst of rapid heartbeats; or a very slow
pulse that a moment earlier had been in training zone (this may occur during
exercise or it may be a delayed reaction).

Pain or pressure in the middle of the chest or in the arm or throat. This can
occur during or after exercise.

*Dizziness, lightheadedness, sudden loss of coordination, confusion, cold sweat,
glassy stare, pallor, blueness, or fainting.* In this case, stop exercise—don't try
to cool down—and lie with feet elevated or sit and put head down between legs
until symptoms pass.

Group 2

Try the suggested remedy briefly; if no help results, consult a doctor.

Persistent rapid heart action. This can occur when you're near training zone and 5 to 10 min after exercise. To correct, keep heart rate at lower end of zone or below and increase very slowly. Consult physician if persistent.

Flare-up of arthritic conditions. Rest and don't resume exercise until condition subsides. If you have no relief with usual remedies, consult physician.

Group 3

These usually can be remedied without medical consultation, though you may wish to report them to your doctor.

Nausea or vomiting after exercise. Exercise less vigorously and take a more gradual cool-down period.

Extreme breathlessness lasting more than 10 min after stopping exercise. Stay at lower end of training zone or below. Be sure you're not too breathless to speak during exercise; if you are, stop exercising. Consult doctor.

Prolonged fatigue. If you are tired 24 hr after exercising or have insomnia not present before starting exercise program, stay at lower end of training zone or below and increase level gradually.

Side stitch (diaphragm spasm). Lean forward while sitting, attempting to push the abdominal organs up against the diaphragm.

Exercise Problems

Previously inactive adults often encounter problems when they begin exercise. You'll avoid such problems if you vow to *make haste slowly*. It may have taken you 10 years to get in the shape you're in and you won't be able to change it overnight. Plan now to make gradual progress. At the start, too little may be better than too much. After several weeks, when your body has begun to adjust to the demands of vigorous effort, you'll be able to increase your exercise intensity. Another way to avoid exercise problems is to warm up before each exercise session. Careful attention to preexercise stretching and warming eliminates many of the nagging complications that plague less patient individuals. Never forget to cool down after each workout. Use good equipment (e.g., shoes and socks), don't start out on hard surfaces, and get plenty of rest. In short, prevention is the most effective way to deal with exercise problems. When problems do arise the next rule is to treat the cause, not just the symptom. If your knee hurts put ice on it, but don't stop there. Find out why it hurts and correct the problem once and for all.

Minor Problems

Blisters.   Foot blisters are really minor burns caused by friction. Blisters may be prevented by using good quality, properly fitted footwear. Runners, as well as tennis and handball players, should consider the tube sock with no heel, which seems to reduce the incidence of blisters. Hikers or skiers can wear thin inner liners with their heavy wool socks. Use Vaseline on potential hot spots.

At the first hint of a blister, cover the skin with some moleskin or a large bandage. Advanced cases can be treated with a sterilized hollow needle. Release the accumulated fluid, treat with an antiseptic, cover with gauze, circle with foam rubber, and go back to work. It is wise to keep the items needed for blister prevention in your locker or gym bag. Always carry a blister prevention kit on hiking trips.

Muscle Soreness.   Soreness usually develops some 24 hr after exercise. It occurs in the muscles involved and may be due to microscopic tears in the muscle or connective tissue or to localized contractions of muscle fibers. Any professional baseball player will say that it is almost impossible to avoid soreness at the beginning of the season. You can minimize the pain and stiffness of muscle soreness by phasing into a program or sport gradually and by engaging in mild stretching exercises when soreness does occur. Stretch the affected muscles gradually. These stretching movements can be used to relieve the discomfort of soreness or as a warm-up for exercise on the following day. Massage and warm muscle temperatures also seem to minimize the discomfort of soreness.

Muscle Cramps.   The cramp is a powerful involuntary contraction. Normally, we tell our muscles when to contract and when to relax. Cramps result when, for some reason, the muscle refuses to relax. In fact, normal control mechanisms fail and the contraction often becomes maximal. Immediate relief comes when the cramped muscle is stretched and massaged. However, that does not remove the underlying cause of the contraction. Salt and calcium are both involved in the chemistry of contraction and relaxation. Cold muscles seem to cramp more readily. It is always wise to warm up sufficiently before vigorous effort and to attend to fluid and electrolyte replacement during hot weather.

Bone Bruises.   Hikers and joggers sometimes get painful bruises on the bottoms of their feet. Such bruises can be avoided by careful foot placement and by quality footwear. Cushioned inner soles also help; air sole shoes or shock-absorbing inner soles help reduce the shocks that cause soreness, bruises, and other side effects of running on hard surfaces. A bad bruise can linger, delaying your exercise program many weeks. There's no instant cure once a bruise has developed, so prevention seems the best advice. Ice may help to lessen discomfort and hasten healing. Padding may allow exercise in spite of the bruise.

Ankle Problems.   A sprained ankle should be iced immediately. Immersion in a bucket of ice water in the first few minutes may allow you to work the next day. A serious sprain should be examined by a physician. High-topped gym shoes reduce the risk of ankle sprains in games such as basketball and handball; low-cut shoes with thick soles invite sprains in such games. Ankle wraps, lace-on supports, or tape allow exercise after a sprain, but again, prevention is a more prudent course. First aid for sprains includes RICE.

Rest

Ice

Compression

Elevation

Achilles Tendon.   Achilles tendon injuries have become quite common. Some high-backed shoes have been implicated in the rash of bursa injuries. The bursa is located beneath the tendon and serves to lubricate its movements. When rubbed long enough, the bursa becomes inflamed. Once inflamed, it may take weeks to return to normal. Ice helps, but continued activity is often impossible for several weeks. Rupture of the Achilles tendon seems to be more frequent in recent years. Partial rupture occurs when some of the fibers of the tendon are torn. Complete rupture results when the tendon, which connects the calf muscles to the heel, is completely detached. Prevention is the only approach to these problems, because surgery is the only cure. An inflammation of the tendon could lead to partial or complete rupture if abused or left untreated. Also, individuals with high serum uric acid levels seem prone to Achilles tendon injuries. Those with high levels should have ample warm-up before exercising and should avoid sudden starts, stops, and changes of direction during their exercise.

Shin Splints.   Pains on the front portion of the shin bone are known as shin splints. They can be caused by a lowered arch, irritated membranes, inflammation of the tibial periosteum, tearing of the tibialis anterior muscle from the bone, a muscle spasm due to swelling of that muscle, hairline fracture of the tibia or fibula, muscle imbalance, or other factors. Rest is the best cure for shin splints, although taping or a sponge heel pad seem to help some cases. Preventive measures include gradual adjustment to the rigors of strenuous training, stretching, avoidance of hard running surfaces, occasional reversal of direction when running on a curved track, and use of the heel-to-toe footstrike, which is the least tiring and least wearing on the rest of the body. Surgery can sometimes relieve the problem when the tibialis muscle outgrows its connective tissue compartment.

Knee Problems.   As knee injuries and subsequent knee operations become more common in sport, more adults will be plagued with knee problems during exercise. The trauma of an injury often leads to early signs of arthritis. Thus, a high school football injury may lead to signs of arthritis in the 20s or early 30s. These degenerative changes often restrict the ability to run, ski, or engage in other vigorous activities. The problems of prevention are being studied by specialists in sports medicine. Possibilities include rule changes, better cleats and playing surfaces, and considerable attention to preseason conditioning. I will mention some potentially dangerous knee exercises in a subsequent section. Those of you with established problems should consult your physician for ways to relieve the limitations imposed by knee problems. Some people have found that aspirin effectively suppresses the inflammation and pain often associated with exercise. If you forget to take the aspirin, ice helps to reduce the inflammation and speed the return to activity. Maintenance of thigh and hamstring strength helps stabilize the knee (try cycling as well as weight training).

Distance runners often develop knee problems for no apparent reason. Runner's knee and some other disturbing problems may result from a condition known as pronation, where the foot rolls to the inside. The problem arises when you engage in a considerable amount of exercise, such as distance running. Foot, knee, and even back problems may result from the structural and postural adjustments required. If you have experienced runner's knee or some other problem, correct the cause, not the symptom.

A variety of do-it-yourself treatments are available. Plastic heel cups, arch supports, or foam rubber pads or doughnuts help solve a number of problems. A good pair of shoes may help. (Two good pairs are better yet—get one pair with thick soles to wear when your feet are sore, another with flexible soles to wear when your legs are sore). If these treatments don't help, consult an experienced athletic trainer or a podiatrist. Specialists may recommend special supports to help the problem, but try the low-cost solutions before you resort to orthotics, cortisone injections, or surgery.

Overuse Syndromes

Don't be alarmed by these overuse syndromes, which we all suffer at one time or another. If you go too far or too fast too soon, if you forget to do your stretching, if you have serious muscle imbalances, if one leg is shorter than the other, or if you have weak feet, you are bound to have problems now and then. You will soon become adept at first aid. Muscle pulls and bruises get ice for several days. Ice helps relieve shin splints and heel spurs, an inflammation of the tissue of the plantar ligament, which fans outward from the heel to the toes. In fact, when in doubt use ice to relieve pain and swelling. You can also use it after exercise to minimize subsequent swelling. I keep an ice "popsicle" frozen in a small soup can. Just tape a tongue depressor upright in the can of water and put it in the freezer. When you need ice just take out your popsicle and go to work. Ice works best when you use it several times a day, rubbing the problem area until it becomes numb. You'll be amazed by the quick results.

Aspirin

I have found that judicious use of aspirin can minimize many nagging problems. With my doctor's advice I have taken one pill a day for 15 years to quiet a painful knee, the result of a high school football injury and a later operation. In recent years we have learned that one pill a day reduces the clotting and little strokes (transient ischemic attacks) that become more prevalent with age. Aspirin also seems to reduce the risk of subsequent heart attacks. Now we are learning that aspirin may have additional benefits for those engaged in vigorous exercise.

Aspirin reduces pain and inflammation by inhibiting the production of cell hormones called prostaglandins. Exercise causes prostaglandin production that may lead to soreness and fatigue. Because prostaglandins cause the breakdown of muscle protein during an infection, they may be involved in the soreness and breakdown associated with prolonged vigorous effort, such as a long distance run.

I have found that a single aspirin tablet before exercise (with lots of water) is worth many more after soreness develops. Aspirin is especially helpful on long downhill runs that are a sure bet to cause soreness. Of course you should know that some people are allergic to aspirin, and that it causes some stomach irritation. In large doses it could even alter enzyme activity. But small doses in advance of exercise reduce the need for larger doses afterward. And aspirin keeps many of us aging athletes active long after others give up.

Exercise Hazards

Regular, moderate physical activity is an established aid to health, fitness, weight control, and perhaps longevity. The term *regular* is easily understood by all, but the concept of *moderate* requires further definition. Moderate exercise for the athlete may be hazardous for the sedentary adult. Moderate activity for the unfit individual could be less than a warm-up for the distance runner. We define moderate as a level of exercise likely to bring about a training effect and improved fitness, without exposing the individual to the hazards of more strenuous effort. The heart rate training zone is an excellent guide to moderate exercise, as is the talk test.

Sudden Vigorous Exercise. Failure to warm up before vigorous exercise results in electrocardiogram abnormalities, regardless of the fitness or age of the subjects. Dr. R.J. Barnard of the UCLA School of Medicine found such abnormalities in 31 of 44 healthy firemen tested on a vigorous treadmill test. The findings indicated inadequate blood flow in the coronary arteries and a lack of oxygen to the heart muscle. This momentary lack of oxygen could account for the occurrence of heart attacks in those with normal coronary arteries. A warm-up consisting of an easy 4- to 5-min jog prevented the occurrence of the oxygen deficit and the electrocardiogram abnormalities (Barnard, Gardner, Diaco, & Kattus, 1982).

Athletes and coaches have long appreciated the contribution of the warm-up to the quality of performance in sport. We are now beginning to realize the value of warm-up for a variety of workers such as firemen, policemen, or even factory and construction workers. A law enforcement officer may not be able to warm up before jumping from the cruiser to chase a suspect, but there is no reason why assembly line employees cannot do calisthenics before beginning work. Calisthenics are common among factory workers in some European countries and in Japan.

That classic victim of the heart attack, the snow shoveler, should also heed the results of Dr. Barnard's experiment. In addition to being a common variety of sudden vigorous exercise, snow shoveling has several other drawbacks that suggest the need for prudence and an adequate warm-up. The snow shoveler leaves the warmth of the house to attack the enemy. He or she wants to finish quickly and return to an easy chair and a cup of coffee. The cold air constricts the blood vessels of the skin and causes a minor increase in blood pressure. The lifting of heavy, wet snow often requires a near-maximal effort. During this exertion blood pressure and heart rate increase dramatically, thus increasing the oxygen needs of the heart. At the same time, the breath holding common to maximal lifting restricts the return of blood to the chambers of the heart and to the coronary arteries as well. Thus, the heart may not get enough oxygen to meet the demands of the activity. A warm-up before and frequent rest periods during the task should help reduce the frequency of heart attacks recorded during this activity. Furthermore, a smaller shovel and avoidance of maximal lifting and breath holding will also be beneficial. Finally, I recommend that the problem be approached as a training exercise, and that the training heart rate be employed as an index of exercise intensity.

Stressful Exercise.   Physiologically speaking, stress is something that is perceived as a threat by the individual. We react to the threat by secreting a group of hormones that assist the mobilization of energy sources and prepare the body for combat or retreat (fight or flight). Many things can be perceived as physical or psychological threats to the body. The body does not differentiate between physical and mental threats, but reacts similarly to each. A difficult exam or an important job interview may be stressful to a student. Swimming or a canoe trip may be stressful to a nonswimmer, and unfamiliar exercise can be stressful to unfit or uncoordinated individuals.

One interesting reaction to stress is an acceleration of the clotting time of the blood. A faster clotting time is undoubtedly useful to a soldier on the battle field or a fighter in the ring, but to an adult with advanced atherosclerotic pathology, with already developed blockage of the blood vessels of the heart, a blood clot could be fatal. Thus, it is important to recognize the types of exercise that accelerate clotting time.

Unfamiliar Exercise. The first experience on a treadmill or in some other unfamiliar situation may be threatening. Studies show that the first exposure to a treadmill test is stressful, and that continued exposure to the situation results in a removal of the threat. One of these studies (Whiddon, Sharkey, & Steadman, 1969) indicated that blood clotting accelerated during the early phase of the study. The clotting time returned to normal when the test was no longer perceived as a threat.

Although little data has been collected to prove the point, it is likely that other unfamiliar or threatening exercise situations may also prove stressful. The first experience on skis, the first parachute jump, white water in a canoe, rappelling, and other obvious examples come to mind. For the previously inactive adult, the first trip to the health club, gym, or pool could also be stressful.

Exhaustive Exercise. Japanese researchers conducted an interesting experiment with dogs indicating that exhaustive exercise can be stressful (Suzuki, 1967). The dogs were taken for runs of various intensities and durations. They ran along the paths of a park with a bike-riding attendant. Postexercise hormone analyses indicated that only the exhaustive runs were stressful. The researchers concluded that nonexhaustive exercise need not be stressful.

Competitive Exercise. Some years ago, researchers at the Harvard University School of Medicine studied the stress responses to various types of competition in rowing (eight-oar crew). Crew members did not perceive the strenuous effort of a practice session as a threat, but did have increased hormone levels after a time trial and an actual competitive race. The nonexercising coxswain also exhibited a stress response after the competitive event. The researchers concluded that exercise, by itself, was not stressful, but that the excitement of competition did elicit the stress response—with or without exercise (Hill, Goetz, & Fox, 1956).

The hormones of the stress response are required for the full mobilization of resources and the optimal performance of the athlete. No one would suggest the need for healthy young men or women to avoid the excitement of competitive sport. However, for the sedentary adult, stress poses additional problems.

Does this mean that adults must avoid the excitement of the unfamiliar, the challenge of the exhaustive, or the thrill of competition? It does not. Your perception of exercise or any other event or consequence can be modified. Over a period of gradual exposure, the exercise neophyte becomes familiar with the demands of an activity. After several months the sedentary adult becomes more fit and finds a particular exercise less exhaustive. With months and years of practice and play the athletic adult learns to live with the physical and psychological requirements of competition.

Adults can and do engage in potentially stressful activities. For many, the excitement of sport keeps them regularly active. Those who seem to thrive on challenge, excitement, or exhaustion do so after a long period of preparation. The first men to scale Mount Everest engaged in years of physical and mental preparation. Aging but successful professional athletes must continue to practice and train if they are to remain competitive. If you desire to return to competitive tennis, softball, golf, or handball, give yourself time to adjust to the demands of competition. Improve your fitness and skill as you prepare for your first casual competition. Set reasonable competitive goals, and by all means, never, never, never take the results too seriously.

Problem Exercises

I have discussed the problems associated with maximal strength exercises and exhaustive training and have considered the potential dangers of highly competitive, exhaustive, or unfamiliar exercise. Now let's consider some common calisthenic-type exercises that may do more harm than good.

Toe Raises.   Do toe raises allow the development of excessive power in the calf, a situation that could lead to Achilles tendon rupture? This is one muscle group where muscle imbalance is impossible to avoid. However, problems can be minimized by stretching the tendon and by turning the toes inward during the exercise. Standing with the balls of the feet on a 2-in. platform insures the stretch of the tendon.

Knee Bends.   Deep knee bends tend to stretch the ligaments of the joint and lead to instability. You would be unwise to practice full knee bends. The muscular strength of the quadriceps (and the hamstring muscles) aids joint stability as well as performance in many activities. The half knee bend (until the thighs are parallel to the floor) is a safe and acceptable way to exercise for quadriceps strength or endurance.

Abdominal Exercises.   The leg lift is often recommended for abdominal development. This exercise should be avoided unless the lower back can be kept on the floor to prevent forward rotation of the pelvis, which tends to aggravate lower back pain. The ever-popular sit-up also tends to lead to lower back problems unless it is performed with the knees bent as in an inverted "V" or hook position. The outmoded straight leg sit-up develops the psoas muscle. This powerful hip flexor tilts the pelvis forward unless it is counteracted by abdominal or other muscle groups. The curl-up is another good abdominal exercise, and the basket hang is useful for advanced abdominal training.

Toe Touches.   Toe touches have been used with the erroneous belief that they exercise the abdominal muscles. As a hamstring or back muscle stretcher, toe touches are all right as long as you curl down slowly, avoid bouncing, and bend your knees. The slow, sitting toe touch is probably a better way to stretch the muscles on the back of the thigh, and the chair-sit toe touch may be a safer way to stretch tight back muscles.

Special Considerations

This section provides a brief summary for those with special exercise needs. Consult specific references, community services, or your physician for additional information.

Senior Citizens

With age comes an increasing need for muscular fitness. Seniors should undertake exercises to develop and maintain muscular endurance and—if needed—strength. Because strength training takes longer in older subjects, it would seem prudent to increase strength to needed levels before loss of strength limits self-sufficiency.

Women

The exercise prescriptions in this book work for men and women. However, women should consider a few specifics. Young women need to know that vigorous prepubertal training may delay the onset of the menstrual cycle; however, early training also seems to reduce the incidence of sex-related cancers in later years. Excess endurance training in young women could reduce mineralization of bones, cause stress fractures, and pose future problems. Strength training strengthens bones and leads to improved strength *and* to increases in muscle mass (hypertrophy). During pregnancy, exercise habits can be continued with physician approval. Most recommend eliminating high-impact aerobics and keeping the heart rate below 140 beats during exercise. Postmenopausal women should be certain to include exercises that put a moderate degree of stress on the muscles and bones of the upper body as well as the legs, to minimize the threat of osteoporosis. Women of all ages need to be aware of their special nutritional needs (e.g., iron and calcium) and make sure they get adequate amounts.

Blacks

A recent series of articles on blacks and exercise (Lubell, 1988) documented the greater prevalence of hypertension among blacks. One in every three black adults has hypertension, compared with one in four nonblacks, and blacks are 2 times more likely to have moderate hypertension and 3 times more likely to have severe hypertension than whites. Although black people will benefit from aerobic and other activities, individuals with hypertension should avoid exercises with an isometric component, such as weight lifting. Aerobic exercise and weight loss will help lower blood pressure, but people with hypertension should undergo a thorough preexercise medical evaluation.

Handicapped

Each handicap carries its own special restrictions, but each has potential as well. Diabetics compete in international competition, but only after establishing control over their condition. Those with multiple sclerosis find that moderate activity, like swimming, expands their potential. Wheelchair athletes compete in marathons and play basketball, and now they can fish at handicapped access sites. Handicapped individuals have learned to ski, to kayak, to do just about anything, and more opportunities are becoming available. For more information contact your recreation department or community service organizations.

Children

Children are not miniature adults; their bones are still being formed and their capacity for exercise in certain circumstances is different from adults. Moreover, the value of prepubertal strength or endurance training is still far from established. Therefore it is wise to encourage but not force participation. Avoid heavy training, prolonged hard work in hot environments, and excess competition (if only to prevent later burnout). Give children the freedom to develop their own games, to play, to explore, and to be kids. Don't impose an adult model or adult goals and objectives on children.

Low Back Fitness

These simple tests, developed and tested at the Sun Valley Health Institute, will help identify areas that need additional attention. Take the tests again after several months to monitor your progress.

Abdominal Muscle Strength

Curl-Up. Lie on your back and bend your knees to a 90° angle. Using one of the following arm positions, slowly curl up to a sitting position; don't swing your arms or allow your feet to come off the floor. If successful, try a more difficult position (higher number); if not try an easier one (lower number). Your score is the highest number achieved.

1. Arms at side, unable to curl up without aid of partner
2. Arms at side, hands pull back of thighs
3. Arms at side
4. Arms folded across chest
5. Hands behind neck
6. Arms extended overhead, fingers intertwined with arms pressing against ears

This test indicates abdominal muscle strength and flexibility of back muscles. If you can't do Number 5 you need more than a maintenance program. Do repetitions of 3 and 4 to achieve 5.

Leg Lift.   This test evaluates the strength of the lower abdominal muscles. Lie on your back, head on floor, legs straight, hands under the hollow of your back. Flatten your back, then attempt to raise both feet 10 in. and hold the position for 10 s.

1. Unable to lift both legs
2. Back raises immediately
3. Back raises after several seconds
4. Able to hold back flat

If you can't do Number 4 you need more abdominal tone. Use the basket hang exercise to improve abdominal tone (see Appendix C).

Flexibility

Sit and Reach.   This is a test of lower back flexibility. Sit with legs flat on floor. With one hand over the other and toes pointing to ceiling, reach forward and try to touch your toes or beyond. Hold for several counts. Score as follows after several warm-up trials.

1. Well short of toes (more than 3 in. short)
2. Touch toes (or come within 2 in.)
3. Touch well beyond toes (more than 3 in. beyond)

Although extreme flexibility isn't necessary for a healthy back, the lower back and leg muscles need adequate flexibility. A 2 is adequate; with practice you may be able to score a 3.

Hip Flexion.   Lie supine on the floor with your legs straight and flat on floor. Keep your head on the floor throughout the test. Bend your right leg and pull your knee to your chest. Test both sides and score as follows.

1. Knee to chest but left leg completely off floor
2. Knee to chest but left leg lifts somewhat
3. Knee completely to chest with left leg flat on floor

Tight hip flexors may cause an exaggerated lumbar curve, which predisposes the back to injury. Do this test and other stretching exercises to improve flexibility of the hip flexors. In time you should be able to score a 3.

APPENDIX

F

LIFESTYLE

- **Fitness Trail**
- **Principles of Training**
- **Fallacies of Training**

Fitness Trail

The fitness trail is an exercise circuit designed to improve the aerobic and muscular fitness of men, women, and children. It was inspired by the popular Swiss exercise trails, the Vita Parcours. With the financial backing of the Vita Insurance Co., more than 400 parcours (French for track or course) have been built in Switzerland. The idea spread quickly to much of Europe, where most segments of the population are now able to enjoy parcours.

The Fitness Trail was especially designed for the U.S. Forest Service.[1] The trail has become so popular that many have been constructed on city or county park land and on school land made available for the general public.

The Fitness Trail consists of seven dual-purpose exercise areas (14 total stations) along a 1/4-mi jogging path. Participants walk or jog between stations, complete the exercise, and continue until they've finished the course. Signs describe and illustrate each exercise.

The trail can fit on 2 acres of land and requires about $500 worth of materials. Where space permits, an additional loop for distance running is recommended. If you don't have the space to construct the entire trail, you can still use some of the stations for muscular fitness training.

The Fitness Trail is versatile. It's ideal for individual or group training. It offers safe, healthful exercise regardless of age or condition. Progress at your own rate and do as few or as many repeats of the exercises as you wish. You may jog the trail, ignoring the exercises. The trail extends an enjoyable physical challenge that encourages the fitness habit.

Training on the trail can take many forms: formal or informal, group or individual. Emphasize muscular fitness training Monday, Wednesday, and Friday,

---

[1]For further information write: Forest Service, U.S. Department of Agriculture, Missoula Technology & Development Center, Missoula, MT 59801.

performing as many repetitions of each exercise as possible at the stations. To increase progress, do a set of exercises, rest, and repeat the set. Stress jogging or running on Tuesday, Thursday, and Saturday or Sunday. Jog some after Monday, Wednesday, and Friday muscular fitness training. Here are some suggested distances.

Fitness level	M-W-F	T-Th-S or Su
Low	1-2 mi	2-3 mi
Medium	2-3 mi	3-5 mi
High	3-4 mi	4-6 mi

Use the distance loop for longer runs.

Welcome to the Fitness Trail

The Fitness Trail offers a physical challenge regardless of age or conditioning and the chance to improve fitness and health while having fun.

The trail has 14 exercise stations along a 1/4-mi jogging path. Jog on the trail to strengthen heart, lungs, and legs. Build muscle strength by performing the exercises. Or do both for all-around fitness. Remember to include warm-ups and cool-downs in your exercise on the Fitness Trail.

Warm-Up

A 4- or 5-min warm-up prepares your body for exercise. Begin with easy stretching, then move to more vigorous calisthenics. Pay attention to stretching your lower back, stretching hamstrings and calf muscles, and increasing exercise tempo gradually.

Cool-Down

A gradual cool-down is vital to avoid sore muscles. Walk or jog slowly after completing exercise to continue the pumping action of muscles, promote circulation, and speed recovery. A few minutes of leg stretching also may help prevent soreness.

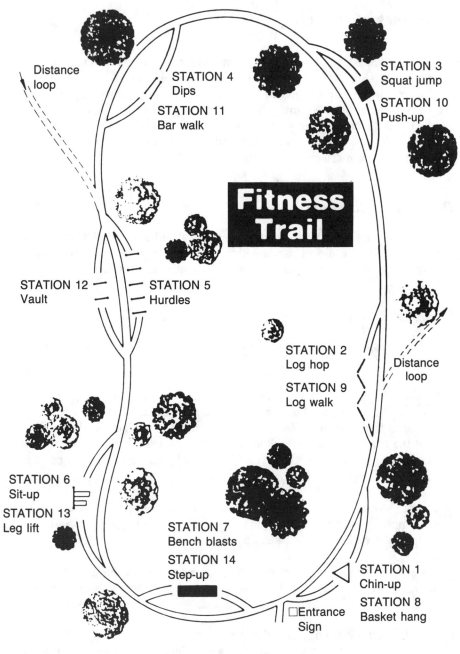

Distance loop

STATION 4
Dips

STATION 11
Bar walk

STATION 3
Squat jump

STATION 10
Push-up

Fitness Trail

STATION 12
Vault

STATION 5
Hurdles

STATION 2
Log hop

STATION 9
Log walk

Distance loop

STATION 6
Sit-up

STATION 13
Leg lift

STATION 7
Bench blasts

STATION 14
Step-up

STATION 1
Chin-up

STATION 8
Basket hang

Entrance
Sign

START/FINISH

Principles of Training

This section[2] introduces important physiological principles that you must follow in order to make steady progress in your training and to avoid illness and injury. I present these principles of training so you can see the basis upon which successful programs are constructed. Several principles explain why individuals respond differently to training, some point out how and why training influences the body, a few describe important elements of daily programs, and several explain the long-term effects of training or detraining.

Principle 1: Readiness

The value of training depends on the physiological and psychological readiness of the individual. Readiness comes with maturation, so prepubertal individuals lack the physiological readiness to respond completely to training.

Principle 2: Individual Response

Individuals respond differently to the same training for some of the following reasons.

Heredity. Physique, muscle fiber characteristics, heart and lung size, and other factors may be inherited. But although we inherit certain characteristics, environmental factors such as diet and training also influence the eventual expression of the characteristic. So although factors associated with aerobic fitness and endurance may be approximately 25% genetically determined, the remainder is subject to change.

Maturity. More mature bodies can handle more training. Less mature athletes don't respond as well to training, and they need more energy for growth and development (see Principle 1: Readiness).

Nutrition. Training involves changes in tissues and organs, changes that require protein and other nutrients. Without proper nutrition, the best training program will fail. Remember to eat adequate protein when you lose weight during training.

Rest and Sleep. Although young athletes may require 8 hr or more of sleep, adults often get by with less. However, when training gets tough, it is wise to get more sleep or to take short naps. Inadequate rest minimizes the gains associated with training.

---

[2]Adapted from Sharkey (1986, pp. 10-17).

Level of Fitness. Improvement due to training is most dramatic when the level of fitness is low. Later, when fitness is high, long hours of effort are needed to achieve small improvements. Less fit individuals fatigue easily and are more prone to illness or injury.

Environmental Influences. Factors in the physical and psychological environment influence the response to training. Psychological factors might include emotional stress at work, home, or school, and physical factors include heat, cold, altitude, and air pollution. Learn to recognize your own ability to tolerate environmental stressors and slow down when conditions are severe.

Illness or Injury. Of course, illness or injury will influence your response to training. The problem is to spot the problem before it becomes serious. Many problems are first noticed during hard effort, and coaches or exercise partners may be the first to notice a problem. Try to listen to your body's signals, and be certain you have recovered before returning to practice.

Motivation. Individuals work harder and gain more when they are motivated and when they see the relationship of hard work to their personal goals. Your training will be easier if you are involved for personal reasons.

Principle 3: Adaptation

Training induces subtle changes as the body adapts to the added demands. Dr. Ned Fredrick, a friend and noted sport scientist, calls training for sport a gentle pastime in which we coax subtle changes from the body. The day-to-day changes are so small as to be unmeasurable, and weeks and even months of patient progress are required to achieve measurable adaptations. Try to rush the process and you risk illness, injury, or both.

Typical adaptations include

- increased enzyme activity or contractile protein,
- improved respiration, heart function, circulation, and blood volume,
- improved muscular endurance, strength, or power, and
- tougher bones, ligaments, tendons, and connective tissue.

The principle of adaptation tells us that training can't be rushed. The best you can do is to follow a sensible program and be satisfied with the results. Trying to do it all in one season is likely to do more harm than good.

Principle 4: Overload

The legendary tale of Milo, a warrior in ancient Greece, illustrates the overload principle. Milo started lifting a young calf, and as the calf grew, so did Milo's strength. Eventually he was able to lift the full-grown animal. Training must place a demand on the body system if desired adaptations are to take place. To begin, training must exceed the typical daily demand. As you adapt to increased loading, you should add more load. The rate of improvement is related to three factors, which you will remember with the acronym FIT.

Frequency
Intensity
Time (duration)

The overload principle is used in all kinds of training. We gradually add more weight to the barbell to achieve increases in strength. Endurance athletes increase training time and intensity to improve race performances. The overload stimulates changes in the muscles and other systems, changes designed to help the body cope with future demands. These changes involve the nervous system, which learns to recruit muscle fibers more effectively; the circulation, which becomes better able to send more blood to the working muscles; and the muscles themselves, where the overload stimulates the production of new protein to help meet future exercise demands.

Principle 5: Progression

To achieve adaptations using the overload principle, training must follow the principle of progression. When the training load is increased too quickly, the body cannot adapt and instead breaks down. Progression must be observed in terms of increases in FIT.

Frequency
  Sessions per day, week, month, or year
Intensity
  Training load per day, week, month, or year
Time
  Duration of training in hours per day, week, month, or year

But progression does not imply inexorable increases, without time for recovery. The body requires periods of rest in which adaptations take place.

MAKE HASTE SLOWLY!

The principle of progression has other implications. Training should also progress from

the general . . . . *to the specific,*
the part . . . . *to the whole, and*
quantity . . . . *to quality.*

Principle 6: Specificity

Exercise is specific. When you jog you recruit certain muscle fibers, energy pathways, and energy sources. If you jog every day you are training, and the adaptations will take place in the muscle fibers used during the exercise. The adaptations to endurance training are different than adaptations to strength training. Endurance training elicits improvements in oxidative enzymes and the muscle's ability to burn fat and carbohydrate in the presence of oxygen. Strength training leads to increases in the contractile proteins actin and myosin, but only in the muscles exercised.

This means that the type of training you undertake must relate to the desired results. Specific training brings specific results. You won't get much stronger with endurance training, and you won't improve endurance much with strength training. Cycling is not the best preparation for running, or vice versa. Performance improves most when the training is specific to the activity.

Of course, every rule or principle can be taken to the extreme. Specificity *does not mean* you should avoid training opposite or adjacent muscles. In fact, you should train other muscles to avoid muscle imbalances that could predispose the body to injury. And you can train adjacent muscles to help you adapt to changes in conditions and to provide a backup when the primary muscle fibers become fatigued. So some cycling may be good for a runner; it will provide muscle balance, train adjacent fibers, and provide some relief from the pounding of running.

Principle 7: Variation

The training program must be varied to avoid boredom and to maintain your interest. The principle of variation embraces two basic concepts.

▌ Work/Rest . . . and . . . Hard/Easy

Adaptation comes when work is followed by rest, when the hard is followed by the easy. Failure to include variation leads to boredom, staleness, and poor performance. Successive sessions of hard work, if not followed by adequate time for rest and recovery, are certain to hinder progress in training.

Achieve variation by changing training routine and drills. When possible, conduct workouts in different places or under different conditions. Follow a long workout with a short one, an intense session with a relaxed one, or high speed with easy distance. When workouts become dull, do something different. Use variety to diminish monotony and to lighten the physical and psychological burdens of heavy training.

Principle 8: Warm-Up/Cool-Down

A warm-up should always precede strenuous activity to

- increase body temperature,
- increase respiration and heart rate, and
- guard against muscle, tendon, and ligament strains.

The warm-up should consist of stretching, calisthenics, and gradually increasing exercise intensity. Stretching may be more effective after the warm-up.

The cool-down is just as important as the warm-up. Abrupt cessation of vigorous activity leads to pooling of the blood, sluggish circulation, and slow removal of waste products. It may also contribute to cramping, soreness, or more serious problems. High levels of the hormone norepinephrine are present immediately after vigorous exercise, making the heart more subject to irregular beats. The cool-down helps remove excess norepinephrine and lower the body temperature. Light activity and stretching continue the pumping action of muscles on veins, helping the circulation in the removal of metabolic wastes.

Principle 9: Long-Term Training

Changes resulting from the gradual overload of body systems lead to impressive improvements in performance. But it takes years of effort to approach high-level performance capability. Long-term training allows for growth and development, gradual progress, acquisition of skills, learning of strategies, and a fuller understanding of the sport. So don't rush the process; too much training too soon may lead to mental and physical burnout and early retirement from the sport. Excellence comes to those who persist with a well-planned, long-term training program.

Principle 10: Reversibility

Most of the adaptations achieved from months of hard training are reversible. In general, it takes longer to gain endurance than it does to lose it. With complete bed rest, fitness can decline at a rate of almost 10% per week! Strength declines more slowly, but lack of use will eventually cause atrophy of even the best-trained muscles. To avoid this problem, maintain a year-round program, with periods of hard work followed by periods of relative rest and variety.

Principle 11: Moderation

This principle applies to all aspects of life; too much of anything can be bad for your health. Temper dedication with judgment and moderation. Train too hard, too long, or too fast, and the body begins to deteriorate. Practice moderation in all things.

Principle 12: Potential

- Every individual has a potential maximal level of performance.
- Most of us never come close to that potential performance.
- The highest potential performances are still to be achieved.
- Regular participation in physical activity will help you achieve your potential and improve the quality of daily living.

Fallacies of Training

Before I close this section on principles, let me add some popular fallacies or misconceptions concerning training. These often quoted "principles" are untrue and have no basis in medical or scientific research.

Fallacy 1: No Pain, No Gain

Although serious training is often difficult and sometimes unpleasant, it shouldn't hurt. In fact, well-prepared athletes can perform difficult events in a state of euphoria, free of pain and oblivious to discomfort. Marathon winners sometimes seem to finish full of vitality, whereas the losers appear near collapse. Pain is not a natural consequence of exercise or training; it is a sign of a problem that shouldn't be ignored. During exercise the body produces natural opiates, called endorphins, that can mask discomfort during exercise. If you experience real pain during training, you should back off. If the pain persists, have the problem evaluated.

Discomfort, on the other hand, can accompany difficult aspects of training such as heavy lifting, intense interval training, or long-distance effort. Discomfort is a natural consequence of the acidity that accompanies the anaerobic effort of lifting or intervals or of the muscle fatigue, microtrauma, and soreness that come with long-distance training. I would accept this statement: **no discomfort no excellence**. Overload sometimes requires working at the upper limit of strength, intensity, or endurance, and that can be temporarily uncomfortable. If exercise results in pain, it is probably excessive. The next two fallacies are associated with the "no pain no gain" misconception.

Fallacy 2: You Must Break Down Muscle to Improve

Microtrauma sometimes occurs in muscle during vigorous training and competition, but it isn't a necessary or even a desirable outcome of training. Runners have shown significant trauma at the end of a marathon with long downhill stretches that require eccentric muscular contractions (contractions of a lengthening muscle). Eccentric contractions are a major cause of muscle soreness, which is associated with muscle trauma, reduced force output, and a prolonged (4 to 6 weeks) period of recovery. Excessive trauma doesn't help training; it stops it.

Weight lifters can traumatize muscle with excess weight or repetitions, but that is not a necessary stage in the development of strength. The most authoritative book on the topic, with over 350 references to the scientific literature concerning resistance training, makes no mention of tearing the muscle down to achieve development (Fleck & Kraemer, 1987). Neither pain not injury are normal consequences of training, and you should avoid both.

Fallacy 3: Go for the Burn

This popular statement is often heard among body builders who do numerous repetitions and sets to build, shape, and define muscles. The burn they describe is probably due to the increased acidity associated with elevated levels of lactic acid in the muscle. Although this sensation isn't dangerous, it isn't a necessary part of a strength program designed to improve performance.

Fallacy 4: Lactic Acid Causes Muscle Soreness

This fallacy has been around for years, without any basis in fact. Although lactic acid may be produced in contractions that lead to soreness, the lactic acid isn't the cause of the soreness. Lactic acid is cleared from muscle and blood within an hour of the exercise. Soreness comes 24 hr or more after the effort, long after the lactic acid has been removed or metabolized. Soreness comes after unfamiliar exertion or after a long layoff and is probably associated with microtrauma to muscle and connective tissue and the swelling that results thereafter. After recovery, additional exposure to the activity will yield less soreness.

Fallacy 5: Muscle Turns to Fat (or Vice Versa)

Another common misconception is that when an athlete stops training, muscle can turn to fat. Muscle will no more turn to fat than fat will turn to muscle. Both are highly specialized tissues with specific functions. Muscles are composed of long, spaghettilike fibers with contractile proteins designed to exert force. Fat cells are round receptacles designed to store fat. Training increases the size of muscle fibers (hypertrophy), and detraining reduces their size (atrophy). Excess caloric consumption causes fat cells to grow in size as they store more fat. The cells shrink when you burn more calories than you eat. But long thin muscle fibers never change into spherical fat cells, or vice versa.

Fallacy 6: I Ran Out of Wind

Athletes often have this sensation when they run too fast for their level of training. The sensation comes from the lungs and reflects another discomfort of exertion. However, the sensation is more likely to be due to an excess of carbon dioxide than a lack of oxygen or air. Carbon dioxide is produced during oxidative metabolism and is the primary stimulus for respiration. So when carbon dioxide levels are high, as they are during vigorous effort, they cause distress signals in the lungs. The respiratory system thinks it is more important to rid the body of excess CO_2 than it is to bring in more O_2. Excess CO_2 is a sign that you have exceeded your lactate threshold, that you are working above your level of training. Become familiar with the sensation and what it is telling you—ignore it and you will soon become exhausted.

APPENDIX

G

CONVERSION TABLES

- Pounds to Kilograms
- Feet to Centimeters
- Miles to Kilometers
- Fahrenheit to Celsius
- Metabolic Conversions

Table G.1   The Conversion of Pounds (lb) to Kilograms (kg)

lb	kg	lb	kg	lb	kg
70	32	150	68	230	104
75	34	155	70	235	107
80	36	160	73	240	109
85	39	165	75	245	111
90	41	170	77	250	113
95	43	175	79	255	116
100	45	180	82	260	118
105	48	185	84	265	120
110	50	190	86	270	122
115	52	195	88	275	125
120	54	200	91	280	127
125	57	205	93	285	129
130	59	210	95	290	132
135	61	215	98	295	134
140	64	220	100	300	136
145	66	225	102		

Table G.2 The Conversion of Feet (ft) to Centimeters (cm)

ft	cm	ft	cm
3′	91	5′	152
3′2″	97	5′2″	157
3′4″	102	5′4″	163
3′6″	107	5′6″	168
3′8″	112	5′8″	173
3′10″	117	5′10″	178
4′	122	6′	183
4′2″	127	6′2″	188
4′4″	132	6′4″	193
4′6″	137	6′6″	198
4′8″	142	6′8″	203
4′10″	147	7′	208

Table G.3 The Conversion of Miles (mi) to Kilometers (km)

mi	km
3.1	5
6.2	10
9.3	15
12.4	20
15.5	25
18.6	30
21.7	35
24.8	40
28.0	45
31.0	50

Table G.4 The Conversion of Fahrenheit (F) to Celsius (C)

°F	°C
−40	−40
0	−18
32	0

°F	°C
50	10
72	22
85	30
98.6*	37
212	100

*Normal body temperature

Metabolic Conversions

It is easy to convert from total calories to calories per minute (cal/min) to aerobic capacity (L/min) to aerobic power (ml/[kg × min]) to metabolic equivalents (METs). To convert from one unit to another, simply carry out the calculation in the direction indicated by the arrow.

For example, if you use 1 L of oxygen per minute (1 L/min) in a brisk walk, you'll burn 5 cal/min (1 L × 5 = 5 cal/min).

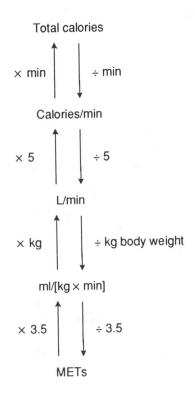

GLOSSARY/INDEX

acclimatization—Adaptation to an environmental condition such as heat or altitude; 223, 228, 231

actin—Muscle protein that works with the protein myosin to produce movement; 24, 272-273

adenosine triphosphate (ATP)—High-energy compound formed from oxidation of fat and carbohydrate. Used as energy supply for muscle and other body functions; the energy currency; 16, 276-279

adipose tissue—Tissue in which fat is stored; 33

aerobic—In the presence of oxygen; aerobic metabolism utilizes oxygen; 2, 15

aerobic fitness—Maximum ability to take in, transport, and utilize oxygen; 2, 15, 25, 39

agility—Ability to change direction quickly while maintaining control of the body; 68

alveoli—Tiny air sacs in the lungs where O_2 and CO_2 exchange takes place; 282

amino acids—Chief components of proteins; different arrangements of the 22 amino acids form the various proteins (muscles, enzymes, hormones, etc.); 130-131

anaerobic—In the absence of oxygen; nonoxidation metabolism; 2, 16, 276-279

anaerobic threshold—More properly called the lactate threshold, the point at which lactic acid produced in muscles begins to accumulate in the blood. Defines the upper limit that can be sustained aerobically; 16-18, 42, 244-245

angina pectoris—Chest pain (also called neck tie pain) associated with narrowed coronary arteries and lack of O_2 to heart muscle during exertion; 181

anorexia nervosa—An eating disorder characterized by excessive dieting and subsequent loss of appetite; 154

arrhythmia—Irregular rhythm or beat of the heart; 171

asymptomatic—Without symptoms; 167

atherosclerosis—Narrowing of coronary arteries by cholesterol build up within the walls; 181

atrophy—Loss of size of muscle; 63

balance—Ability to maintain equilibrium while in motion; 68

behavior therapy—A system of record keeping and motivation designed to help change a behavior (e.g., overeating); 143-145

blood pressure—Force exerted against the walls of arteries; 291-292

body composition—The relative amount of fat and lean tissue; 34, 105-106, 111, 366

bronchiole—Small branch of airway; sometimes undergoes spasm making breathing difficult, as in exercise-induced asthma; 282

buffer—Substance in blood that soaks up hydrogen ions to minimize changes in acid-base balance (pH); 285

bulimia—An eating disorder characterized by alternate bouts of gorging and purging; 154

calorie—Amount of heat required to raise 1 kg of water 1 °C; same as kilocalorie; 100, 351

capillaries—Smallest blood vessels (between arterioles and venules) where oxygen, foods, and hormones are delivered to tissues and carbon dioxide and wastes are picked up; 288

carbohydrate—Simple (e.g., sugar) and complex (e.g., potatoes, rice, beans, corn, and grains) foodstuff that we use for energy; stored in liver and muscle as glycogen—excess is stored as fat; 97, 132-133

cardiac—Pertaining to the heart; 287-288

cardiac output—Volume of blood pumped by the heart each minute; product of heart rate and stroke volume; 288-289

cardiorespiratory endurance—Synonymous with aerobic fitness or maximal oxygen intake; 15, 25, 39

cardiovascular system—Heart and blood vessels; 29, 285-290

central nervous system (CNS)—The brain and spinal cord; 271

cholesterol—Fatty substance formed in nerves and other tissues. Excessive amounts in blood have been associated with increased risk of heart disease; 121-123, 194-196

Clo units—The insulating value of clothing; 229

concentric—Contraction that involves shortening of the contracted muscle; 79

contraction—Development of tension by muscle; concentric—muscle shortens; eccentric—muscle lengthens under tension; static—contraction without change in length; 76-77

cool-down—Postperformance exercise used to dissipate heat, maintain blood flow, and aid recovery of muscles; 404

coronary arteries—Blood vessels that originate from the aorta and branch out to supply oxygen and fuels to the heart muscle; 180, 288

coronary prone—Having several risk factors related to early development of heart disease; 182

creatine phosphate (CP)—Energy-rich compound that backs up ATP in providing energy for muscles; 276-279

defibrillator—Device that applies strong electric shock to stop irregular heart action and restore normal heart rhythm; 171

dehydration—Loss of essential body fluids; 220

delayed muscle soreness—Muscle soreness that peaks 24 to 48 hr after unfamiliar exercise or vigorous eccentric contractions; 79, 385, 406

deoxyribonucleic acid (DNA)—The source of the genetic code housed in the nucleus of the cell; 72

diastolic pressure—Lowest pressure exerted by blood in artery; occurs during resting phase (diastole) of heart cycle; 291-292

duration—Distance or length of time (or calories burned in the case of the exercise prescription); 45

eccentric—Contraction that involves lengthening of a contracted muscle; 79

electrocardiogram (ECG)—A graphic recording of the electrical activity of the heart; 168-171

electrolyte—Solution of ions (sodium, potassium) that conducts electric current; 221

endurance—The ability to persist or to resist fatigue; 64-65, 75, 89-92

energy balance—Balance of caloric intake and expenditure; 97-103

enzyme—An organic catalyst that accelerates the rate of chemical reactions; 276-277

epinephrine (adrenaline)—Hormone from the adrenal medulla and nerve endings of the sympathetic nervous system; secreted during times of stress and to help mobilize energy; 33

ergometer—A device, such as a bicycle, used to measure work capacity; 302-303

evaporation—Elimination of body heat when sweat vaporizes on surface of skin. Evaporation of 1 L of sweat yields a heat loss of 580 calories; 220

fartlek—Swedish term meaning speed play; a form of training where participants vary speed according to mood as they run through the countryside; 245

fat—Important energy source; stored for future use when excess calories are ingested; 32-33, 98, 118-119, 130, 276-279

fatigue—Diminished work capacity, usually short of true physiological limits. Real limits in short intense exercise—factors within muscle (muscle pH, calcium), in long duration effort—glycogen depletion, or CNS fatigue due to low blood sugar; 279

fitness—A combination of aerobic capacity and muscular strength and endurance that enhances health and the quality of life; 2-12

flexibility—Range of motion through which the limbs or body parts are able to move; 66, 78-80

frequency—Number of times per day or week (in the case of the exercise prescription); 46

glucose—Energy source transported in blood; essential energy source for brain and nervous tissue; 207, 276

glycogen—Storage form of glucose; found in liver and muscles; 276-279

heart attack—Death of heart muscle tissue that results when atherosclerosis blocks oxygen delivery to heart muscle; also called a myocardial infarction; 179

heart rate—Frequency of contraction, often inferred from pulse rate (expansion of artery resulting from beat of heart); 44

heart rate range—The difference between the resting and maximal heart rates; 44

heat stress—Temperature-humidity combination that leads to heat disorders such as heat cramps, heat exhaustion, or heat stroke; 217-244

hemoglobin—Iron-containing compound in red blood cell that forms loose association with oxygen; 286

high-density lipoprotein (HDL) cholesterol—A carrier molecule that takes cholesterol from the tissue to the liver for removal. Inversely related to heart disease risk; 121, 195

hypoglycemia—Low blood sugar (glucose); 207

hypothermia—Life-threatening heat loss brought on by rapid cooling, energy depletion, and exhaustion; 227

inhibition—Opposite of excitation in the nervous system; 62, 272

insulin—Pancreatic hormone responsible for getting blood sugar into cells; 133

intensity—The relative rate, speed, or level of exertion; 43

interval training—Training method that alternates short bouts of intense effort with periods of active rest; 246-247

ischemia—Lack of blood to specific area like heart muscle; 180

isokinetic—Contraction against resistance that is varied to maintain high tension throughout range of motion; 64, 77, 86

isometric—Contraction against immovable object (static contraction); 64, 76

isotonic—Contraction against a constant resistance; 63, 77, 86

lactic acid—A by-product of anaerobic glycolysis that also serves as a metabolic intermediate that transports energy from muscle to muscle and from muscle to the liver. High levels in muscle poison the contractile apparatus and inhibit enzyme activity; 33, 276, 277, 307

lean body weight—Body weight minus fat weight; 105, 241

lipid—Fat; 32-33, 98, 120-122

speed of movement—The sum of reaction time (time from stimulus to start of movement) and movement time (time to complete the movement); 66-67, 80, 92

strength—Ability of muscle to exert force; 59-64, 74, 84-89

stroke volume—Volume of blood pumped from ventricle during each contraction of heart; 288-289

synapse—Junction between neurons; 271

systolic pressure—Highest pressure in arteries that results from contraction (systole) of the heart; 291-292

tendon—Tough connective tissue that connects muscle to bone; 74

testosterone—Male hormone; 62

threshold—The minimal level required to elicit a response; 42

tonus—Muscle firmness in absence of a voluntary contraction; 93

training stimulus—The type of exercise that elicits the desired adaptation to training; 71-72

training zone—The heart rate zone within which training is likely to produce the desired effect; 43, 52

triglycerides—A fat consisting of three fatty acids and glycerol; 121, 192

Valsalva maneuver—Increased pressure in abdominal and thoracic cavities caused by breath holding and extreme effort; 87

variable (or accommodating) resistance—A machine or system that matches resistance to the capability of the muscle group; 64

velocity—Rate of movement or speed; 67

ventilation—The amount of air inhaled per minute; the product of tidal volume and frequency; 283

ventricle—Chamber of heart that pumps blood to lungs (right ventricle) or to the rest of body (left ventricle); 287

warm-up—A preperformance activity used to increase muscle temperature and to rehearse skills; 331, 404

weight control—See energy balance; 97-103, 113-116, 125-129

weight training—Progressive resistance exercise using weight for resistance; 86

wellness—A conscious and deliberate approach to an advanced state of physical, psychological, and spiritual health; 4

wind chill—Cooling effect of temperature and wind; 225-226

work capacity—The ability to achieve work goals without undue fatigue and without becoming a hazard to oneself or co-workers; 238-241

REFERENCES

Adams, W.C., Bernauer, E.M., Dill, D.B., & Bomar, J.B., Jr. (1975). Effect of equivalent sea level and altitude training on $\dot{V}O_2$max and running performance. *Journal of Applied Physiology*, **39**, 262-268.

American College of Sports Medicine (1986). *Guidelines for graded exercise testing and exercise prescription*. Philadelphia: Lea & Febiger.

American Heart Association. (1988). *Heart facts*. Dallas: Author.

Anderson, T., & Kearney, J. (1982). Effects of three resistance training programs on muscular strength and absolute and relative endurance. *Research Quarterly for Exercise Science and Sport*, **53**, 1-7.

Ardell, D. (1984). *The history and future of wellness*. Pleasant Hills, CA: Diablo Press.

Åstrand, P.O., & Rodahl, K. (1977, 1986). *Textbook of work physiology: Physiological bases of exercise* (2nd, 3rd eds.). New York: McGraw-Hill.

Balke, B. (1963). *A simple field test for the assessment of physical fitness*. [Report no. 63-6]. Oklahoma City: Civic Aeronautic Research Institute, Federal Aviation Agency.

Balke, B. (1968). Variation in altitude and its effects on exercise performance. In H.B. Falls (Ed.), *Exercise physiology*. New York: Academic Press.

Barham, J. (1960). *A comparison of the effectiveness of isometric and isotonic exercise when performed at different frequencies per week*. Unpublished doctoral dissertation, Louisiana State University, Baton Rouge.

Barnard, R.J., Gardner, G.W., Diaco, N., & Kattus, A.A. (1972). *Ischemic response to sudden strenuous exercise*. Paper presented at the annual meeting of the American College of Sports Medicine, Philadelphia.

Benson, H. (1975). *The relaxation response*. New York: Harper & Row.

Blair, S., & Kohl, H. (1988). Physical activity or physical fitness: Which is more important for health? *Medicine and Science in Sports and Exercise*, **20**, S8.

Blomqvist, C.G., & Saltin, B. (1983). Cardiovascular adaptations to physical training. *Annual Review of Physiology*, **45**, 169-185.

Boileau, R., McKeown, B., & Riner, W. (1981). The influence of cardiovascular and metabolic parameters on arm and leg $\dot{V}O_2$max. *Medicine and Science in Sports and Exercise*, **13** (Suppl.), p. 27.

Borensztajn, J. (1975). Effect of exercise on lipoprotein lipase activity in rat heart and skeletal muscle. *American Journal of Physiology*, **229**, 394-400.

Borg, G. (1973). Perceived exertion: A note on history and methods. *Medicine and Science in Sports*, **5**, 90-93.

Bouchard, C. Hollmann, W., Venrath, H., Herkenrath, G., & Schlussel, H. (1966). *Minimal amount of physical training for the prevention of cardiovascular disease.* Paper presented at the 16th World Conference for Sports Medicine, Hanover, Germany.

Boyer, J.L., & Kasch, F.W. (1970). Exercise therapy in hypertensive men. *Journal of the American Medical Association*, **211**, 1668-1671.

Bray, G. (1983). The energetics of obesity. *Medicine and Science in Sports and Exercise*, **15**, 32-40.

Breslow, L., & Enstrom, J. (1980). Persistence of health habits and their relationship to mortality. *Preventive Medicine*, **9**, 469-483.

Brooks, G. (1988, May). *Lactate as a metabolic intermediate.* Symposium presented at the annual meeting of the American College of Sports Medicine, Dallas.

Brown, M., & Goldstein, J. (1984). How LDL receptors influence cholesterol and atherosclerosis. *Scientific American*, **233**, 58-67.

Brownell, K., Greenwood, M., Stellar, E., & Shrager, E. (1986). The effects of repeated cycles of weight loss and regain in rats. *Physiology and Behavior*, **38**, 459-464.

Bruce, R.A., & Kluge, W. (1971). Defibrillatory treatment of exertional cardiac arrest in coronary disease. *Journal of the American Medical Association*, **216**, 653-658.

Brynteson, P., & Sinning, W. (1973). The effects of training frequencies on the retention of cardiovascular fitness. *Medicine and Science in Sports*, **5**, 29-33.

Butterfield, G. (1987). Whole-body protein utilization in humans. *Medicine and Science in Sports and Exercise*, **19**, S157-S165.

Caspersen, C.J. (1987). Physical inactivity and coronary heart disease. *The Physician and Sportsmedicine*, **15**, 43-44.

Cattell, R.B., Eber, H.W., & Tatsuoka, M.M. (1970). *Handbook for the Sixteen Personality Factor Questionnaire.* Champaign, IL: Institute for Personality and Ability Testing.

Centers for Disease Control. (1987). *Protective effect of physical activity on coronary heart disease.* MMWR, **36**, 426-430.

Christensen, E.H., & Hansen, O. (1939). Arbeitsfähigkeit und shrnährung [Working capacity and diet]. *Scandinavian Archives of Physiology*, **81**, 160-172.

Collingswood, T., Bernstein, I., & Blair, S. (1987). The interrelation of coronary heart disease risk factors: A factor analysis of 23 variables. *Journal of Cardiac Rehabilitation*, **7**, 234-236.

Comfort, A. (1979). *The biology of senescence.* New York: Elsevier.

Consolazio, C.F., Johnson, R.E., & Pecora, L.J. (1963). *Physiological measurements of metabolic functions in man.* New York: McGraw-Hill.

Cooper, K.H. (1968). *Aerobics.* New York: Bantam.

Cooper, K.H. (1970). *The new aerobics.* New York: Bantam.

Cooper, K.H., Purdy, J.G., White, S.R., Pollock, M.L., & Linnerud, A.C. (1975). Age-fitness adjusted maximal heart rates. In D. Brunner & E. Jokl (Eds.), *The role of exercise in internal medicine* (Medicine and Sport, Vol. 10). Basel, Switzerland: Karger.

Cooper, K.H., Pollock, M.L., Martin, R.P., White, S.R., Linnerud, A.C., & Jackson, A. (1976). Physical fitness levels vs. selected coronary risk factors: A cross sectional study. *Journal of the American Medical Association*, **236**, 166-169.

Costill, D., Saltin, B., Soderberg, M., & Jansson, L. (1973). *Factors limiting the ability to replace fluids during prolonged exercise.* Paper presented at the annual meeting of the American College of Sports Medicine, Seattle, WA.

Costill, D., Verstappen, F., Kuipers, H., Janssen, E., & Fink, W. (1984). Acid-base balance during repeated bouts of exercise: Influence of HCO_3. *International Journal of Sports Medicine*, **5**, 228-231.

Coyle, E., Hemmert, M., & Coggan, A. (1986). Effects of detraining on cardiovascular responses to exercise: Role of blood volume. *Journal of Applied Physiology*, **60**, 95-99.

Crews, D., Landers, D., O'Conner, J., & Clark, J. (1988). Psychosocial stress response following training. *Medicine and Science in Sports and Exercise*, **20**, S85.

Cureton, T.K. (1969). *The physiological effects of exercise programs upon adults.* Springfield, IL: Thomas.

Davis, P., & Starck, A. (1980). Age and performance in a police population. *Law Enforcement Bulletin*, Washington, DC: Federal Bureau of Investigation, 15-21.

DeLorme, T., & Watkins, A. (1951). *Progressive resistance exercise.* New York: Appleton-Century Crofts.

Demopolus, H., Santomier, J., Seligman, M., Pietrogro, D., & Hogan, P. (1986). Free radical pathology: Rationale and toxicology of antioxidants and other supplements in sports medicine and exercise science. In F. Katch (Ed.), *Sport, health and nutrition: 1984 proceedings of the Olympic Scientific Congress* (pp. 139-189). Champaign, IL: Human Kinetics.

deVries, H.A. (1986). *Physiology of exercise* (4th ed.). Dubuque, IA: Brown.

deVries, H.A., & Adams, G.M. (1972). Electromyographic comparison of single doses of exercise and meprobromate as to effects on muscular relaxation. *American Journal of Physical Medicine*, **51**, 130-141.

Dintiman, G., & Ward, R. (1988). *Sportspeed.* Champaign, IL: Human Kinetics.

Dishman, R. (Ed.) (1988). *Exercise adherence.* Champaign, IL: Human Kinetics.

Docktor, R., & Sharkey, B.J. (1971). Note on some physiological and subjective reactions to exercise and training. *Perceptual and Motor Skills*, **32**, 233-234.

Eckstein, R. (1957). Effect of exercise and coronary artery narrowing on coronary collateral circulation. *Circulation Research*, **5**, 230-238.

Ehrlich, N. (1971). Acquisition rates of competitors and performers: A note on the theory of athletic performance. *Perceptual and Motor Skills*, **33**, 1066.

Ekblom, L.A., Goldbarg, A., & Gullbring, B. (1973). Response to exercise after blood loss and reinfusion. *Journal of Applied Physiology*, **35**, 175-180.

Enos, W.F., Beyer, J.C., & Holmes, R.H. (1955). Pathogenesis of coronary disease in American soldiers killed in Korea. *Journal of the American Medical Association*, **158**, 912-917.

Fleck, S., & Kraemer, W. (1987). *Designing resistance training programs*. Champaign, IL: Human Kinetics.

Folk, G.E. (1974). *Environmental physiology*. Philadelphia: Lea & Febiger.

Food and Nutrition Board. (1968). *Recommended daily allowances* (7th ed.). Washington, DC: National Academy of Sciences.

Frederick, E.C. (1973). *The running body*. Mountain View, CA: World Publications.

Friedman, M., & Rosenman, R. (1973). Instantaneous and sudden death. *Journal of the American Medical Association*, **22**, 1319-1328.

Fries, J., & Crapo, L. (1984). *Vitality and aging*. San Francisco: W.H. Freeman.

Froelicher, V.F. (1972). Animal studies of effect of chronic exercise on the heart and atherosclerosis: A review. *American Heart Journal*, **84**, 496-501.

Froelicher, V.F. (1984). *Exercise testing and training*. Chicago: Year Book Medical.

Gibbons, L.W., Cooper, K.H., Martin, R.P., & Pollock, M.L. (1977). Medical examination and electrocardiographic analysis of elite distance runners. In P. Milvy (Ed.), *The marathon*. New York: New York Academy of Sciences.

Glasser, W. (1976). *Positive addiction*. New York: Harper & Row.

Gollnick, P.D., & King, D.W. (1969). Effect of exercise and training on mitochondria of rat skeletal muscle. *American Journal of Physiology*, **216**, 1502-1509.

Gollnick, P.D., Peihl, K., Saubert, C.W., Armstrong, R.B., & Saltin, B. (1972). Diet, exercise, and glycogen changes in human muscle fibers. *Journal of Applied Physiology*, **33**, 421-425.

Gordon, E.E. (1967). Anatomical and biochemical adaptations of muscle to different exercises. *Journal of the American Medical Association*, **201**, 755-758.

Greenleaf, J.E., Greenleaf, C.J., VanDerveer, D., & Dorchak, K.J. (1976). *Adaptation to prolonged bedrest in man: A compendium of research*. Washington, DC: National Aeronautics and Space Administration.

Gwinup, G. (1970). *Energetics*. New York: Bantam.

Hammond, E. (1964). Smoking in relation to mortality and morbidity. *Journal of the National Cancer Institute*, **4**, 1161-1170.

Haymes, E.M., Harris, D.V., Beldon, M.D., Loomis, J.L., & Nicholas, W.C. (1972). *The effect of physical activity level on selected hematological variables in adult women*. Paper presented at the annual meeting of the American Association for Health, Physical Education, and Recreation, Houston, TX.

Hempel, L., & Wells, C. (1985). Cardiorespiratory cost of the Nautilus express circuit. *The Physician and Sportsmedicine*, **13**, 82-97.

Hermansen, L., & Wachtlova, M. (1971). Capillary density of skeletal muscle in well trained and untrained men. *Journal of Applied Physiology*, **30**, 860-863.

Hettinger, T., & Müller, E.A. (1953). Muscle strength and training. *Arbeitsphysiologie*, **15**, 111-126.

Hickson, R. (1980). Interference of strength development by simultaneously training for strength and endurance. *Journal of Applied Physiology*, **45**, 255-263.

Hill, S.R., Goetz, F.C., & Fox, H.M. (1956). Studies on adrenocortical and psychological responses to stress in man. *Archives of Internal Medicine*, **97**, 269-298.

Hoeger, W. (1989). *Lifetime physical fitness and wellness*. Englewood, CO: Morton.

Holloszy, J.O. (1967). Biochemical adaptations in muscle: Effects of exercise on mitochondrial oxygen uptake and respiratory enzyme activity in skeletal muscle. *Journal of Biological Chemistry*, **242**, 2278-2282.

Holloszy, J.O. (1973). Biochemical adaptations to exercise: Aerobic metabolism. In J.H. Wilmore (Ed.), *Exercise and sports sciences reviews* (Vol. 1). New York: Academic Press.

Holloszy, J.O., Dalsky, G., Nemeth, P., Hurley, B., Martin, W., & Hagberg, J. (1986). Utilization of fat as a substrate during exercise: Effect of training. In B. Saltin (Ed.), *Biochemistry of exercise IV* (pp. 183-190). Champaign, IL: Human Kinetics.

Horvath, S., & Horvath, E. (1973). *The Harvard Fatigue Laboratory: Its history and contributions*. Englewood Cliffs, NJ: Prentice-Hall.

Hultman, E. (1971). Muscle glycogen stores and prolonged exercise. In R.J. Shephard (Ed.), *Frontiers of fitness*. Springfield, IL: Thomas.

Hurley, B., Hagberg, J., & Goldberg, A. (1988). Resistance training can reduce coronary risk factors without altering VO_2max or percent body fat. *Medicine and Science in Sports and Exercise*, **20**, 150-154.

Ikai, M. (1970). *Training of muscle strength and power in athletes*. Paper presented at F.I.M.S. Congress, Oxford, England.

Ikai, M., & Steinhaus, A.H. (1961). Some factors modifying the expression of human strength. *Journal of Applied Physiology*, **16**, 157-163.

Ismail, A.H., & Young, R.J. (1977). Effects of chronic exercise on the personality of adults. In P. Milvy (Ed.), *The marathon*. New York: New York Academy of Sciences.

Issekutz, B., & Miller, H. (1962). Plasma free fatty acids during exercise and the effect of lactic acid. *Proceedings of the Society of Experimental Biology and Medicine*, **110**, 237-239.

Jackson, C., & Dickinson, A. (1988). Adaptations of skeletal muscle to strength or endurance training. In W. Grana, J. Lombardo, B. Sharkey, & J. Stone (Eds.), *Advances in sports medicine and fitness* (pp. 45-59). Chicago: Year Book Medical.

Jackson, C., & Sharkey, B. (1988). Altitude training and human performance. *Sports Medicine*, **6**, 279-284.

Jackson, J., Sharkey, B.J., & Johnston, L.P. (1968). Cardiorespiratory adaptations to training at specified frequencies. *Research Quarterly*, **39**, 295-300.

Jacobson, E. (1938). *Progressive relaxation*. Chicago: University of Chicago Press.

Jenkins, D., Taylor, R., & Wolever, T. (1982). The diabetic diet, dietary carbohydrate and differences in digestibility. *Diabetologia*, **23**, 477-485.

Kanehisa, H., & Miyashita, M. (1983). Specificity of velocity in strength training. *European Journal of Applied Physiology*, **52**, 104-110.

Kasari, D. (1976). *The effects of exercise and fitness on serum lipids in college women*. Unpublished master's thesis, University of Montana.

Katch, F., & McCardle, W. (1983). *Nutrition, weight control and exercise*. Philadelphia: Lea and Febiger.

Kearney, J., & Van Handel, P. (1989). Economy: A physiologic perspective. In W. Grana, J. Lombardo, B. Sharkey, & J. Stone (Eds.), *Advances in sports medicine and fitness* (pp. 57-89). Chicago: Year Book Medical.

Kenrick, M.M., Ball, M.F., & Canary, J.J. (1972). *Exercise and fat loss in obese patients*. Paper presented at the annual meeting of the American Academy of Physical Medicine and Rehabilitation, San Juan, Puerto Rico.

Kenyon, G. (1968). Six scales for assessing attitudes toward physical activity. *Research Quarterly*, **37**, 566-574.

Keul, J. (1971). Myocardial metabolism in athletes. In B. Pemow & B. Saltin (Eds.), *Muscle metabolism during exercise*. New York: Plenum.

Klissouras, V. (1976). Heritability of adaptive variation. *Journal of Applied Physiology*, **31**, 338-344.

Komi, P. (1986). The stretch-shortening cycle in human power output. In N.L. Jones, N. McCartney, and A.J. McComas (Eds.), *Human muscle power*. Champaign, IL: Human Kinetics.

Komi, P., & Buskirk, E.R. (1972). Effect of eccentric and concentric muscle conditioning on tension and electrical activity of human muscle. *Ergonomics*, **15**, 417-422.

Kramsch, D., Aspen, A., Abramowitz, B., Kreimendahl, T., & Hood, W. (1981). Reduction of coronary atherosclerosis by moderate conditioning exercise in monkeys on an atherogenic diet. *New England Journal of Medicine*, **305**, 1483-1489.

Kraus, H., & Raab, W. (1961). *Hypokinetic disease*. Springfield, IL: Thomas.

Leaf, A. (1973). Getting old. *Scientific American*, **229**, 45-55.

Lemon, P. (1987). Protein and exercise: Update 1987. *Medicine and Science in Sports and Exercise*, **19**, 179-190.

Leon, A., Connett, J., Jacobs, D., & Rauramaa, R. (1987). Leisure-time physical activity levels and risk of coronary heart disease and death: The multiple risk factor intervention trial. *Journal of the American Medical Association*, **258**, 2388-2395.

Lieber, C.S. (1976). The metabolism of alcohol. *Scientific American*, **234**, 25-33.

Lopez, S.A., Vial, R., Balart, L., & Arroyave, G. (1974). Effects of exercise and physical fitness on serum lipids and lipoproteins. *Atherosclerosis*, **20**, 1-9.

Lubell, A. (1988). Blacks and exercise. *The Physician and Sportsmedicine*, **16**, 162-176.

Markoff, R., Ryan, P., & Young, T. (1982). Endorphins and mood changes in long-distance running. *Medicine and Science in Sports and Exercise*, **14**(1), 11-15.

Maslow, A.H. (1954). *Motivation and personality*. New York: Harper.

Massey, B.H., Nelson, R.C., Sharkey, B.J., & Comden, T. (1965). Effects of high-frequency electrical stimulation on the size and strength of skeletal muscle. *Journal of Sports Medicine*, **5**, 136-144.

Mayer, J., & Bullen, B.A. (1974). Nutrition, weight control and exercise. In W.R. Johnson & E.R. Buskirk (Eds.), *Science and medicine of exercise and sport*. New York: Harper & Row.

McCafferty, W. (1981). *Air pollution and athletic performance*. Springfield, IL: Charles C Thomas.

Mitchell, J.H., Reardon, W., McCloskey, D.I., & Wildnethal, K. (1977). Possible roles of muscle receptors in the cardiovascular response to exercise. In P. Milvy (Ed.), *The marathon* (pp. 232-252). New York: New York Academy of Sciences.

Móle, P.A., Baldwin, K.M., Terjung, R.L., & Holloszy, J.O. (1973). Enzymatic pathways of pyruvate metabolism in skeletal muscle: Adaptations to exercise. *American Journal of Physiology*, **224**, 50-54.

Móle, P.A., Oscai, L.B., & Holloszy, J.O. (1971). Adaptation of muscle to exercise: Increase in levels of palmityl CoA synthetase, carnitine palmityl-transferase, and palmityl CoA dehydrogenase, and in the capacity to oxidize fatty acids. *Journal of Clinical Investigation*, **50**, 2323-2329.

Móle, P.A., Stern, J., Schultz, C., Bernauer, E., & Holcomb, B. (1989). Exercise reverses depressed metabolic rate produced by severe caloric restriction. *Medicine and Science in Sports and Exercise*, **21**, 29-33.

Morgan, W.P., & Goldston, S. (1987). *Exercise and mental health*. New York: Hemisphere.

Morgan, W.P., Roberts, J.A., Brand, F.R., & Feinerman, A.D. (1970). Psychological effects of chronic physical activity. *Medicine and Science in Sports*, **2**, 213-218.

Morganroth, J., & Maron, B.J. (1977). The athlete's heart syndrome: A new perspective. In P. Milvy (Ed.), *The marathon*. New York: New York Academy of Sciences.

Morris, J., & Crawford, M. (1958). Coronary heart disease and physical activity of work. *Journal of the British Medical Association*, **2**, 1485-1496.

Morris, J.N., Heady, J., & Raffle, P. (1956). Physique of London busmen. *Lancet*, **2**, 569-574.

Morris, J.N., Heady, J., Raffle, P., et al. (1953). Coronary heart disease and physical activity of work. *Lancet*, **2**, 1053-1057.

Morris, J.N., Raffle, P. (1954). Coronary heart disease in transport workers. *British Journal of Industrial Medicine*, **11**, 260-272.

Moxley, R.T., Brakman, P., & Astrup, T. (1970). Resting levels of fibrinolysis in blood in inactive and exercising men. *Journal of Applied Physiology*, **28**, 549-552.

Nadel, E.R. (Ed.) (1977). *Problems with temperature regulation during exercise*. New York: Academic Press.

Nadel, E.R. (1988). New ideas for rehydration during and after exercise in hot weather. In D. Lamb (Ed.), *Sports science exchange* (Vol. 1, No. 3; pp. 1-4). Chicago: Gatorade Sports Science Institute.

Naisbitt, J. (1984). *Megatrends*. New York: Warner Books.

Narum, J. (1983). *The effect of circuit weight training on strength, maximal oxygen intake, anaerobic threshold, and work output during simulated cross-country ski movements*. Unpublished master's thesis, University of Montana.

Newham, D. (1988). The consequences of eccentric contractions and their relationship to delayed onset muscle pain. *European Journal of Applied Physiology*, **57**, 353-359.

Nikkila, E., Taskinen, M., Rehunen, S., & Harkonen, M. (1978). Lipoprotein lipase activity in adipose tissue and skeletal muscle of runners: Relationship to serum lipoproteins. *Metabolism*, **27**, 1661-1667.

Oscai, L.B., & Holloszy, J.O. (1969). Effects of weight changes produced by exercise, food restriction or overeating on body composition. *Journal of Clinical Investigation*, **48**, 2124-2128.

Paffenbarger, R.S. (1978). Physical activity as an index of heart disease risk in college alumni. *American Journal of Epidemiology*, **108**, 161-172.

Paffenbarger, R.S., & Hale, W.E. (1975). Work activity and coronary heart mortality. *The New England Journal of Medicine*, **292**, 455-464.

Paffenbarger, R.S., Hyde, R., & Wing, A. (1986). Physical activity, all-cause mortality, and longevity of college alumni. *New England Journal of Medicine*, **314**, 605-613.

Pashkow, F., Pashkow, P., & Schafer, M. (1988). *Successful cardiac rehabilitation*. Loveland, CO: Heart Watchers Press.

Passmore, R., & Durnin, J. (1955). Human energy expenditure. *Physiology Review*, **35**, 801-824.

Pate, R.R., & Ross, J.G. (1987). Factors associated with health-related fitness. *Journal of Physical Education, Recreation and Dance*, **58**(9), 93-95.

Pette, D. (1984). Activity induced fast to slow transitions in mammalian muscle. *Medicine and Science in Sports and Exercise*, **16**, 517-528.

Pipes, T., & Wilmore, J.H. (1975). Isokinetic vs. isotonic strength training in adult men. *Medicine and Science in Sports*, **7**, 262-274.

Pollock, M.L. (1973). The quantification of endurance training programs. In J.H. Wilmore (Ed.), *Exercise and sports sciences reviews* (Vol. 1). New York: Academic Press.

Pollock, M.L., Dimmick, J., Miller, H., Kendrick, Z., & Linnerud, A. (1975). Effects of mode of training on cardiovascular function and body composition of middle-aged men. *Medicine and Science in Sports*, **7**, 139-145.

Pollock, M.L., Wilmore, J., & Fox, S. (1984). *Exercise in health and disease*. Philadelphia: W.B. Saunders.

Pomerleau, O., Scherzer, H., Grunberg, N., Pomerleau, C., Judge, J., Fertig, J., & Burleson, J. (1987). The effects of acute exercise on subsequent cigarette smoking. *Journal of Behavioral Medicine*, **10**(2), 117-127.

Powel, K., & Paffenbarger, R. (1985). Workshop on epidemiologic and public health aspects of physical activity and exercise: A summary. *Public Health Reports*, **100**, 118-126.

President's Council on Physical Fitness and Sport. (1973, May). National adult physical fitness survey. *PCPF&S Newsletter*, pp. 1-27.

Pritikin, N. (1979). *The Pritikin program for diet and exercise*. New York: Bantam Press.

Raab, W. (1965). Prevention of ischaemic heart disease. *Medical Services Journal of Canada*, **21**, 719-734.

Radcliffe, J., & Farentinos, R. (1985). *Plyometrics: Explosive power training*. Champaign, IL: Human Kinetics.

Ross, J.G., Dotson, C.O., & Gilbert, G. (1985). Are kids getting appropriate activity? *Journal of Physical Education, Recreation and Dance*, **56**(1), 40-43.

Roth, E.M. (Ed.) (1968). *Compendium of human responses to the aerospace environment III*. Washington, DC: National Aeronautic and Space Administration.

Ryder, H.W., Carr, H.J., & Herget, R. (1976). Future performance in footracing. *Scientific American*, **234**, 109-116.

Saltin, B. (1977). The interplay between peripheral and central factors in the adaptive response to exercise and training. In P. Milvy (Ed.), *The marathon* (pp. 224-231). New York: New York Academy of Sciences.

Saltin, B., Blomqvist, G., Mitchell, J.H., Johnson, R.L., Jr., Wildenthal, K., & Chapman, C.B. (1968). Response to exercise after bed rest and after training. *Circulation*, **38**(Suppl. 7), 1-78.

Saltin, B., Henriksson, J., Nygaard, E., & Andersen, P. (1977). Fiber types and metabolic potentials of skeletal muscles in sedentary men and endurance runners. In P. Milvy (Ed.), *The marathon*. New York: New York Academy of Sciences.

Seltzer, C.C., & Mayer, J. (1965). A simple criterion of obesity. *Postgraduate Medicine*, **38**, A101-A106.

Selye, H. (1956). *The stress of life*. New York: McGraw-Hill.

Sharkey, B.J. (1970). Intensity and duration of training and the development of cardiorespiratory endurance. *Medicine and Science in Sports*, **2**, 197-202.

Sharkey, B.J. (1974). *Physiological fitness and weight control*. Missoula, MT: Mountain Press.

Sharkey, B.J. (1975). *Physiology and physical activity*. New York: Harper & Row.

Sharkey, B.J. (1977). *Fitness and work capacity*. Washington, DC: U.S. Government Printing Office.

Sharkey, B.J. (1979). *Heat stress*. Missoula, MT: U.S. Department of Agriculture/Forest Service Equipment Development Center.

Sharkey, B.J. (1984). *Training for cross-country ski racing*. Champaign, IL: Human Kinetics.

Sharkey, B.J. (1986). *Coaches guide to sport physiology*. Champaign, IL: Human Kinetics.

Sharkey, B.J. (1987). Functional vs chronological age. *Medicine and Science in Sports and Exercise*, **19**, 174-178.

Sharkey, B.J. (1988a). Specificity of exercise. In S. Blair et al. (Eds.), *Resource manual for guidelines for exercise testing and prescription*. Philadelphia: Lea and Febiger.

Sharkey, B.J. (1988b). Specificity of testing. In W. Granna, J. Lombardo, B. Sharkey, & J. Stone (Eds.), *Advances in sports medicine and fitness* (pp. 25-43). Chicago: Year Book Medical.

Sharkey, B.J., & Holleman, J.P. (1967). Cardiorespiratory adaptations to training at specified intensities. *Research Quarterly*, **38**, 398-404.

Sharkey, B.J., Jukkala, A., & Herzberg, R. (1978). *The fitness trail*. Missoula, MT: USDA Forest Service.

Sharkey, B.J., Jukkala, A., Putnam, T., & Tietz, J. (1978). *Fitness and work capacity: Wildland firefighting*. Missoula, MT: USDA Forest Service.

Sharkey, B.J., Simpson, C., Washburn, R., & Confessore, R. (1980). HDL-cholesterol. *Running*, **5**, 38-41.

Sharkey, B.J., Wilson, D., Whiddon, T., & Miller, K. (1978, Sept.). Fit to work? *Journal of Health, Physical Education and Recreation*, pp. 18-21.

Siscovick, D., LaPorte, R., & Newman, J. (1985). The disease-specific benefits and risks of physical activity and exercise. *Public Health Reports*, **100**, 180-188.

Sleamaker, R. (1989). *Serious training for serious athletes*. Champaign, IL: Human Kinetics.

Smith, M., & Sharkey, B. (1984). Altitude training: Who benefits? *The Physician and Sportsmedicine*, **12**, 48-62.

Spain, D.M. (1966). Atherosclerosis. *Scientific American*, **215**, 48-56.

Stamler, J., Wentworth, D., & Neaton, J. (1986). Is relationship between serum cholesterol and risk of premature death from coronary heart disease continuous and graded? *Journal of the American Medical Association*, **256**, 2823-2828.

Stevenson, J., Felek, V., Rechnitzer, P., & Beaton, J. (1964). Effect of exercise on coronary tree size in rats. *Circulation Research*, **15**, 265-270.

Stray-Gunderson, J. (1986). The effect of pericardiectomy on maximal oxygen consumption and cardiac output in untrained dogs. *Circulation Research*, **58**, 523-529.

Stunkard, A., Foch, T., & Hrubec, V. (1986). A twin study of human obesity. *Journal of the American Medical Association*, **256**, 51-54.

Superko, R. (1988). The atherosclerotic process. In S. Blair, P. Painter, R. Pate, L.K. Smith, & C.B. Taylor (Eds.), *Resource manual for guidelines for exercise testing and prescription* (pp. 101-110). Philadelphia: Lea and Febiger.

Tesch, P., Thorsson, A., & Kaiser, P. (1984). Muscle capillary supply and fiber type characteristics in weight and power lifters. *Journal of Applied Physiology*, **56**, 35-38.

Tobin, J., Miller, K., Sharkey, B., & Coladarci, T. (1982). *Prediction of VO₂max from a bicycle field test*. Missoula, MT: University of Montana Human Performance Lab.

Tutko, T., & Tosi, U. (1976). *Sports psyching*. New York: Hawthorn.

U.S. Department of Health and Human Services. (1980). *Promoting health/preventing disease: Objectives for the nation*. Washington, DC: U.S. Government Printing Office.

U.S. Department of Labor. (1968). *Dictionary of occupational titles*. Washington, DC: U.S. Government Printing Office.

U.S. Public Health Service. (1987). *The 1990 health objectives for the nation: A midcourse review*. Washington, DC: U.S. Government Printing Office.

Van Aaken, E. (1976). *Van Aaken method*. Mountain View, CA: World Publications.

Van Linge, B. (1962). The response of muscle to strenuous exercise. *Journal of Bone and Joint Surgery*, **44**, 711-721.

Vega deJesus, R., & Siconolfi, S. (1988). Fat mobilization and utilization during exercise at lactates of 2 and 4 mm. *Medicine and Science in Sports and Exercise*, **20**, (Suppl. 71).

Washburn, R., Sharkey, B., Narum, J., & Smith, M. (1982). Dryland training for cross-country skiers. *Ski Coach*, **5**, 9-12.

Watson, P., Srivastava, A., & Booth, F. (1983). Cytochrome C synthesis rate is decreased in the 6th hour of hindlimb immobilization in the rat. In J. Knutgen, J., Vogel, & J. Poortmans (Eds.), *Biochemistry of exercise* (Vol. 13; pp. 378-384). Champaign, IL: Human Kinetics.

Weltman, A. (1989). The lactate threshold and endurance performance. In W. Grana, J. Lombardo, B. Sharkey, & J. Stone (Eds.), *Advances in sports medicine and fitness* (pp. 91-115). Chicago: Year Book Medical.

Wenger, B. (1988). Human heat acclimatization. In K. Pandolf, M. Swaka, & R. Gonzalez (Eds.), *Human performance physiology and environmental medicine at terrestrial extremes*. Indianapolis: Benchmark Press.

Wenger, H., & Bell, G. (1986). The interaction of intensity, duration and frequency of exercise training in altering cardiorespiratory fitness. *Sports Medicine*, **3**, 346-356.

Whiddon, T.R., Sharkey, B.J., & Steadman, R.J. (1969). Exercise, stress and blood clotting in men. *Research Quarterly*, **40**, 431-434.

Williams, P. (1974). *Low back and neck pain*. Springfield, IL: Charles C Thomas.

Wilmore, J.H. (1983). *Athletic training and physical fitness*. Boston: Allyn & Bacon.

Wilson, P.K., Castelli, W., & Kannel, W. (1987). Coronary risk prediction in adults (The Framingham Study). *American Journal of Cardiology*, **59**, 91-94.

Wilson, P., Fardy, P., & Froelicher, V. (1981). *Cardiac rehabilitation, adult fitness and exercise testing*. Philadelphia: Lea and Febiger.

Wood, P. (1975). Middle-aged joggers slow healthy lipoprotein pattern. *Medical Tribune*, **38**, 27.

Wood, P., Stefanick, M., Dreon, D., Frey-Hewitt, B., et al. (1988). Changes in plasma lipids and lipoproteins in overweight men during weight loss in dieting as compared with exercise. *New England Journal of Medicine*, **318**, 1173-1179.

Zauner, C.W., Burt, J.J., & Mapes, D.F. (1968). The effect of strenuous and mild premeal exercise on postprandial lipemia. *Research Quarterly*, **39**, 395-401.

Zukel, W., Lewis, R.H., & Enterline, P. (1959). A short-term community study of the epidemiology of coronary heart disease. *American Journal of Public Health*, **49**, 1630-1638.

Zuti, W.B., & Golding, L. (1976). Comparing diet and exercise as weight reduction tools. *The Physician and Sportsmedicine*, **4**, 59-62.